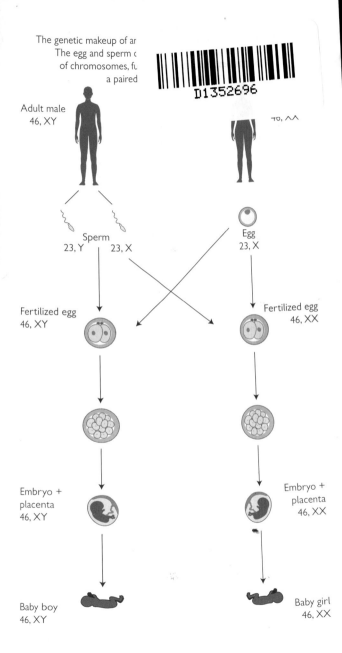

The genetic makeup of ar
The egg and sperm c
of chromosomes, fL
a paired

Adult male
46, XY

Sperm
23, Y   23, X

Egg
23, X

Fertilized egg
46, XY

Fertilized egg
46, XX

Embryo +
placenta
46, XY

Embryo +
placenta
46, XX

Baby boy
46, XY

Baby girl
46, XX

OXFORD MEDICAL PUBLICATIONS

Oxford Handbook of
Genetics

Published and forthcoming Oxford Handbooks

Oxford Handbook of Acute Medicine 3/e
Oxford Handbook of Anaesthesia 2/e
Oxford Handbook of Applied Dental Sciences
Oxford Handbook of Cardiology
Oxford Handbook of Clinical and Laboratory Investigation 2/e
Oxford Handbook of Clinical Dentistry 4/e
Oxford Handbook of Clinical Diagnosis 2/e
Oxford Handbook of Clinical Examination and Practical Skills
Oxford Handbook of Clinical Haematology 3/e
Oxford Handbook of Clinical Immunology and Allergy 2/e
Oxford Handbook of Clinical Medicine—Mini Edition 7/e
Oxford Handbook of Clinical Medicine 7/e
Oxford Handbook of Clinical Pharmacy
Oxford Handbook of Clinical Rehabilitation 2/e
Oxford Handbook of Clinical Specialties 8/e
Oxford Handbook of Clinical Surgery 3/e
Oxford Handbook of Complementary Medicine
Oxford Handbook of Critical Care 3/e
Oxford Handbook of Dental Patient Care 2/e
Oxford Handbook of Dialysis 3/e
Oxford Handbook of Emergency Medicine 3/e
Oxford Handbook of Endocrinology and Diabetes 2/e
Oxford Handbook of ENT and Head and Neck Surgery
Oxford Handbook of Expedition and Wilderness Medicine
Oxford Handbook for the Foundation Programme 2/e
Oxford Handbook of Gastroenterology and Hepatology
Oxford Handbook of General Practice 3/e
Oxford Handbook of Genitourinary Medicine, HIV and AIDS
Oxford Handbook of Geriatric Medicine
Oxford Handbook of Infectious Diseases and Microbiology
Oxford Handbook of Key Clinical Evidence
Oxford Handbook of Medical Sciences
Oxford Handbook of Nephrology and Hypertension
Oxford Handbook of Neurology
Oxford Handbook of Nutrition and Dietetics
Oxford Handbook of Obstetrics and Gynaecology 2/e
Oxford Handbook of Occupational Health
Oxford Handbook of Oncology 2/e
Oxford Handbook of Ophthalmology 2/e
Oxford Handbook of Paediatrics
Oxford Handbook of Palliative Care 2/e
Oxford Handbook of Practical Drug Therapy
Oxford Handbook of Pre-Hospital Care
Oxford Handbook of Psychiatry 2/e
Oxford Handbook of Public Health Practice 2/e
Oxford Handbook of Reproductive Medicine and Family Planning
Oxford Handbook of Respiratory Medicine 2/e
Oxford Handbook of Rheumatology 2/e
Oxford Handbook of Sport and Exercise Medicine
Oxford Handbook of Tropical Medicine 3/e
Oxford Handbook of Urology 2/e

Oxford Handbook of
Genetics

Guy Bradley-Smith

GP Principal,
Honorary Clinical Lecturer,
Peninsula College of Medicine and Dentistry,
Exeter, Devon, UK

Sally Hope

GP Principal,
Woodstock, Oxon;
Honorary Research Fellow in Women's Health,
University of Oxford,
Oxford, UK

with

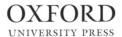

Helen V. Firth

Consultant in Clinical Genetics,
Addenbrooke's Hospital,
Cambridge, UK

Jane A. Hurst

Consultant in Clinical Genetics,
Oxford Radcliffe Hospitals,
Oxford, UK

OXFORD
UNIVERSITY PRESS

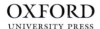

OXFORD
UNIVERSITY PRESS

Great Clarendon Street, Oxford OX2 6DP

Oxford University Press is a department of the University of Oxford.
It furthers the University's objective of excellence in research, scholarship,
and education by publishing worldwide in

Oxford New York

Auckland Cape Town Dar es Salaam Hong Kong Karachi
Kuala Lumpur Madrid Melbourne Mexico City Nairobi
New Delhi Shanghai Taipei Toronto

With offices in

Argentina Austria Brazil Chile Czech Republic France Greece
Guatemala Hungary Italy Japan Poland Portugal Singapore
South Korea Switzerland Thailand Turkey Ukraine Vietnam

Oxford is a registered trade mark of Oxford University Press
in the UK and in certain other countries

Published in the United States
by Oxford University Press Inc., New York

British Library Cataloguing in Publication Data
Data available

Library of Congress Cataloging-in-Publication-Data
Data available

Typeset by Cepha Imaging Private Ltd., Bangalore, India
Printed in China
on acid-free paper by
Asia Pacific Offset

ISBN 978–0–19–954536–0

10 9 8 7 6 5 4 3 2 1

Foreword

'Primary care practitioners don't need to bother with genetics—it's all too scientific and the conditions are too rare'. So said a colleague in primary care. 'But you do genetics all the time', I replied, 'by taking a family history and considering its impact'. Indeed, primary care has been doing so for many years as recognized by the Royal College of General Practitioners in a 1998 report. And genetic conditions are common: a 2004 study in general practice indicated that a minimum of one in ten patients has a disorder with a genetic component.

It is particularly important to identify families with single gene disorders which cause considerable ill health and premature mortality, such as familial hypercholesterolaemia, Marfan syndrome, inherited cardiomyopathies, and arrhythmias. Taking a family history may also identify families with a predisposition to common diseases such as cancer, cardiovascular disease, and diabetes, genetic information adding to risks associated with lifestyle, in considering referral, management, and treatment. Primary care physicians may also deal with the genetic aspects of results from the antenatal and newborn screening programmes.

In the future, some believe that tests may identify genetic responses to drug metabolism and susceptibility for common disorders to result in interventions—medical or lifestyle—tailored to a person's genetic makeup.

The NHS National Genetics Education and Development Centre therefore asked colleagues in general practice what they thought their roles were in the pathway for patients with genetic conditions. General practitioners felt that their role was to identify and refer patients, and to treat and manage the condition when advice had been received from hospital colleagues. They also felt that they had a role in explaining the implications of the genetic condition for the patient and the wider family, offering support and referring as appropriate. These three key themes—identifying patients, clinical management, and communicating genetic information—form the basis of curriculum statement 6, 'Genetics in Primary Care', of the Royal College of General Practitioners.

Primary care practitioners are skilled in counselling, screening, and health promotion and have a special understanding of the impacts of health and disease on patients and families. To extend these skills to genetic conditions, then, 'just in time information' is needed.

This book provides such information in abundance—ready for that moment during a consultation when a vital piece of information is required to assist in diagnosis, management, or referral. The book's contents are based firmly in general practice, highlighting consultation and management plans, clinical implications, and necessary genetic information for nearly 100 conditions or clinical situations. These are then followed by investigations or management expected to be undertaken by secondary care. There are sections on appropriate general genetic concepts, such as patterns of inheritance, genetic investigations, and when and how to refer to specialized genetic services. The writers are two primary care physicians and two clinical geneticists; they have combined their experiences of genetics in practice to produce a book with information specifically tailored for genetics in a primary care setting.

Primary care physicians (and specialty trainees) are not expected to act as genetics specialists, but this book will assist in determining whether a condition has a genetic component which may affect management and/or require referral and as a quick review of genetics concepts to answer patients' questions.

Peter Farndon MSc MD FRCP DCH
Director
NHS National Genetics Education and Development Centre
Professor of Clinical Genetics and Consultant Clinical Geneticist
Birmingham, UK

Preface

We have enjoyed writing this new handbook. One of the biggest lessons we have learnt during this project is the complementary nature of the skills of primary care practitioners (PCP) and clinical geneticists. Genetic diseases are often chronic, life-long, and sometimes life-limiting, so caring for the patient and his/her family in the long term and being alert to the potential complications of the diagnosis (medically, socially, and emotionally) falls upon the PCP and his/her team. Similarly, the primary care team, with their intimate knowledge of the individual and his/her family, is often best placed to recognize who may be at risk for a genetic disorder and ensure timely referral. We also recognize that both the long-term nature of primary care and the portability of primary care records when patients move areas, can be a strength in managing genetic disease and helping to identify those at risk.

Because precise diagnosis is the cornerstone of accurate genetic advice, clinical genetics services are resourced to validate diagnoses (i.e. obtain the primary documentation, for example the histology report or cytogenetics report), which may be very difficult from primary care. Clinical genetics services are also networked and resourced to work across extended families where different branches may be living in different regions of the country, which may create obstacles for primary care teams. In addition, clinical geneticists have expertise in the diagnosis of rare disorders and in risk analysis that is not available in primary care. As a result, caring for patients with genetic disorders requires a partnership between primary care and regional genetics services. We hope this book will help that partnership to develop and grow.

We are now in an era where the knowledge gained from the human genome project, to sequence the human genome, is beginning to impact on patient care and management. We hope this handbook will give you a taste of these developments and help you to recognize which patients may benefit from referral to a clinical geneticist. We also hope that it will provide you with sufficient insight into the investigation and management of genetic disorders to support your patient and his/her family through this process and afterwards. Most of all, we trust that that this book will equip you for the changes to practice that our growing understanding of genomic medicine will undoubtedly bring, and give you sufficient knowledge and information to bring the benefits to your patients. If so, we will be participating in the Human Genetics Commission's vision that there 'should be a well-funded NHS genetics service supported by a genetically literate primary care work force'.

Guy Bradley-Smith
Sally Hope
Helen V. Firth
Jane A. Hurst

Acknowledgements

We would like to thank the many colleagues who have helped us in the preparation of this book including Michael Parker, Jacqueline Hodgkinson, Serena Nik-Zainal, Sarah Downing, Soo-Mi Park, Sue Kenwrick, Catherine Bennett, Julia Rankin, Kate Cushing, David Kernick and Peter Miller. In addition, we would particularly like to acknowledge Professor Ian Young whose textbook *Essential Medical Genetics* has been a core resource, and Professor Diana Eccles for her advice on the Cancer chapter.

Our thanks are also due to Anna Winstanley and Kate Wanwimolruk from Oxford University Press.

Most of all we would like to thank our families for their support and encouragement during the writing of this book.

Guy Bradley-Smith
Sally Hope
Helen V. Firth
Jane A. Hurst

Confirmation of the precise diagnosis is essential before giving genetic advice (📖 see Referral to a genetics service, p. 80). Regional genetic services will routinely obtain this documentation before providing advice to patients. Unless PCPs are clear, either from previous recent genetic department advice held in their patient's record, or from their own knowledge, genetic risk assessment should be done by genetics professionals.

Contents

Detailed contents

7 Cancer   **229**

Symbols and abbreviations

📖	cross reference
✍	referral
☎	telephone
🖰	website
3C	craniocerebellocardiac (dysplasia)
ABI	Association of British Insurers
AC	abdominal circumference
AC2	Amsterdam criteria 2 (diagnosis of HNPCC)
ACE	angiotensin-converting enzyme
ACMG	American College of Medical Genetics
ACTH	adrenocorticotrophic hormone
AD	autosomal dominant
ADO	allele drop-out
ADPKD	autosomal dominant polycystic kidney disease (adult PKD)
ADRP	autosomal dominant retinitis pigmentosa
AFAP	attenuated familial adenomatous polyposis
AFP	alpha-fetoprotein
AFO	ankle–foot orthosis
AID	artificial insemination by donor
AIDS	acquired immune deficiency syndrome
ALT	alanine transaminase
AML	angiomyolipoma
APC	activated protein C
APECED	autoimmune polyendocrinopathy–candidiasis–ectodermal dystrophy
APOE	apolipoprotein E
APTT	activated partial thromboplastin time
AR	autosomal recessive
ARC	Antenatal Results and Choices
ARH	autosomal recessive hypercholesterolaemia
ARND	alcohol-related neurodevelopmental disorder
ARPKD	autosomal recessive polycystic kidney disease (infantile PKD)
ART	assisted reproductive technology
ARVC	arrhythmogenic right ventricular cardiomyopathy
ARVD	arrhythmogenic right ventricular dysplasia

AS	ankylosing spondylitis
ASBAH	Association for Spina Bifida and Hydrocephalus
ASD	atrial septal defect
ASHG	American Society of Human Genetics
AST	aspartate transaminase
AZF	azoospermia factor
BAAF	British Association for Adoption and Fostering
BAV	bicuspid aortic valve
BAPP	β-amyloid precursor protein
BBS	Bardet–Biedl syndrome
BMD	Becker muscular dystrophy
BMI	body mass index
BMT	bone marrow transplantation
BOR	branchio-oto-renal (syndrome)
bp	base pair
BP	blood pressure
BPD	biparietal diameter
BPES	blepharophimosis–ptosis–epicanthus inversus syndrome
BPNH	bilateral periventricular nodular heterotopia
BRCA	breast cancer (gene)
BSHG	British Society for Human Genetics
BSO	bilateral salpingo-oophorectomy
BWS	Beckwith–Wiedemann syndrome
CA125	cancer antigen 125
CADASIL	cerebral autosomal dominant arteriopathy with subcortical infarcts and leukoencephalopathy
CAH	congenital adrenal hyperplasia
CAIS	complete androgen insensitivity syndrome
CAL	*café au lait* (spot)
CAUV	congenital absence of the uterus and vagina
CBAVD	congenital bilateral absence of the vas deferens
CCAM	congenital cystic adenomatoid malformation
CD	coeliac disease
CDH	congenital dislocation of the hip
cDNA	coding DNA
CDP	chondrodysplasia punctata
CEMRI	contrast-enhanced magnetic resonance imaging
CF	cystic fibrosis
CFC	cardiofaciocutaneous syndrome
cffDNA/RNA	cell-free fetal DNA/RNA
CFTR	cystic fibrosis transmembrane conductance regulator (gene)

CGH	comparative genomic hybridization
CGRP	calcitonin-gene related peptide
CHD	congenital heart disease
CHRPE	congenital hypertrophy of the retinal pigment epithelium
CHT	congenital hypothyroidism
CI	confidence interval
CJD	Creutzfeldt–Jakob disease
CK	creatine kinase
CLDT	Community Learning Disability Team
CLE	congenital lobar emphysema
CL/P	cleft lip/palate
cM	centimorgan
CML	chronic myelogenous leukaemia
CMT	Charcot–Marie–Tooth (disease)
CMMR-D	constitutional mismatch-repair deficiency syndrome
CMV	cytomegalovirus
CNS	central nervous system
COCH	coagulation factor C homologue
COX-2	cyclooxygenase 2
CPN	community psychiatric nurse
CPVT	catecholaminergic polymorphic ventricular tachycardia
CRC	colorectal cancer
CRL	crown–rump length
CRS	congenital rubella syndrome
CSF	cerebrospinal fluid
CT	computerized tomography
CVD	cerebrovascular disease
CVS	chorionic villus sampling
CXR	chest X-ray
DCM	dilated cardiomyopathy
DDAVP	1-deamino-8-D-arginine vasopressin
dNTP	deoxynucleotide
ddNTP	dideoxynucleotide
DH	Department of Health (UK)
DIDMOAD	diabetes insipidus–diabetes mellitus– optic atrophy–deafness (syndrome)
DLA	disablility living allowance
DM	diabetes mellitus
DMD	Duchenne muscular dystrophy
DMSA	dimercaptosuccinic acid
DNA	deoxyribonucleic acid

DOAS	do once and share
DR	detection rate
DRD	dopa-responsive dystonia
DRE	digital rectal examination
DSS	Department of Social Security (UK)
DWP	Department of Work and Pensions (UK)
DVLA	Driver and Vehicle Licensing Agency (UK)
DWM	Dandy–Walker malformation
DXA	dual-energy X-ray absorptiometry
DZ	dizygotic (twin)
ECG	electrocardiogram
EDS	Ehlers–Danlos syndrome
EDTA	ethylenedinitrilotetraacetate
EEG	electroencephalogram
EMA	endomysial antibodies
ENT	ear, nose, and throat
ENTIS	European Teratology Information Services
EPL	early pregnancy loss
ERG	electroretinography
ESRF	end-stage renal failure
EUA	examination under anaesthesia
FACS	fetal anticonvulsant syndrome
FAP	familal adenomatous polyposis
FAS	fetal alcohol syndrome
FBC	full blood count
FBS	fetal blood sampling
FDB	familial defective apoB-100
FDR	First-degree relative
Fe	iron
FEV_1	forced expiratory volume in 1 second
ffDNA	free fetal DNA
FGF	fibroblast growth factor
FH	familial hypercholesterolaemia
FHSA	Family Health Services Authority
FISH	fluorescent *in situ* hybridization
FLAIR	fluid-attenuated inversion recovery (sequence in MRI)
FMRP	FMR protein
FMTC	familial medullary thyroid cancer
FOB	faecal occult blood
FOQ	family origin questionnaire
FRAX	fragile X (syndrome)

FRAXA	variant of fragile X syndrome
FRAXE	variant of Fragile X syndrome
FRDA	Friedreich's ataxia
FSH	follicle-stimulating hormone
FXTAS	fragile X tremor ataxia syndrome
G6PD	glucose-6-phosphate dehydrogenase (deficiency)
GAD	glutamic acid decarboxylase
GAG	glycosaminoglycan
GAIC	Genetics and Insurance Committee
GAP	GTPase-activating protein
GC	genetic counsellor
GEFS(+)	generalized epilepsy with febrile seizures
GEEPS	Gastroschisis, Exomphalos, Extrophies Parents' Support Group
GH	growth hormone
GIG	Genetic Interest Group
GMC	General Medical Council (UK)
GnRH	gonadotrophin-releasing hormone
GPSI	General Practitioner with a Special Interest
GTT	glucose tolerance test
Hb	haemoglobin (HbA, HbH, HbF, etc.)
HbA1c	glycated haemoglobin
HC	head circumference
hCG	human chorionic gonadotrophin
HCM	hypertrophic cardiomyopathy
HD	Huntington disease
HDGC	hereditary diffuse gastric cancer
HDL	high-density lipoprotein
HDN	haemolytic disease of the newborn
Hep B/C	hepatitis B/C
HFEA	Human Fertilization and Embryology Authority (UK)
HGC	Human Genetics Commission
HGAC	Human Genetics Advisory Committee
HH	hereditary haemochromatosis
HIV	human immunodeficiency virus
HJV	hemojuvelin
HLA	human leucocyte antigen
HLH	hypoplastic left heart
HLHS	hypoplastic left heart syndrome
HMG-CoA	hydroxymethylglutaryl coenzyme A
HMPS	hereditary mixed polyposis syndrome

HMSN	hereditary motor sensory neuropathy
HNF-1β	hepatocyte nuclear factor-1β
HNPCC	hereditary non-polyposis colorectal cancer
HNPP	hereditary neuropathy with liability to pressure palsies
HOCM	hypertrophic obstructive cardiomyopathy
HPA	human platelet antigen
HPE	holoprosencephaly
HPFH	hereditary persistence of fetal haemoglobin
HPJT	hyperparathyroidism, jaw tumour (syndrome)
HPLC	high-performance liquid chromatography
HR	hazard ratio
HRC	HNPCC-related cancer
HRT	hormone replacement therapy
HSMN	Hereditary Motor and Sensory Neuropathy
HSP	hereditary spastic paraplegia
HV	health visitor
IAM	internal auditory meatus
ICA	intracranial aneurysm
ICD	implantable cardioverter defibrillator
ICSI	intracytoplasmic sperm injection
IDDM	insulin-dependent diabetes mellitus
IDMs	infants of diabetic mothers
IgA	immunoglobulin A
IgG	immunoglobulin G
IgM	immunoglobulin M
IHC	immunohistochemistry
IHD	ischaemic heart disease
IL-1	interleukin-1
IM	intramuscular
INR	International normalized ratio
IOP	intra-ocular pressure
IP	interphalangeal (joints)
IQ	intelligence quotient
IRT	immunoreactive trypsinogen
IUD	intrauterine (fetal) death
IUGR	intrauterine growth retardation
IV	intravenous
IVF	in vitro fertilization
JPS	juvenile polyposis
JVP	jugular venous pressure
kb	kilobase

KS	Kallmann syndrome
LAM	lymphangiomyomatosis
LD	Learning Disability
LDL	low-density lipoprotein
LDP	Local Delivery Plan
LEOPARD	(syndrome comprising) lentigines–ECG abnormalities–ocular hypertelorism–pulmonary stenosis–abnormal genitalia–retardation of growth–deafness
LFT	liver function test
LH	luteinizing hormone
LHON	Leber hereditary optic neuropathy
LOD	logarithm of the odds ratio (score)
LOF	loss of function
LSCS	lower segment Caesarean section
LV	left ventricle/left ventricular
LVH	left ventricular hypertrophy
Mb	megabase
MCADD	medium-chain acyl-CoA dehydrogenase deficiency
MCDK	multicystic dysplastic kidney
MCH	mean corpuscular haemoglobin
MCP	metacarpophalangeal (joint)
MCUG	micturating cysturethrogram
MCV	mean corpuscular volume
MD	myotonic dystrophy
MDT	multidisciplinary team
MELAS	mitochondrial myopathy–encephalopathy–lactic acidosis–stroke-like episodes
MEN	multiple endocrine neoplasia (MEN1 and MEN2)
MFS	Marfan syndrome
MH	malignant hyperthermia
MHC	major histocompatibility complex
MLPA	multiplex ligation-dependent probe amplification
MMIH	megacystis–microcolon–intestinal hypoperistalsis (syndrome)
MMR	measles, mumps, rubella (vaccine)
MMRep	mismatch-repair (genes)
MMSE	Mini-Mental State Examination
MODY	maturity-onset diabetes of the young
MoM	multiple of the median
MPNST	malignant peripheral nerve sheath tumour
MPS	mucopolysaccharide (disorders)
MRA	magnetic resonance angiography

MRI	magnetic resonance imaging
mRNA	messenger RNA
MSI	microsatellite instability
MSU	mid-stream urine specimen
mSv	millisievert
MTC	medullary thyroid carcinoma
mtDNA	mitochondrial DNA
MTHFR	5,10-methylenetetrahydrofolate reductase (gene)
MURCS	Müllerian duct anomalies–renal aplasia–cervicothoracic somite dysplasia (Klippel–Feil anomaly)
MVP	mitral valve prolapse
MZ	monozygotic (twin)
NAIT	neonatal alloimmune thrombocytopenia
NAS	National Autistic Society
NBS	National Blood Service
NCV	nerve conduction velocity (test)
NF	neurofibromatosis (NF1 and NF2)
NGEDC	National Genetics Education and Development Centre
NHL	non-Hodgkin's lymphoma
NHS	National Health Service
NHSP	newborn hearing screening programme (UK)
NICE	National Institute of Clinical Excellence (UK)
NIDDM	non-insulin-dependent diabetes mellitus
NOR	nucleolar organizing region
NOS	National Osteoporosis Society (UK)
NS	Noonan syndrome
NSAIDs	non-steroidal anti-inflammatory drugs
NSKPU	National Society for phenylketonuria
NT	nuchal translucency
NTD	neural tube defect
NTIS	UK National Teratology Information Service
OCP	oral contraceptive pill
OEIS	(combination of) omphalocele–exstrophy of the cloaca–imperforate anus–spinal defects
OFC	occipital–frontal circumference
OFD	oral–facial–digital (syndrome; OFD1, OFD2, etc.)
O&G	obstetrics and gynaecology
OGD	oesophagogastroduodenoscopy
OHSS	ovarian hyperstimulation syndrome
OI	osteogenesis imperfecta
OMIM	Online Mendelian Inheritance in Man (database)

OR	odds ratio
ORL	oto-rhino-laryngology
OTC	over the counter medicines
OTIS	Organization of Teratology Information Services (US)
PAPP-A	pregnancy-associated plasma protein A
PAR	pseudoautosomal region
PCGS	Primary Care Genetics Society
PCR	polymerase chain reaction
PCP	primary care practitioner
PCT	Primary Care Trust (UK)
PDA	patent ductus arteriosus
PDSA	Platelet Disorder Support Association
PEGASUS	Professional Education for Genetic Assessment and Screening
PESA	percutaneous epididymal sperm aspiration
PET	pre-eclampsia
PGD	pre-implantation genetic diagnosis
PGH	pre-implantation genetic haplotyping
PGS	pre-implantation genetic screening
PHQ	Patient Health Questionnaire
PJS	Peutz–Jeghers syndrome
PKU	phenylketonuria
PMA	Personal Medical Attendant
PNET	primitive neuroectodermal tumour
POAG	primary open-angle glaucoma
POC	product of conception
POF	premature ovarian failure
PPH	postpartum haemorrhage
PRS	Pierre–Robin sequence
PSA	prostate-specific antigen
PT	prothrombin time
PUBS	periumbilical blood sampling
PUJ	pelvi-ureteral junction
PUV	posterior urethral valve
PVNH	periventricular nodular heterotopia
QFPCR	quantitative fluorescence polymerase chain reaction
QoF	Quality and outcomes Framework (UK)
QT_c	QT interval corrected for heart rate
RB	retinoblastoma
RCAD	renal cysts and diabetes
RCGP	Royal College of General Practitioners (UK)
RCOG	Royal College of Obstetricians and Gynaecologists (UK)

RFA	requirements for accreditation
RFT	renal function test
RhD	rhesus D
RNA	ribonucleic acid
RP	retinitis pigmentosa
RR	relative risk (or risk ratio)
SAH	subarachnoid haemorrhage
SBE	subacute bacterial endocarditis
SCA	spinocerebellar ataxia
SCD	sudden cardiac death
SD	standard deviation
SDR	second-degree relative
SEGA	subependymal giant cell astrocytoma
SEN	subependymal nodule
SENCO	Special Educational Needs Co-ordinator
SERMS	selective oestrogen receptor modulators
SGB	Simpson–Golabi–Behmel (syndrome)
SLE	systemic lupus erythematosus
SLO	Smith–Lemli–Opitz (syndrome)
SMA	spinal muscular atrophy
SNOMED CT	Systematized Nomenclature of Medical Clinical Terms
SNP	single-nucleotide polymorphism
SpR	Specialist Registrar
SPR	screen positive rate
SSD	Social Service Department
STS	steroid sulphatase
SUD	sudden unexplained death
SUDEP	sudden unexplained death in epilepsy
T1D	type 1 diabetes
T2D	type 2 diabetes
TA	transabdominal
TAMBA	Twins and Multiple Births Association
TC	transcervical
TD	thanatophoric dysplasia
TEV	talipes equinovarus
TFT	thyroid function test
TGA	transposition of the great arteries
TIA	transient ischaemic attack
TNF	tumour necrosis factor
TOP	termination of pregnancy

TORCH	(screen for) toxoplasmosis–other (including syphilis, varicella zoster, parvovirus)–rubella–cytomegalovirus–herpes simplex virus
TRAP	twin reverse arterial perfusion sequence
tRNA	transfer RNA
TRUS	transrectal ultrasound
TS	Turner syndrome
TSC	tuberous sclerosis
UBOs	unidentified bright objects (in MRI scan)
uE$_3$	unconjugated oestriol
UKFOCSS	UK Familial Ovarian Cancer Screening Study
UKHCDO	UK Haemophilia Centre Doctor's Organization
USS	ultrasound scan
UTI	urinary tract infection
VACTERL	(combination of) vertebral defects–anal atresia–cardiac anomalies–tracheo-oesophageal fistula–(o)esophageal atresia–renal anomalies–limb defects
VATER	(combination of) vertebral defects–anal atresia–tracheo-oesophageal fistula–(o)esophageal atresia–renal anomalies
VHL	von Hippel–Lindau (disease)
VMA	vanillylmandelic acid
VSD	ventricular septal defect
VTE	venous thromboembolism
VUR	vesico-ureteral reflux
VWD	Von Willebrand disease
VWF: Ag	Von Willebrand factor antigen
VWF: RiCof	ristocetin cofactor of Von Willebrand factor
VZV	varicella zoster virus
WHO	World Health Organization
WWS	Walker–Warburg syndrome
X-HMSN	X-linked hereditary motor and sensory neuropathies
Xic	X-chromosome inactivation centre
XL	X-linked (inheritance)
XLD	X-linked dominant
XLI	X-linked ichthyosis
XLR	X-linked recessive
XLRP	X-linked retinitis pigmentosa
ZIG	zoster immune globulin

The impact of genetic disease on families

Introduction

In primary care, the concept of *family* underpins and sustains much of what practitioners do. This was acknowledged previously when the name of the service that managed primary care services (in the UK) was the 'Family Health Services Authority' (FHSA).

However, during the 21st century, the members of a 'family' have become slightly harder to define. Now, the people grouped by our computer systems at any one address, may be:

• Parents, step-parents, partners.
• Children, step-children, adopted children, foster children, children from donor gamete conceptions, etc.
• Extended family members.

It is possible that PCPs will think of some family members as being 'close' and some being more 'divided'. We are likely to know of families' inter-relatedness by birth or co-habitation, and are likely to have cared for many of our patients for a long period.

This knowledge, together with our medical skills, often informs what we do and how we act, but:

> The implications of the concept of 'family' for our understanding, investigation, and management of genetic disease are significant and should not be underestimated.

This chapter will explore both the positives of our long-term care of a population and some of the dangers to which we are exposed unless we challenge some of our thinking and behaviour. It will also examine some of the difficulties that face patients who have been diagnosed with a genetic problem.

Adoption

Introduction

Adoption is the legal transfer of parental responsibility from the birth family to a new adoptive family. In the UK the Adoption Act 1976 states that to be eligible for adoption the child must be under the age of 18yrs and there must be no possibility of continuing in the care of his/her birth parents. Should the child be married, or have been married, he/she cannot be adopted. In the UK, an Adoption Order severs all legal ties with the birth family and confers parental rights and responsibilities on the new adoptive family. The birth parents no longer have any legal rights over the child and they are not entitled to claim him/her back. The child becomes a full member of the adoptive family; he/she takes the surname and assumes the same rights and privileges as if he/she had been born to his/her adoptive parents, including the right of inheritance.

Adoption continues to provide an important service for children, offering a positive and beneficial outcome. Research shows that, generally, adopted children make very good progress through their childhood and into adulthood and do considerably better than children who have remained in the care system throughout most of their childhood.

Fostering is an agreement to offer a temporary home to children whose parents are unable to care for them. It is usually organized by social workers working for local authorities. The authority pays for the children's accommodation and food.

An adoption agency is the organization that has arranged the adoption and has had contact with the birth and adoptive parents. The agency may be a state-run organization, a charity, or a profit-making company. The agencies have a statutory obligation to keep records of the adoption process.

Confidentiality. In the UK when an adopted individual reaches the age of 18 he/she can request the original birth certificate that will contain the mother's name and address at the time of the birth. A birth parent is not able to obtain details of the child's new family and name, although some contact between the birth and adoptive parents is more common now.

Consultation plan in primary care

PCPs are most likely to be involved in the adoption process by:
- Requests from an adoption agency for a medical report on prospective adoptive parents.
- Receipt of the medical records of a newly adopted child which should have had all previous surname data removed by the notifying authority.

Management in primary care

Given the complexity of the genetic issues outlined below, PCPs should discuss any genetic issues, with one or more of the following:
- The medical officer of the adoption agency.
- A community paediatrician with responsibility for adoption.
- A clinical geneticist.

Genetic issues relating to adoption

Genetic information given to adoptive parents

Family history

The birth parents are asked to give information about medical problems in the family. Often there is no contact with the father and this limits the information that can be given.

In the USA, the American Society of Human Genetics (1991) endorsed a statement concerning the importance of including a genetic history as part of the adoption process. Their recommendations are as follows and were written to encourage state and private agencies to collect helpful genetic histories.

- Every person should have the right to gain access to his or her medical record, including genetic data that may reside therein.
- A child entering foster care or the adoption process is at risk of losing access to relevant genetic facts about himself or herself.
- The compilation of an appropriate genetic history and the inclusion of genetic data in the adoptee's medical files should be a routine part of the adoption process.
- Genetic information should be obtained, organized, and stored in a manner that permits review, including periodic updating, by appropriate individuals.
- When medically appropriate, genetic data may be shared among the adoptive parents, biological parents, and adoptees. This should be done with the utmost respect for the right to privacy of the parties. The sharing of information should be bidirectional between the adoptive and biological parents until the child reaches an appropriate age to receive such information himself/herself.
- The right to privacy includes the right of any party to refuse to enter into, or cease to participate in, the process of gathering genetic information.

Known genetic disease prior to adoption

When there is a known genetic condition in the family (e.g. single gene or chromosomal disorder) the question of whether to test a healthy child for the condition may arise prior to adoption. 'It should not be assumed that genetic (predictive or carrier) testing will be required before a suitable placement can be achieved. In each case, we would advise discussion between the medical adviser to the adoption agency and a clinical geneticist. The important factors other than the possible laboratory test results need to be identified for future attention in advance of any test being performed' (Clinical Genetics Society 1994).

Genetic disorder diagnosed in child after adoption

The geneticist may be involved in the diagnosis of a genetic condition in an adopted individual that may be of importance to his/her birth family.

Some adopted adults are in contact with their birth families but in most the route to passing on this information is through the adoption agency. The geneticist may write a brief letter stating the name of the condition that has been diagnosed in the adopted child and that this is a condition that could have genetic implications for the biological family, and recommending referral to their local genetic service. The medical advisor to the agency can assess the information and it may be feasible for them then to contact the birth family. Records made many years ago are less complete and for individuals >18yrs old these may not be adequate to enable contact to be made with the birth family.

Genetic disorder diagnosed in birth family after a child has been adopted out

The geneticist may be involved in the diagnosis of a genetic condition or carrier status in the biological parent of a child who has been adopted out of the family. In most situations the route to passing on this information is through the adoption agency. The geneticist may write a brief letter stating the name of the condition that has been diagnosed in the biological family and that it could have genetic implications for the adopted child, and recommending referral to their local genetic service. The medical adviser to the agency can assess the information and, for those who are still <18yrs of age, should have the information to contact the parents of the adopted child. Records made many years ago are less complete and it may be more difficult to trace an individual, adopted as a child, who is now an adult.

Genetic testing

When a child is being considered for adoption the guidelines for genetic testing should be followed as for other children. The American Society of Human Genetics (ASHG) and the American College of Medical Genetics (ACMG) recommend the following:

- All genetic testing of newborns and children in the adoption process should be consistent with the tests performed on all children of a similar age for the purposes of diagnosis or of identifying appropriate prevention strategies.
- Because the primary justification for genetic testing of any child is a timely medical benefit to the child, genetic testing of newborns and children in the adoption process should be limited to testing for conditions that manifest themselves during childhood or for which preventive measures or therapies may be undertaken during childhood.
- In the adoption process, it is not appropriate to test newborns and children for the purpose of detecting genetic variations of or predispositions to physical, mental, or behavioural traits within the normal range.

Further information

American College of Medical Genetics (ACMG) 🖱 www.acmg.net
American Society of Human Genetics 🖱 www.ashg.org
British Association for Adoption and Fostering: 🖱 www.baaf.org

Support group

Adoption UK: 🖱 www.adoption.org.uk

Confidentiality and consent

Introduction

Confidentiality is a major issue for all healthcare employees and conflicts in the duty of confidentiality are common in all areas of medicine. There are some particular difficulties associated with genetic diagnosis and genetic testing because of the potential implications for other family members.

- PCPs usually care for several family, and extended family, members.
- PCPs are the only holders of a patient's *entire medical record*.

PCPs must be particularly on their guard against the potential for breaching confidentiality when dealing with genetic issues.

Disclosure

The general duty to maintain the confidential nature of personal genetic information is not an absolute one. The Human Genetics Commission (HGC) note circumstances where it *may* be appropriate to disclose personal information. Wherever possible, this will be with the consent of the patient, and will be in the interest of the patient, of relatives, or of the wider public. The HGC recognizes that, exceptionally:

'Disclosure of sensitive personal genetic information without consent may be justified in rare cases where a patient refuses to consent to such disclosure but the benefit to other family members or the wider public substantially outweighs the need to respect confidentiality.'

As far as courts are concerned, some in the US have begun to support decisions that direct clinicians to tell family members on a 'right to know' basis about adverse genetic information. One court case in the UK has agreed that a clinician *could* breach confidentiality in order to prevent serious harm, but did not establish a duty in law so to do. The Data Protection Act 1998 (UK) concerns the responsibilities of all who hold individuals' personal data. This clearly includes the information held on patients by healthcare professionals but has no direct content that relates to genetic information.

The General Medical Council (GMC) in the UK has published recent guidance on both confidentiality and consent and does accept that there may be circumstances in which confidentiality may be breached, without consent, in the disclosure of genetic information.

If a PCP decides to disclose confidential information, he/she must be prepared to explain and justify that decision. In practice, such cases are rare and will usually be discussed and/or implemented in conjunction with a Clinical Genetics department so that the decision about the balance of interests is shared and agreed.

Coding of primary care computer records (📖 *see also Ethics, p. 18*)

History

Although many PCPs were using electronic coding for entries in patients' records from ~1990, the introduction of the Quality and Outcomes Framework to the UK GP contract in 2004 necessitated GPs recording much of their computerized patient records as READ codes. Whereas these codes are accurate for most day-to-day medical note-keeping, there are two technical problems when PCPs seek to apply them to genetic diagnoses:

- There are *not enough codes* to permit accurate coding of all genetic information, e.g. 'FH:Chromosomal anomaly' will require free text supplementation with further details.
- Coding may be about to change; the standard terminology for the NHS Care Records service will be SNOMED CT (the Systematized Nomenclature of Medical Clinical Terms).

Implementation

The British Society for Human Genetics (BSHG) has considered the holding of personal information to aid clinical care and diagnosis within genetics departments, and noted that 'Family records are held in addition to individual patient records to facilitate clinical care. The heritable nature of genetic conditions means that it is considered good practice to hold genetic medical records for an indefinite period.'

This advice confirms what is held to be usual practice in primary care records which commonly retain patient-reported data, such as 'Family history of ischaemic heart disease', recorded if, for example, a son reports that his father has had a recent myocardial infarction. Important in this example is:

- The son has been made aware of his father's problem either directly (i.e. his father told him) or indirectly (i.e. he obtained the information from another source).
- The diagnosis is not substantiated unless the PCP also looks after the son's father.
- No consent has been obtained from the father for this information to be put in his son's clinical record.

The question to be addressed is whether or not the same practice should be applied to information about genetic diagnoses? Is genetic information a special case?

Clearly, an individual can give consent to a geneticist to pass on genetic information to his PCP, which can then be recorded on his/her own medical record; but what of the coding of other family members?

Given both the sensitive and the very specific nature of most genetic diagnoses, a general approach might be that:

- The affected individual is encouraged (by their geneticist) to consent to the sharing of their personal genetic information with appropriate family members.

The Joint Committee on Medical Genetics in their report of April 2006, *Consent and confidentiality in genetic practice:*

> ... strongly support the good practice of confirming and documenting that it is acceptable to an individual that his or her information may be shared and samples used for the benefit of other family members.

- The genetics team may then contact family members, giving them the information to which the affected individual has consented and asking them to either pass that information to their PCP or to allow the genetics team to contact the PCP directly.
- The PCP can then code other family members' notes with as accurate a code as is possible.
- Parents may give consent for their children's notes to be appropriately coded.

In practice, most families agree in principle to the sharing of information, though in reality it may remain within the immediate family unless there is considerable effort on the part of the health professionals to help disseminate the information. See the start of this topic for a reminder about disclosure without consent.

Children

In 1985, in England, Gillick challenged the right of a doctor to prescribe contraception to a girl under the age of 16yrs without obtaining the consent of the girl's parents. This became an important case in English law and Lord Scarman gave the following ruling in the House of Lords, 'As a matter of law the parental right to determine whether or not their minor child below the age of 16 will have medical treatment terminates if and when the child achieves sufficient understanding and intelligence to enable him to understand fully what is proposed.' It is a matter for a doctor to judge whether a child aged under 16yrs is 'Gillick competent', i.e. is competent to make judgements about their own medical care. Furthermore, if a child is deemed 'Gillick competent' a doctor can only disclose information to the parent with the child's consent, regardless of parental responsibility.

In the non-Gillick competent child, authority must be given by whoever has parental responsibility under the provisions of the Children's Act 1989. In deciding whether to disclose information, the practitioner's overriding consideration must always be what is in the *best interests of the child*.

A child's biological parents both have parental responsibility if they were married at the time of the child's birth. In such circumstances a practitioner will normally disclose all information concerning a young child to either parent without the other's consent. When such parents are separated or divorced, information may still be disclosed to either parent irrespective of who has custody, unless a court has removed parental responsibility from one or other parent.

With parents who were unmarried at the time of the child's birth, only the mother automatically has legal parental responsibility. Her consent is therefore required before information may be disclosed to the father, unless he has been given parental responsibility either by agreement with the mother or by a court order.

Deceased patients

Consent in such circumstances should be sought from the next of kin or executors of the deceased's estate. The Human Genetics Commission recognizes that 'There may be some clinical situations where genetic information about the dead is needed *in order to assess the risk to a living relative*. This information may be obtained by testing samples removed from an individual during life. The approach we favour is that a presumption should be made that the dead person would have consented in his or her lifetime to such testing and that this justifies post-mortem testing.'

Refusal of consent

While privacy and the right to refuse consent is an important proposition, it is not an absolute principle and it can be overridden if the harm to others outweighs the importance to the individual concerned, e.g. if the refusal of consent is capricious or vindictive.

Useful websites

General Medical Council (GMC):
🖰 http://www.gmc-uk.org/news/articles/Consent_guidance.pdf
🖰 http://www.gmc-uk.org/guidance/current/library/confidentiality.asp
British Society for Human Genetics: 🖰 www.bshg.org.uk

Further reading

Hope, T., Savulescu, J., and Hendrick, J. (2008). *Medical Ethics and Law: The Core Curriculum*, 2nd edn. Churchill Livingstone, Edinburgh.

Consanguinity

Introduction

A consanguineous relationship is one between individuals who are second cousins or closer. Consanguineous marriage is customary, for example, in the Middle East, parts of South Asia including Pakistan, in some Jewish communities, and amongst Irish travellers. Although the custom is often perceived to be associated with Islam, it is (usually) independent of religion.

In a birth study amongst northern European children (0.4% of parents related), the prevalence of recessive disorders was 0.28%, compared with British Pakistani children (69% of parents related) in whom the prevalence of recessive disorders was 3.0–3.3%. The effect is particularly marked for rare recessive disorders. The proportion of nuclear genes shared for a given degree of relationship is given in Table 1.1.

Table 1.1 Proportion of nuclear genes shared as a function of degree of relationship

Relationship	Proportion of nuclear genes shared
Monozygotic twins	1 (100%)
First-degree relatives (siblings, parent:child, dizygotic twins)	1/2 (50%)
Second-degree relatives (half-sibs, double first cousins, uncle/aunt:nephew/niece)	1/4 (25%)
Third-degree relatives (first cousins, half-uncle/aunt:niece/nephew)	1/8 (12.5%)

There is no measurable increase in the rate of spontaneous abortion or infertility in populations with a high incidence of customary consanguineous marriage.

Terminology for relationships

- **First cousin.** Individuals are first cousins if one of each set of parents are siblings (A and B in Fig. 1.1).
- **Double first cousin.** Individuals are double first cousins if both of each set of parents, respectively, are siblings (E and F in Fig. 1.1).
- **First cousin once removed.** 'Removed' indicates a difference in generations, e.g. a first cousin once removed is the child of a first cousin (A and D in Fig. 1.1; also B and C).
- **Second cousins.** Individuals are second cousins if a paternal grandparent is sibling to a maternal grandparent, i.e. the offspring of first cousins are second cousins (☐ see C and D in Fig. 1.1).

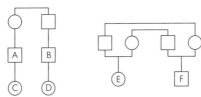

Fig. 1.1 Diagram illustrating the terminology of relationships. A and B are first cousins. A and D and also B and C are first cousins once removed, E and F are double first cousins. C and D are second cousins. (Reproduced from Firth, Hurst and Hall, (2005). *Oxford Desk Reference—Clinical Genetics*, with permission from Oxford University Press.)

Consultation plan in primary care

History

- A detailed three-generation family tree including details of younger generations, i.e. cousins, nephews, and nieces.
- Where there is multiple consanguinity, drawing a family tree becomes complex and it may be helpful to supplement it by documenting in words the stated relationships in the family.
- If there is a family member with a known recessive disorder, or a potentially recessive disorder (e.g. microcephaly), highlight that individual as the proband in the family tree.

Management in primary care ✍

Given the complexity of the family histories and the relatively increased risk of significant genetic disease, a referral should be made to Clinical Genetics. This is especially important if there is a family history of a genetic disorder.

Possible investigations in secondary care

The geneticist will ascertain if there is a specific genetic test relevant to the family. Autosomal recessive disorders with a known high carrier rate in a given ethnic group include:

- **Northern European/Caucasian:** Cystic fibrosis (CF) carrier testing.
- **Mediterranean**: Haemoglobinopathy screen (thalassaemia and sickle cell disorders) and CF carrier testing.
- **Ashkenazi Jewish:** Tay–Sachs carrier testing (carrier risk ~1/30 in Ashkenazim) and CF carrier testing (including W1282X) (📖 see Chapter 5, Cystic fibrosis, p. 104).
- **African-American/African-Caribbean/African:** Haemoglobinopathy screen (sickle).
- **Indian/South-East Asian:** Haemoglobinopathy screen (thalassaemia and sickle cell disorders) and CF carrier testing. As a result of consanguineous marriage, the birth prevalence of children with CF is approximately the same amongst British Pakistanis as it is amongst northern Europeans (despite the lower CF carrier rate in the Pakistani population).

Genetics

Inheritance and recurrence risk

This will be determined initially by whether or not there is a known, or possible, autosomal recessive (AR) condition in the family.

> If there is a known or possible recessive disorder in the family, other consanguineous relationships within the extended family are at **high** genetic risk for that disorder.

In a family with no known AR disorder then empiric data can be used to estimate the genetic risk.
- The birth prevalence of serious congenital and genetic disorders diagnosed by 1yr for children of unrelated parents is 2.0–2.5%. For children of first-cousin parents the risk is doubled at 4.0–4.5%.
- Longer-term studies that include conditions diagnosed later in childhood (neurological disorders, thalassaemia, etc.) give an overall 4.0% risk for children of unrelated parents, with an approximate doubling of this risk to 8.0% in offspring of first cousins.

Carrier detection

Carrier detection for many metabolic disorders by conventional biochemical methods is problematic due to an overlap in values between heterozygotes (carriers) and normals. Where accurate carrier detection is not feasible by DNA mutation analysis or linkage studies, the clinical geneticist will calculate a risk from the pedigree and may offer additional ultrasound surveillance.

> ⮞ If there is a family history of a genetic disorder, offer to refer consanguineous couples to Clinical Genetics prior to pregnancy.

Prenatal diagnosis

Detailed fetal anomaly ultrasound scanning (USS) will detect structural anomalies that occur in a small percentage of pregnancies affected by severe recessive disorders (e.g. cystic kidneys, congenital heart disease, structural anomalies of the brain).
- Most severe recessive disorders will remain undetected as the great majority of metabolic disorders and neurodevelopmental disorders (leucodystrophies, etc.) will *not* be detectable by fetal USS.
- Detailed fetal anomaly USS will usually be offered to first-cousin relationships and closer, but the couple will be informed of the limitations.
- In the absence of a family history, routine obstetric USS is appropriate for relationships less close than first cousins.
- Prenatal diagnosis is available for most metabolic disorders that have been characterized previously in the family, using various sampling techniques, e.g. cultured/uncultured chorionic villus sampling (CVS) cells, amniotic fluid, amniocytes, DNA.

Effects of genetic disease on families

The confirmation of the presence, or absence, of a genetic diagnosis can, as in all areas of medical practice, produce both positive and negative responses. PCPs are well used to both breaking bad news (e.g. a diagnosis of cancer) and also to reassuring patients that they do not have a medical problem (e.g. diabetes). Genetic diagnoses have the added dimension that most results may not only affect the individual concerned, but potentially their siblings, their children, and their, as yet, unborn children.

> Unless PCPs are clear, either from previous genetic department advice held in the GP records, or from their own knowledge, genetic risk assessment should be done by genetics professionals.

Genetic diseases may evoke:

Fear

Individuals may be fearful at every stage:
- Approaching their PCP.
- Awaiting the initial contact with Genetics.
- Deciding whether or not to have genetic tests.
- Awaiting relevant results.
- Discussing the diagnosis with family and friends.
- Deciding whether to have (more) children.

Practitioners need to be gentle, supportive, clear, and concise in their explanations, checking back that those explanations are understood. They will need to allow time, maybe over several consultations, for patients' fears to be explored as much as they require them to be. However, PCPs must ensure that family members, for whom they care, have their fears dealt with in a way that does not compromise confidentiality.

Guilt

Parents tend to feel guilty when adverse events (e.g. illness, accidents) happen to their children. The knowledge that one may have passed on an illness, or the susceptibility to an illness, to a child can lead to an abiding, and often painful, sense of guilt. This may arise at the time of diagnosis and again around the time when parents want to inform their children of their genetic inheritance. Discussion with the local Genetics department may be helpful in this situation.

Depression

The knowledge that an individual has a genetic problem and may have passed it on to the next generation, the decision to not have children, the decision to opt for the termination of an affected fetus all have the potential to trigger a depressive response of varying severity. Warning signs may include a patient's description of their sense of *hopelessness* or *inevitability*. PCPs should use their normal screening tools (e.g. Patient Health Questionnaire (PHQ)) in the diagnosis of depression, and use local mental health services where required, but also be aware of the help that may be provided by genetic counsellors.

Relationship jeopardy

People in any relationship occasionally have to deal with the discovery of secrets from their past or their present, difficulties in communication, differences of opinion over whether to have children or not. The diagnosis of a genetic problem in the family may precipitate tension. The relationships potentially at risk are those between:

- A couple in their reproductive years
- Parent/child
- Inter-sibling

A known or potential genetic problem may jeopardize a relationship:

- **In the present.** Genetics professionals routinely, and expertly, counsel patients through the investigation/diagnostic pathway, but PCPs may well be approached for further support by those finding their personal journey difficult as their partner/parent/siblings struggle with the implications for themselves or their family members.
- **In the future.** There will be some individuals who need extra support when their diagnosis, possibly made in childhood or early adult life, needs further discussion as they embark on a relationship with child-bearing in mind. Couples may initially present to PCPs to discuss this following diagnosis of a genetic condition.

  This is the more likely event than the other possibility of non-disclosure of a diagnosis. Individuals may well wrestle with their own conscience in keeping back information and seek support from their PCP.

Other family members may feel distress following the diagnosis of a genetic problem in their family. They may be fearful of its consequences or simply need further information. PCPs can recommend a referral to Clinical Genetics for advice. (📖 see Referral to a genetics service, p.80 and Family history of a possible genetic disorder, p. 202).

Unless genetic issues are dealt with sensitively, confidentially, and with appropriate consent, the patient's relationship with their PCP may be jeopardized.

Stigmatization

Intolerant attitudes may cause distress to those with obvious genetic conditions such as achondroplasia. Better education on genetic issues in schools and the media may help to replace stigmatization with understanding.

Support groups for genetic disorders can: (i) provide peer and family support; (ii) provide information and advice; and (iii) help affected individuals and their families feel less isolated.

Financial

In spite of the current UK insurance moratorium and employment law, affected individuals may have fears about the impact of their genetic diagnosis on both their income and the affordability of insurance. While it is outside the remit of PCPs to give financial advice, some background information may be helpful—📖 see Financial issues, p. 22.

Ethics

Defined by the *Oxford English Dictionary* as 'the science of morals in human conduct', most practitioners in medicine or nursing will be aware of the four overarching principles of ethics: autonomy, beneficence, justice, and confidentiality. These are discussed in turn below.

Autonomy

This is the expectation that individuals have personal freedom and the ability, therefore, to determine outcomes for themselves. Within medicine, this would include the ability to make their own choices about the medical care they wish to receive. Responsible practitioners must therefore give patients the right information, at the right time, in the right (i.e. understandable) way. If information is delivered in such a way, the patient facing an intervention (e.g. genetic testing) will be better able to give *informed consent*. They may ask for guidance, as well as information, and here the clinician (doctor, nurse, counsellor) may have to make a judgement on how much guidance to give.

As genetic advice is sometimes difficult to explain and the ramifications of a genetic diagnosis may be extensive, advice to patients following a new genetic diagnosis will usually be offered in the first instance by the Clinical Genetics department. PCPs who are approached by patients or their relatives for guidance will need to recognize when they can provide advice and when they should refer their patient to the Clinical Genetics department (📖 see Effects of genetic disease on families, p. 16).

Beneficence

Can be best exemplified by its counterpart, *non-maleficence*, enshrined in the oath traditionally taken by physicians and believed to have been written by Hippocrates, the father of medicine, in the 4th century BC:

> *I will prescribe regimens for the good of my patients according to my ability and my judgment and never do harm to anyone.*

It is the doctor's duty to leave the patient in a better, rather than a worse, state after treatment. In genetics, there are situations in which good may be done for one person, for example by agreeing to their request for non-disclosure of a diagnosis to other family members, which may in turn harm others who thus remain ignorant of their genetic risk as a consequence of the non-disclosure.

> Genetic diagnoses or susceptibilities may place intolerable pressures on some patients, or their families, and members of the primary care team need to be able to recognize when individuals or families are under strain (📖 see Support, p. 30).

Justice

Fairness for all in access and opportunity is an ethic to be applied within the bounds of what is possible within a health service.

An individual's right not to undergo genetic investigations, or not to reveal their results to other at-risk family members, may be viewed either: (i) as their right to autonomy; or (ii) as a denial of an opportunity to others, including their unborn children.

Confidentiality

Confidentiality is regarded as a core principle of healthcare; the issues raised by genetic diagnoses can create conflicts of duty (📖 see Confidentiality and consent, p. 8). Factors to consider when considering annotating the records of other family members with information about a genetic diagnosis in the family include:

- *Avoidance of harm:* some genetic conditions may have serious implications during childhood, e.g. a family history of sensitivity to anaesthetic agents. Where this is the case there are grounds for making sure that the information is noted in the medical record in order to prevent avoidable harm. Because this is not a breach of confidentiality, the harms don't need to meet the standard of 'risk of death or serious harm'. They just need to be harms that the parents and the doctor agree are important and that a child might reasonably wish their health professional to be informed about.

- *Patient expectation:* even where there are no implications in childhood, the avoidance of future harm, the parents' consent, and the child's reasonable expectation that their health professional will be informed, may be sufficient grounds in themselves, for ensuring that the information is available for health professionals and (ultimately) for the child him/herself.

- *Children:* one of the concerns in current practice hinges around the implications of not testing children for diseases of adult onset for which they are at risk or for carrier status (📖 see Genetic testing of children, p. 24). Family contact can be very easily lost as the years pass by. When a parent is told to inform their child and to bring him/her back for testing when she is older, this may not happen in practice— people forget, decide not to tell, or families break up. If there is a note in the child's file (e.g. family history of Duchenne muscular dystrophy), this can be followed up at a later date by his/her doctor, wherever and whoever this is.

- *Seeking the patient's views:* there are other ways of respecting the 'right not to know'. For example, when people first register with a practice (or have their first 'adult' appointment) they could be asked (making it clear that this is a general policy question and not a specific individual question) for their views on being informed about inherited disorders. When would they want to know and when wouldn't they? If the information isn't recorded at all, patients will be deprived of a much more important right—'the right to be informed if they want to be'—and the right to be provided with informed health care. They might otherwise be at risk of serious and avoidable harm caused by ignorance of the family history.

The triple helix of medical ethics

Medical ethics is a vast and controversial area. One can think of genetic medical ethics as a triple helix made up from three backbone strands:

- What you believe is right (after thoughtful contemplation of pros and cons).

- 'Standard practice' amongst clinical geneticists and/or PCPs.
- The law or various rulings/guidelines recommend (see GMC and Ethox websites).

These three strands may be identical, similar, or at odds with each other. They are loosely stuck-together by clinical experience, and communication between you and the family and other professionals involved in a particular case. Professionals must be continually aware of their own prejudices. If you are in doubt, always seek advice.

Useful websites

BSHG: ℗ www.bshg.org.uk

General Medical Council (GMC): ℗ http://www.gmc-uk.org

The Ethox Centre, University of Oxford, is dedicated to enhancing patient care by improving ethical understanding and ethical standards (see Chapter 11, p. 430).

Further reading

Hope, T., Savulescu, J., and Hendrick, J. (2008). *Medical Ethics and Law: the Core Curriculum*, 2nd edn. Churchill Livingstone, Edinburgh.

Financial issues

Most medical diagnoses have implications for an individual's financial status, be that regular payment for prescriptions, lack of pay for periods of time off work, extra outlay to obtain requisite care or mobility needs, etc. From this point of view, genetic diagnoses are the same, although they:

- May cause significant mortality and morbidity from birth.
- May produce systemic illness many years after predictive testing.
- May have financial implications for those outside the immediate family group.

Insurance

Insurance usually operates according to one of two different principles:

Solidarity

The UK National Health Service (NHS) is an example of an organization that, although run by government, essentially operates according to the principle of solidarity. Here, there is *no differentiation between those at low risk or high risk,* with all reaping the benefits of available health care according to their health needs.

Mutuality

A mutual insurance company accepts money from customers at a rate that, from actuarial statistics, will vary according to the customer's health status. They may not wish to insure people who have a high risk of poor health and reduced life expectancy. The contributions, and individuals' risks, are pooled and payments made when necessary, but, over time, enough people survive for the company to make a profit.

PCPs often receive requests for specific health data on a named individual by means of a Personal Medical Attendant (PMA) report from a mutual insurance company.

In recognition of the facts that both the *amount* of genetic investigation of patients is increasing rapidly and that genetic information about any one individual and their family can have huge *significance* for their actuarial risk, a **moratorium** was negotiated in 2006. This voluntary agreement, known as the *Concordat and Moratorium on Genetics and Insurance* was agreed between the Association of British Insurers (ABI) and the UK government, with the assistance of the Genetics and Insurance Committee (GAIC) and Human Genetics Advisory Committee (HGAC). The moratorium has been extended to 2014, with no review planned before 2011.

The essence of the *Concordat* as it affects PCPs is that:

- Patients will not be put under pressure to undergo predictive genetic testing.
- Patients will not be asked to disclose the results of genetic tests performed within their family.
- Insurers may ask patients or their PCPs for their family history and their genetic test results with *their consent.*
- Patients may be asked to disclose predictive genetic test results for (as an example)
  - life policies for >£500 000
  - critical illness policies for >£300 000
  - income protection policies for >£30 000.

- Patients with adverse predictive tests would not be treated unfavourably by their insurer *without justification*.
- The use of predictive genetic tests will be continually reviewed.

PCPs may be put in a difficult position when they are asked to provide a report to an insurer, as they have both a commitment to the insurance company, who are paying for the report, and to their patient. In such a case, it could be good practice to ask to see the patient to discuss the completed report before it is sent, and to explain the content with reference to the moratorium, or to ask the patient to exercise their right to see the report (which few patients actually exercise), again, with an explanation beforehand of the boundaries of the moratorium.

Employment

The issues raised in the debate about the use of genetic information as regards an individual's employment, are similar to the insurance debate above.

Employers increasingly request potential employees to provide medical information before firm offers of employment are made. PCPs may then be approached, with their patient's consent, to elaborate on that information if there is a concern raised about the patient's suitability for employment on the basis of their provided medical history.

'Inside information'

A report from the Human Genetics Commission (HGC) in the UK in 2002 and a follow-up report in 2006 found that:

- There was little evidence to justify the use of genetic testing by employers for health and safety purposes or recruitment decisions, and little evidence that employers had plans to introduce such measures.
- Employees should not be forced to take genetic tests as a pre-condition of their employment.
- Employers should inform the HGC voluntarily if they have plans to introduce predictive personal genetic information pre-employment.

These responses are broadly supported by the UK Disability Discrimination Act of 1995. In the USA, an executive order signed by President Clinton in 2000 forbad the use of genetic information in employment decisions for those in federal departments, and US congress is considering an act aiming to protect all citizens against unwarranted genetic testing.

Progressive genetic conditions, however, can impact on a patient's continuing employment. As with any other medical disorder, PCPs will need to advise patients if they believe them to have a physical or mental risk within their field of work. The affected individual should be encouraged to be open with their employer either directly or through employer's occupational health schemes if they, or their PCP, perceive a risk in the workplace. Health reports subsequently requested can then be clear about the physical or mental aspects of an illness that may have an impact on their work.

Genetic testing of children

The best interests of the child need to direct genetic testing.

In general, predictive genetic testing of children is only undertaken when the potential benefit of testing can reasonably be viewed as outweighing the disadvantages of testing; particularly (i) removing the child's autonomy, when more mature, to be involved in decisions affecting his/her own future; and (ii) the risk of stigmatization. It is usually undertaken when the child is at significant risk for a genetic disorder for which screening is burdensome and effective treatment is possible, e.g. retinoblastoma or familial adeno-matous polyposis (FAP).

PCPs will rarely be asked to test children directly, except for in-surgery paternity testing (📖 see Paternity testing, p. 28), but may find the following guidance from the American Medical Association (1996) useful:

- When a child is at risk for *a genetic condition for which preventative or other therapeutic measures are available*, genetic testing should be offered or, in some cases, required. An example of such a disorder would be cystic fibrosis.
- When a child is at risk for *a genetic condition with paediatric onset for which preventive therapeutic measures are not available*, parents generally should have discretion to decide whether the child should undergo genetic testing.
- When a child is at risk for *a genetic condition with adult onset for which preventive or effective therapeutic measures are not available, genetic testing of children generally should not be performed*. Families should still be informed of the existence of tests and given the opportunity to discuss the reasons why the tests are generally not offered for children. An example of such a disorder would be Huntingdon disease.
- *Genetic testing for carrier status* should be deferred until the child either reaches maturity or needs to make reproductive decisions.
- *Genetic testing of children for the benefit of a family member* should not be performed unless testing is necessary to prevent substantial harm to the family member.
- Consent can be given by a competent young person (📖 see Confidentiality and consent, p. 8).

Holistic care

Both undergraduate medical training and general practice training, championed by the UK Royal College of General Practitioners (RCGP), have endorsed the practice of holistic care for some years.

Centred on the patient

Care that maintains patients at its core will:
• Hear their concerns.
• Examine and investigate them appropriately and considerately.
• Check their understanding of explanations given and options available to them.
• Remain non-directive in further discussion of treatment options while patients make their own decisions.
• Maintain an awareness of their personal, cultural, ethical, and religious beliefs, particularly where these affect attitudes to family systems, fertility issues, pregnancy, etc.
• Give consideration to the psychosocial effects on the individual.
• Explore medicine in relation to their employment.

Confidentiality and consent
See Confidentiality and consent, p. 8.
Although genetic disease has implications for all family members, an individual patient should expect their medical information to be kept confidential until they give their consent for it to be shared. A PCP, who is likely to be caring for other family members of an affected individual, must remember this, and may need to seek advice if conflicts arise.

Clear communication

All PCPs are familiar with the patient who books an appointment to ask 'What did the hospital say?', expecting clarification or confirmation of information given during an outpatient appointment with the genetics service. To provide good care, PCPs must be able to communicate clearly, which means having a basic understanding of:
• Patterns of inheritance (see Chapter 2).
• The tests in use for genetic diagnostic and predictive testing (see Genetic investigations, pp. 74–77).
• The validity and limitations of those tests.
• Principles of risk assessment for genetic disease and common chromosomal anomalies.
• Reproductive options available (see Reproductive options, p. 400)
• Other sources of information and support for patients which clarify or add to the information we are trying to communicate (see Chapter 11, pp. 421 and 422).

Continuity of care

Working with a local population provides the PCP with daily insights into the society for which they care. Primary care is a powerful instrument for the follow-up of patients at risk of a genetic condition, or those who have a genetic condition for which non-specialist surveillance is indicated.

Co-ordination

Genetics crosses many medical specialty boundaries (e.g. paediatrics, obstetrics, oncology, ophthalmology) and many specialist services are established already where clinical geneticists hold joint outpatient clinics with other specialty colleagues. It remains common, however, for primary care to hold a role, for many of their patients, in effectively co-ordinating their care. This skill could be increasingly utilized in the provision of care to patients with a genetic disorder.

Paternity testing

PCPs first began to participate in genetic investigation when paternity testing was introduced several years ago. Such testing is usually performed by a private laboratory at the request of a solicitor, or court, in cases where paternity is disputed. Initially requiring blood tests from the child and both parents, it is now usually performed using DNA extracted from a buccal swab or saliva sample.

Occasionally, one or other parent may ask for a private test to be done on their child, without legal behest. A PCP should consider here whether the test is, or is not, in the child's best interest and whether the result will confer any benefit, or harm, in both the short and the long term. If in doubt, get further advice before participating in the testing.

Disclosure of non-paternity during genetic testing

> Some genetic tests have the potential to reveal non-paternity. Unless this potential is recognized and discussed in advance of testing, a test result revealing non-paternity raises serious ethical dilemmas.

In practice, clinical geneticists try to foresee situations where tests could potentially disclose non-paternity and include discussion of this topic in the pre-test counselling. Occasionally, unusual genetic mechanisms suggest non-paternity, but more thorough analysis reveals parentage to be true.

Examples of genetic tests that may disclose non-paternity include:
- Parental carrier testing, where both mutations have been defined in the affected child.
- Linkage-based tests where haplotypes are determined for different family members—when these results are collated discrepancies may be seen.

Private ('direct to consumer') genetic testing

Genetic screening is coming to the masses.
Sunday Times, 1 March 2008

Introduction

It was inevitable, with the announcement of the sequencing of the human genome in 2003, that personal genome scans would soon be offered by private companies. Genetic testing can be accessed via web-based services such as *'deCODEme'* and *'23andMe'* offering, for ~£500, to assess a person's DNA from a posted buccal swab, and to give a risk assessment for 20 common diseases, such as ischaemic heart disease, diabetes, and prostate cancer. It is still too early for most tests that are based on newly discovered associations to provide stable estimates of genetic risk for many diseases. One of the first genomes to be sequenced in full was that of James Watson (who, with Francis Crick, discovered the structure of DNA).

Currently, the advertising of medicines in the UK is illegal, but the advertising of medical tests is not. Consumers can buy pregnancy or ovulation testing kits, or have their blood cholesterol and glucose tested on the spot, or have their blood pressure measured in the high street. There are calls for the regulation of the testing industry, including genetic testing.

Genes Direct

The Human Genetics Commission (HGC) in the UK published their analysis of the need for regulation in 2003 in *Genes Direct: Ensuring the Effective Oversight of Genetic Tests Supplied Directly to the Public*. In this, the argument was made for a mixture of statutory and voluntary controls for private genetic testing.

- **Statutory regulation** of tests for the diagnosis of genetic disorders was suggested, whereby they could only be administered by health professionals. This is because the results may have physical, mental, and social consequences, both for the individual tested and their family members, and would necessitate expert genetic counselling prior to testing.
- **Voluntary regulation** was suggested for tests that offer a guide to a person's susceptibility to a given disease or range of diseases. Such tests are deemed to be comparable to the blood pressure screening or cholesterol measurements, in that they may be helpful in guiding an individual to consult a health professional for further advice and/or treatment.

With the expectation that it would be a PCP to whom the person would turn for interpretation of their results, the HGC concluded: 'We feel strongly that there should be a well-funded NHS genetics service supported by a genetically literate primary care work force, which can properly manage and allow access to new predictive genetic tests that are being developed.'

Support

The problem with the gene pool is that there is no lifeguard.

The care of people with chronic disease occupies a large part of a PCPs working life. The nature of the long-term relationship with a PCP, the fact that they hold the patient's entire medical record, and both the quality and power of computerized health records, strengthen the availability and appropriateness of that care.

Individuals with a genetic problem may not only have their life affected by a 'chronic disease', but, potentially, the lives of those around them or those yet unborn. The strains put on such lives are not to be underestimated.

Short-term support

Inevitably, the initial support given to people receiving a genetic diagnosis and/or risk assessment will be delivered by those trained for the task, clinical geneticists and genetic counsellors. A small number of patients may exercise their right to refuse the diagnosis being notified to their PCP, but most will allow free communication with their PCP, who will then be clearly informed of both the diagnosis, and the nature of the support that their patient is receiving.

Longer-term support

The PCP needs to maintain as much psychological and physical support as the individual, or family, requires, particularly at such times as:
- Assisted conception involving pre-implantation genetic diagnosis (PGD).
- A new pregnancy facing early genetic diagnosis by CVS , amniocentesis, or USS.
- Termination of an affected pregnancy.
- An unexpected genetic problem at birth.
- The death of an affected child.
- Teenagers discovering an adverse family history for the first time.
- New relationships in adult life.
- Separation/divorce.

At such times, liaison with genetic services may be considered for short-term support, possibly in conjunction with the other support available through local psychological services, or the support groups mentioned throughout this book.

Liaison with other agencies

In a more general sense, PCPs regularly deal with outside agencies, and genetic care may involve the following:

Education
- Nursery care.
- Special Educational Needs Co-ordinators (SENCOs).
- Teaching staff in both mainstream and special education.
- Transition services for learning disabled teenagers moving from education to employment.

Combined social services/health
- Community Learning Disability Teams (CLDTs).
- Physical disability teams.

Department of Work and Pensions (DWP)
- Disability living allowance.
- Carers' allowances.
- Mobility allowances.
- Incapacity benefit.
- 'Permitted work'.

Local councils
- Housing.
- Travel passes.
- Disabled driver parking places and car badges.
- Council tax exemption.
- Proxy voting rights.

Solicitors
- Medical negligence awards.
- Applications for power of attorney (for those who are competent to do so).
- Applications to the court of protection (for those who lack mental capacity).

The caveat in all such dealings for medical and nursing staff is to be sure when their patient's consent is required before information is passed on, e.g. to lawyers, employers, etc. Always ensure that you are acting, where possible, in your patient's best interest.

Support groups
The Genetic Interest Group (GIG) is a national alliance of patient organizations with a membership of over 130 charities which support children, families, and individuals affected by genetic disorders (℞ www.gig.org.uk).

Termination of pregnancy

In the UK, a termination that is performed as a result of genetic testing remains subject to the provisions of the 1967 Abortion Act, which made termination legal in the UK up to 28 weeks' gestation. An amendment made to the Act in 1990 by the Human Fertilization and Embryology Act made it legal only up to 24 weeks, except as outlined below. Thus, as UK law stands at present, termination of a pregnancy can occur provided two doctors sign a document (Certificate A: HSA1) confirming that one of the following pertains:

* The continuance of the pregnancy would involve risk to the life of the pregnant woman greater than if the pregnancy were terminated.
* The termination is necessary to prevent grave permanent injury to the physical or mental health of the pregnant woman.
* The pregnancy has NOT exceeded its 24th week and that the continuance of the pregnancy would involve risk, greater than if the pregnancy were terminated, of injury to the physical or mental health of the woman.
* The pregnancy has NOT exceeded its 24th week and that the continuance of the pregnancy would involve risk, greater than if the pregnancy were terminated, of injury to the physical or mental health of any existing child(ren) of the family of the pregnant woman.
* There is a substantial risk that if the child were born it would suffer from such physical or mental abnormalities as to be seriously handicapped.

In 2005 there were fewer than 200 terminations after 24 weeks, accounting for 0.1% of the total. The act does not extend to Northern Ireland. Abortion is only legal there if the life or the mental or physical health of the woman is at 'serious risk'.

PCPs will be aware of such legislation and most will be experienced in counselling women, or couples, requesting termination of a pregnancy. The moral/ethical arena will continue to resound to arguments on either side of the debate—further liberalization or further restriction, the rights of the unborn against the rights of the mother, the right of a parent to raise a child with problems identified before birth against the rights of society to shoulder the cost of raising such a child. PCPs, in practising holistic care, must find ways to place their patient's beliefs and moral stance to the fore, and keep their own internal struggles to the background.

Maternal risks

It is important to remember that women, particularly with certain dominantly inherited conditions (e.g. myotonic dystrophy, hypertrophic cardiomyopathy, and Marfan syndrome) may be at higher medical risk during termination. The PCP should alert the O&G team.

Late effects of termination

Termination of pregnancy can have both immediate effects (e.g. haemorrhage, uterine perforation, infection), and later, largely psychological repercussions. These may include:

- Depression/anxiety
- Denial
- Social withdrawal
- Relationship difficulties
- Fear of discovery by others of the termination
- Drug or alcohol abuse

Earlier discussion (📖 see Effects of genetic disease on families, p. 16) alluded to some of the difficulties that family members may experience if there is a genetic disease or risk in the family, and the termination of an affected fetus may magnify many of those described difficulties for both the individual who has the termination and other family members. PCPs, in consideration of their patient's needs, may consider referral for supportive counselling for those women suffering psychologically after termination of a pregnancy.

Support group

ARC: Antenatal Results and Choices: 🖑 www.arc-uk.org

Patterns of inheritance

Autosomal dominant (AD) inheritance

AD disorders are encoded on the autosomes (i.e. not the X or Y chromosome) and the disorder manifests in heterozygotes, i.e. when a single copy of the mutant allele is present. AD disorders are characterized by inter- and intrafamilial variability. Factors influencing this variability may include modifier genes (the expression of which can influence a phenotype resulting from a mutation at *another* locus) and environmental exposure.

Examples of AD conditions
- Huntington disease (HD)
- Hereditary non-polyposis colorectal cancer (HNPCC)
- Neurofibromatosis type 1 (NF1)
- Myotonic dystrophy (MD)
- Adult dominant polycystic kidney disease (ADPKD)

Aspects of AD inheritance
- **Penetrance** is the percentage of individuals with a mutation who express the disorder to any degree, from the most trivial to the most severe. Many dominant disorders show age-dependent penetrance, e.g. hereditary motor and sensory neuropathies (HMSN), hereditary spastic paraparesis (HSP), Huntington disease (HD). Features of these conditions are not present at birth, but become evident over time. Some conditions show incomplete penetrance, i.e. not all mutation carriers will manifest the disorder during a natural lifespan, e.g. some individuals who inherit hereditary non-polyposis colorectal cancer (HNPCC) do not develop cancer.
- **Expressivity** is the variation in the severity of a disorder in individuals who have inherited the same disease allele. Many AD conditions show quite striking variation in severity between families (interfamilial variation) and also within families carrying the same mutation (intrafamilial variation). A mildly affected parent can have a severely affected child and vice versa. For example, in tuberous sclerosis a parent with normal development and minimal cutaneous signs may have a child who develops infantile spasms and severe developmental delay.
- **Somatic mosaicism:** A new mutation arising at an early stage in embryogenesis can give rise to a partial phenotype, often present in a dermatomal distribution, e.g. segmental neurofibromatosis type 1 (NF1). If the mutation is also present in the ovary or testis (germline mosaicism) it can be transmitted to future generations (who will inherit it in its non-mosaic form) (📖 see Mosaicism, p. 46).
- **Germline mosaicism** (gonadal mosaicism): A new mutation arising during oogenesis or spermatogenesis may cause no phenotype in the parent unless the somatic cells are involved as well (gonosomal mosaicism), but can be transmitted to the offspring. If a population of germ cells harbours the mutation there may be a significant recurrence risk, e.g. osteogenesis imperfecta (📖 see Mosaicism, p. 46).
- **Reproductive fitness:** Some AD disorders have a reproductive fitness of zero, i.e. mutation carriers do not reproduce. Such a condition is

maintained in the population entirely by new mutation. Many other AD disorders have only modest effects on reproductive fitness.

- **New mutation rate:** The *de novo* mutation rate varies considerably between different AD conditions. It is high in NF1, with as many as 50% of cases representing new mutations; for other conditions, e.g. HD, new mutation is unusual.
- **Paternal age effect:** For a few AD disorders the chance of a new mutation increases with advancing paternal age, e.g. achondroplasia, Apert syndrome.
- **Anticipation** is worsening of disease severity in successive generations. This is a feature of a few AD conditions and characteristically occurs in triplet repeat disorders where there is expansion of the triplet repeat in the maternal or paternal germline, e.g. myotonic dystrophy (maternal), Huntingdon disease (HD) (paternal). In addition to variable expressivity, the mutation itself is unstably transmitted and varies in size between different generations (dynamic mutation).
- Some conditions show incomplete and age-dependent penetrance and these factors can make it difficult to give accurate genetic advice where the familial mutation is unknown.

Genetic advice (📖 see Figs. 2.1 and 2.2)

- Males and females are affected equally.
- Males and females can both transmit the disorder.
- There is a 50% risk to offspring in any pregnancy that they will inherit the mutation (NB depending on penetrance and expressivity, the risk of becoming symptomatic may be less than this).
- The severity of the disorder in the offspring may vary, being similar, more severe, or less severe than in the parent.
- Examine parents very carefully before concluding that they are unaffected. For disorders with incomplete or age-dependent penetrance, apparently unaffected individuals may still be at some risk of transmitting the disorder (see above).

Some AD disorders, particularly cancer susceptibility disorders such as retinoblastoma and von Hippel–Landau disease (VHL) (📖 see Chapter 7, Retinoblastoma and von Hippel–Landau disease, pp. 284 and 288) are recessive at the cellular level. The mutation confers increased susceptibility to tumours because of a heritable mutation in one allele, but cell behaviour appears normal in the heterozygous state. Tumorigenesis requires inactivation of the second allele ('second-hit').

Typical family tree
Autosomal dominant inheritance

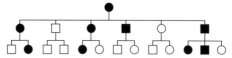

A typical family tree showing autosomal dominant inheritance. An affected parent has a 50% risk of transmitting the condition to each child whether they are male or female.

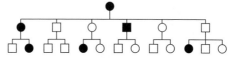

The same family tree showing AD inheritance with incomplete penetrance. In this example the penetrance is reduced from 100% to 67%.

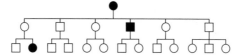

In this example the family tree still shows AD inheritance, but with the penetrance reduced to 33%. The family tree then begins to look suggestive of a disorder following multifactorial inheritance (□ see Multifactorial inheritance, p. 48 for further discussion).

Fig. 2.1 Family trees showing AD inheritance. (Reproduced from Firth, Hurst and Hall (2005). *Oxford Desk Reference—Clinical Genetics,* with permission from Oxford University Press.)

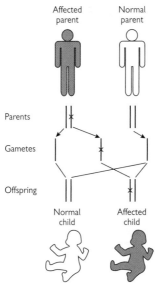

Fig. 2.2 Autosomal dominant inheritance. (Reproduced with permission from Oxford University Press, Firth, Hurst and Hall, *Oxford Desk Reference—Clinical Genetics*, 2005).

Autosomal recessive (AR) inheritance

AR disorders are encoded on the autosomes (i.e. not the X or Y chromosome) and the disorder manifests in homozygotes (two identical mutations) and compound heterozygotes (two different mutations), i.e. when both alleles at a given locus are mutated. Heterozygotes (single mutation) do not manifest a phenotype (e.g. cystic fibrosis (CF)), or if they do, this is very mild in comparison with the disease state (e.g. sickle cell trait vs. sickle cell disease). Affected siblings often follow a broadly similar clinical course which is more similar than for many autosomal dominant (AD) disorders.

Examples of AR conditions
- Cystic fibrosis (CF)
- Sickle cell disease
- Hereditary haemochromatosis (HH) type 1
- Phenylketonuria (PKU)

Aspects of AR inheritance
- **Consanguinity:** AR disorders are far more common in the offspring of consanguineous partnerships (see Chapter 1, Consanguinity, p. 12).
- **Heterozygote advantage:** for common recessive conditions, heterozygote advantage is usually more important than recurrent mutation for maintaining the disease gene at high frequency, e.g. sickle cell disease where heterozygotes are less susceptible than normal individuals to malaria.
- **Founder effect** is a high prevalence of a genetic disorder in an isolated or inbred population due to the fact that many members of the population are derived from a common ancestor who harboured a disease-causing mutation. The affected individuals in a given population are all homozygous for the same mutation (founder mutation). An example of this is congenital Finnish nephropathy, which occurs with disproportionately high incidence in Finland compared with other European populations.
- **Carrier determination:** for a relative of the proband is reasonably straightforward if the mutations in the proband are defined. Determining whether an unrelated partner is a carrier is usually more problematic. Unless the partner has a family history of the disorder, he/she will be at population risk for carrier status. If the disorder is rare, the risk of affected offspring will be low and equivalent to half the carrier risk in the general population. Carrier testing for those at population risk is possible for a few diseases, e.g. CF, spinal muscular atrophy (SMA), sickle cell disease, thalassaemia, in certain circumstances eg. where one parent is a known carrier. Whereas inborn errors of metabolism often show a marked distinction in enzyme activity (or other biochemical markers) between normal and affected, there is often considerable overlap in levels between heterozygotes (carriers) and normals, making assignment of carrier status problematic. Tay–Sachs disease is a notable exception.
- **Population risk for carrier status from disease frequency** can be calculated by geneticists using the Hardy–Weinberg equation.

Genetic advice (📖 see Figs. 2.3 and 2.4)

- Disease expressed only in homozygotes and compound heterozygotes.
- Parents are obligate carriers (spinal muscular atrophy (SMA) is an exception to this rule as there is a significant new mutation rate of 1.7%).
- Risk to carrier parents for an affected child is 25% (1 in 4).
- Healthy siblings of affected individuals have a two-thirds risk of carrier status.
- Risk of carrier status diminishes by one-half with every degree of relationship distanced from parents of affected individual, e.g. second-degree relatives (grandparents and aunts/uncles) and third-degree relatives (first cousins, great-grandparents, great-aunts, and great-uncles).
- All offspring of an affected individual whose partner is a non-carrier are obligate carriers.

Typical family tree

Autosomal recessive inheritance

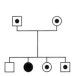 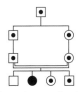

Fig. 2.3 Family trees showing AR inheritance. If both parents are carriers, there is a 25% risk of an affected child in any pregnancy, independent of gender. The diagram on the right illustrates a consanguineous relationship between first cousins (📖 see Consanguinity, p. 12). A common ancestor is a carrier for a recessive mutation that may occur in homozygous form in a descendent as a consequence of consanguinity. (Reproduced from Firth, Hurst and Hall (2005). *Oxford Desk Reference—Clinical Genetics*, with permission from Oxford University Press.)
📖 See Fig. 2.4, p. 42.

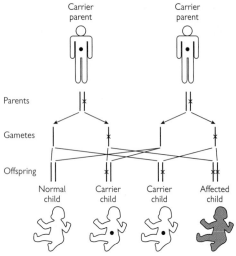

Fig. 2.4 Autosomal recessive inheritance. (Reproduced from Firth, Hurst and Hall (2005) *Oxford Desk Reference—Clinical Genetics*, with permission from Oxford University Press.)

Mitochondrial inheritance

Mitochondrial DNA (mtDNA) has unique genetic features that distinguish it from nuclear DNA. The mtDNA genome of humans is a double-stranded circular DNA, 16.6kb in length and encoding 13 proteins (all subunits of respiratory chain complexes involved in oxidative phosphorylation), two ribosomal RNAs, and 22 transfer RNAs. There are no introns and most of the mitochondrial genome is coding sequence. Mitochondria typically contain several copies of mtDNA and a typical human somatic cell can contain up to 1000 mitochondria (i.e. 5000–10 000 copies of mtDNA) representing >1% of the cell's total DNA. Mature oocytes contain a staggering ~100 000 copies of mtDNA, whereas sperm contain only ~100 copies.

The organs most often affected in mitochondrial disorders are highly energy-demanding tissues, such as the central nervous system (CNS), skeletal and cardiac muscle, pancreatic islets, liver, and kidney.

> Components of the mitochondria are encoded by both mitochondrial and nuclear DNA. Hence some mitochondrial disorders, e.g. Leigh's disease are encoded by the nuclear genome, in which case they usually follow an autosomal recessive pattern of inheritance.

Examples of mitochondrially inherited conditions
- MELAS (Mitochondrial Encephalopathy, Lactic Acidosis and Stroke-like episodes)
- Leber Hereditary Optic Neuropathy (LHON)

Aspects of mitochondrial inheritance
- **Maternal inheritance.** Mitochondrial DNA (mtDNA) is exclusively maternally inherited since paternal mitochondria enter the egg on fertilization (where they constitute 0.1% of the total mitochondria) and they and their mtDNA are rapidly eliminated early in embryogenesis. For the purposes of genetic counselling the risk of paternal inheritance is essentially zero.
- **Mutation rate.** Human mtDNA has a mutation rate 10–20 times that of nuclear DNA, probably due to replication repair systems that are less stringent than those in the nucleus. This characteristic has been utilized by anthropologists to study human migration patterns.

Genetic advice (📖 see Figs. 2.5 and 2.6)
- Inheritance is matrilineal, i.e. the condition can only be transmitted by females in the maternal line.
- Males do not transmit mitochondrially inherited disorders.
- Typically a mitochondrially inherited condition can affect both sexes.
- Correlation between phenotypic severity and level of mutant mtDNA is poor in many mitochondrial diseases.

Typical family tree
Mitochondrial inheritance

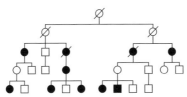

Fig. 2.5 A typical family tree showing mitochondrial inheritance. Offspring of females in the maternal line are at risk; males do not transmit the condition. (Reproduced from Firth, Hurst and Hall (2005). *Oxford Desk Reference—Clinical Genetics*, with permission from Oxford University Press.)

Homoplasmy (all mitochondria with the same genotype)

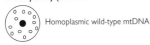

Heteroplasmy (two populations of mitochondria with different genotypes)

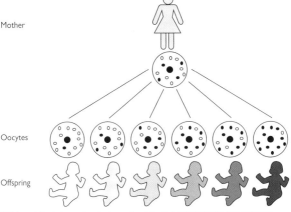

NB. Correlation between phenotypic severity and level of mutant mtDNA is poor in many mitochondrial diseases.

Fig. 2.6 Mitochondrial inheritance. (Reproduced from Firth, Hurst and Hall (2005). *Oxford Desk Reference—Clinical Genetics*, with permission from Oxford University Press.)

Mosaicism

Many genetic disorders result in every cell in the body having the same mutation. However, it is possible, if a somatic mutation occurs early in embryogenesis, for one individual to have two, or more, cell lines that differ in their genetic constitution (📖 see Fig. 2.7). It occurs in two forms:

Somatic mosaicism

This would be suspected in either:
- An individual with a *de novo* single-gene disorder who appears less severely affected than usual.
- An individual with a segmental distribution of a genetic anomaly, e.g. segmental neurofibromatosis type 1 (NF1) where *café au lait* spots and/or cutaneous neurofibromas follow a dermatomal pattern.

Germline mosaicism

An adult with germline mosaicism may appear to be phenotypically normal, but has two or more children with an autosomal dominant disorder, such as tuberous sclerosis. This can be explained by the parent having germline mosaicism with a proportion of his/her sperm or egg cells carrying the gene mutation.

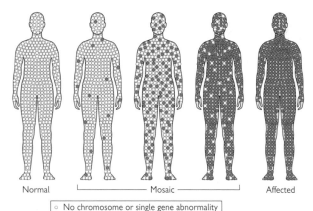

Normal | Mosaic | Affected

- ○ No chromosome or single gene abnormality
- ● Chromosome or single gene abnormality

Fig. 2.7 Figure to show varying degrees of mosaicism.

Multifactorial inheritance

Introduction

From a clinical perspective there is a continuous spectrum of disease from, at the one end, disorders that are strictly genetic and caused by fully penetrant mutations with minimal contribution from the environment to, at the other extreme, those caused predominantly by environmental factors (e.g. teratogens) with minimal contribution from genetic factors. Between these two extremes lie the incompletely penetrant and the polygenic disorders, creating a smooth transition from strictly genetic to multifactorial illnesses (🕮 see Fig. 2.8).

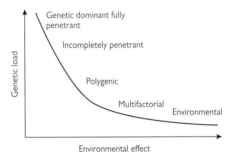

Fig. 2.8 The progression from strictly genetic to strictly environmental causation in the aetiology of disease. (Reproduced from Firth, Hurst and Hall (2005). *Oxford Desk Reference—Clinical Genetics*, with permission from Oxford University Press.)

Examples of multifactorial inheritance

Congenital or childhood
- Cleft lip/palate (isolated)
- Congenital dislocation of the hip (CDH)
- Congenital heart disease (most)
- Neural tube defect (NTD)
- Hirschsprung's disease
- Pyloric stenosis

Later life
- Schizophrenia
- Ischaemic heart disease (IHD)
- Diabetes mellitus
- Alzheimer disease
- Inflammatory bowel disease

Aspects of multifactorial inheritance

The disease processes mentioned above do not generally follow a Mendelian pattern of inheritance, nevertheless they share a tendency to cluster in families, more than would be expected by chance. Many of these conditions probably depend on a mixture of major and minor *genetic* determinants, together with *environmental* factors: *multifactorial inheritance*. Diseases inherited in this manner are termed **complex diseases**. Multifactorial inheritance may involve a small number of loci (oligogenic), many loci (polygenic), or a single major locus with a polygenic background.

In multifactorial inheritance, disease occurrence is attributable to the interaction of the environment with alleles at many loci interspersed throughout the genome. The mapping and identification of these genes, though now a huge research area, is difficult because the disease-associated alleles occur almost as commonly in patients as in healthy individuals; even the highest-risk genotypes confer only modest risk of disease. Thus there are, currently, few susceptibility genes known to play a role in multifactorial diseases.

Complex traits

Traits such as intelligence, behavioural traits, height, and weight approximate to a normal distribution in the general population (⬚ see Fig. 2.9). A large number of loci are involved in determining these characteristics, together with environmental factors. For example, factors influencing height include parental height, nutrition, and chronic illness, and in total >100 genetic loci contribute to height.

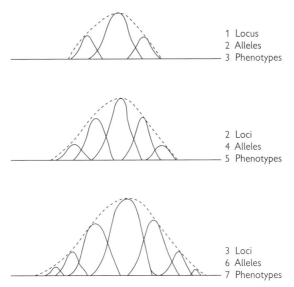

1 Locus
2 Alleles
3 Phenotypes

2 Loci
4 Alleles
5 Phenotypes

3 Loci
6 Alleles
7 Phenotypes

Fig. 2.9 How a trait determined by a small number of loci, each with two different alleles, can assume a continuous distribution of 1:2:1, 1:4:6:4:1 and 1:6:15:20:15:6:1 respectively. (Adapted from McGuffin, P., Owen, M.J., and Gottesman, I.I. (2002). *Psychiatric Genetics and Genomics*, Oxford University Press, Oxford.)

Falconer's polygenic threshold model

This is based on the assumption that liability to a condition is multifactorial and follows a normal distribution in the population, and that the disease occurs when a particular threshold value is exceeded. The normal distribution for liability is shifted in close relatives of an affected individual; hence a greater proportion of them will exceed the critical threshold value and be affected (📖 see Fig. 2.10). For first-degree relatives the expected incidence approximates to the square-root of the population incidence.

For a condition affecting 1/1000 individuals (0.1%), the risk to sibs, parents, and children is ~1/30 (3%), falling to 1/100 (1%) for second-degree relatives, and close to population risk for third-degree relatives. This is fairly close to the figures observed for neural tube defects and cleft palate.

Gender predisposition. For most multifactorial disorders males or females have a greater frequency. If the disorder does occur in the less likely gender then there is a greater recurrence risk implying more genes and/or environmental factors are present in that family.

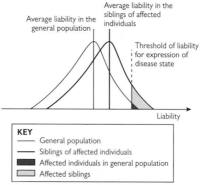

Fig. 2.10 The distribution of liability to a multifactorial trait or disease. (Reproduced from Firth, Hurst and Hall (2005). *Oxford Desk Reference—Clinical Genetics,* with permission from Oxford University Press.)

Typical family tree
Multifactorial inheritance

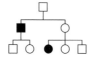

Fig. 2.11 Multifactorial inheritance. (Reproduced from Firth, Hurst and Hall (2005). *Oxford Desk Reference—Clinical Genetics,* with permission from Oxford University Press.)

Genetic advice

Several general principles affect the risk:

- **Relationship to the affected individual.** The risk is greatest amongst close relatives and decreases rapidly with increasing distance of relationship (📖 see Fig. 2.11).
- **Severity of the disorder in the proband.** The risks to relatives are greater if the proband is severely affected, than if the proband is only mildly affected. The average liability in the siblings of affected individuals will be greater (further right-shifted) in such families (📖 see Fig. 2.10).
- **The number of affected individuals in the family.** If two or more close relatives are affected, then risks for other relatives are increased. If there are several affected close relatives, the possibility of an autosomal dominant (AD) disorder with incomplete penetrance should be considered carefully.
- **Gender.** This may affect the risk for disorders such as pyloric stenosis and cleft lip.

Taking a family history

A standard approach to all consultations in which there may be a genetic element, is to take a full family history, going back three generations, also referred to as a 'pedigree' (from the French *pied á grue* = crane's foot). As genetic knowledge increases, the taking of such a history may be indicated in an increasing number of consultations, whether there is an obvious genetic component or not.

Some genetic specialists have access to sophisticated pedigree computer software which enables easy tabulation of the family history, and can be shared with relevant professionals. Despite this, nearly all consultants and genetic counsellors in the UK approach family history taking with pen in hand, and the great majority of genetic consultations in the UK are based on hand-drawn family trees. One approach is shown on the next page (📖 see Fig. 2.12).

PCPs will need a pen and paper, and a working knowledge of both the basic symbols and the correct understanding of genetic nomenclature (📖 see inside back cover).

Genetic nomenclature

The first individual identified in a family tree (pedigree) who has been identified clinically as being affected by a genetic disorder, is known as the **proband**. The individual who is seeking advice is called the **consultand**.

Guidelines for PCPs (e.g. NICE) commonly require the reader to quantify the number of *first-* or *second-degree relatives* with the target condition:

- *First-degree relative:* one who shares half the DNA and is a full sibling, child, or a parent of the individual. This can also be expressed as one meiosis difference.
- *Second-degree relative:* one who is two meioses away from the individual, i.e. their grandparent, grandchild, uncle, aunt, nephew, niece, half-sibling.

Such history-taking has attendant difficulties:

- Evocation of painful memories/experiences, e.g. death of a close relative or pregnancy loss.
- Possible disclosure of non-paternity, extramarital relationships, consanguinity, etc.
- The need to be re-visited over time as medical histories change.

This will require empathic, but focused, responses from the history-taker who must be constantly diplomatic and gentle, and recognize the need for confidentiality.

Useful resources

Useful resources can be found at: 🕸 http://www.geneticseducation.nhs.uk/family_history/Family_History_Series.pdf

(a)

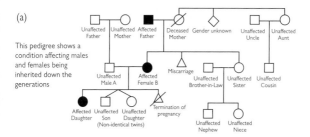

This pedigree shows a condition affecting males and females being inherited down the generations

	How to draw a pedigree

Drawing a pedigree is often a quick and easy way of showing information about medical conditions and genetic relationships in a family.
1. Start with couple being seen Male A and Female B
2. For each person: record names, dates of birth, illnesses, surgery

Ask about miscarriages, stillbirths, deaths

3. Ask about any children with other partners
4. Ask about siblings and their children, then parents
5. Ask whether couples are related

(b)

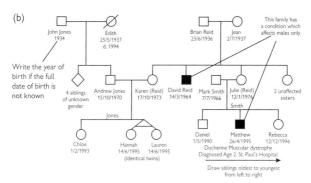

Fig. 2.12 How to draw a pedigree (a, b). Reproduced with kind permission of the National Genetics Education and Development Centre (NGEDC).

X-linked (XL) inheritance

XL disorders are encoded on the X chromosome. An XL recessive (XLR) disorder manifests in males who have one X chromosome, but generally not in carrier females who have two X chromosomes (one normal and one mutated copy). Some X-linked disorders are almost never expressed in females. In some disorders females have symptoms infrequently, e.g. Duchenne muscular dystrophy (DMD)/Becker muscular dystrophy (BMD), whereas for others, e.g. X-linked hereditary motor and sensory neuropathy (X-HMSN) and fragile X syndrome (FRAXA), manifestation in female carriers is fairly common but is usually less severe than in affected males. Disorders, in which heterozygotes commonly manifest, e.g. X-HMSN, may be said to follow **X-linked semi-dominant inheritance**.

X-inactivation

In order to fully understand sex chromosome inheritance patterns, it is important to divert briefly into **epigenetics**. This term means 'on top of genetics'. Epigenetics studies processes, e.g. methylation that turn genes 'on' or 'off'.

The sex chromosomes differ from the autosomes:
- The **Y chromosome** has ~122 genes that code mainly for the processes necessary to turn the fetus into a male.
- The **X chromosome** has >1000 genes, many of which are key to normal growth and development, including genes that:
  - code for dystrophin—a major protein in muscles
  - code for several of the proteins involved in the clotting sequence, e.g. haemophilia A (Factor VIII) and haemophilia B (Factor IX).

A normal male will have a single Y and a single X chromosome, whereas a normal female complement is two X chromosomes. In order to prevent overexpression of the X chromosome in a female, only one copy of the X chromosome is active in a female cell, the other being, *mostly*, inactivated. This process, **X-inactivation**, occurs in every cell in a developing female embryo 1–2 weeks after conception. It is also referred to as **Lyonization** in honour of its proposer, Dr Mary Lyon.

The early events in X-inactivation are under the control of the X-chromosome inactivation centre (Xic). The *XIST* gene (X Inactivation Specific Transcript), located at Xq13.3, plays an essential role in the initiation of X-inactivation by spreading an inactivation signal. Initiation of X-inactivation involves a counting step in which the number of X chromosomes in the cell is counted such that only a single X chromosome is functional per diploid adult cell, i.e. in a female with three X chromosomes (47,XXX), two X chromosomes are inactivated and in a male with two X chromosomes (47,XXY), one is inactivated.

A small region of the inactivated X chromosome remains unaffected by this process and is found at the tip of the short arm—the **pseudoautosomal region** (PAR) (📖 see X-linked dominant inheritance, p. 57).

X-inactivation in the embryo is a random process, which should therefore result in ~50% of cells containing the maternal X inactive and ~50% of cells containing the paternal X inactive.

Significant deviation from a 50:50 inactivation pattern is a feature of some X-linked disorders, a phenomenon referred to as *skewed X-inactivation*. Skewing of X-inactivation is occasionally observed among normal females in the population.

Examples of XL recessive conditions
- Duchenne (DMD) and Becker (BMD) muscular dystrophy
- Haemophilia A and B
- Glucose-6-phosphate dehydrogenase (G6PD) deficiency
- Red–green colour blindness

Aspects of XL recessive inheritance
- ***Manifesting carriers***. Unfavourable skewing of X-inactivation in key tissues may be a major factor in determining whether or not an XLR disorder is expressed in heterozygotes. As noted, the penetrance in heterozygotes shows wide variation between different XLR disorders.
- ***Germline mosaicism***. A number of XLR disorders—most notably DMD/BMD—have a substantial risk of germline mosaicism (i.e. oocytes or sperm with a mixture of chromosomal material). For the mother of an affected boy with a known mutation that is not present in the mother's genomic DNA, there is a 1 in 5 (20%) risk to a future son who inherits the same X chromosome as his affected brother (i.e. there is an overall 5% risk to future pregnancies), hence prenatal diagnosis should be offered (see Chapter 5, Duchenne and Becker muscular dystrophy, p. 112).

Typical family tree
X-linked recessive inheritance

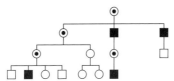

Fig. 2.13 A typical family tree showing X-linked recessive inheritance. The condition is expressed in males, but not in females. For a carrier female, on average, 50% of her sons will be affected and 50% of her daughters will be carriers. All daughters of an affected male are obligate carriers and none of his sons inherit the condition. (Reproduced from Firth, Hurst and Hall (2005) *Oxford Desk Reference—Clinical Genetics*, with permission from Oxford University Press.)

X-linked recessive inheritance

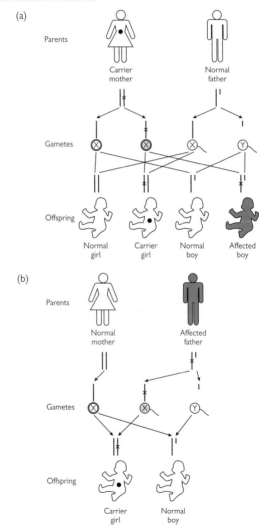

Fig. 2.14 X-linked recessive inheritance. (a) Offspring of a carrier mother. (b) Offspring of an affected father. (Reproduced from Firth, Hurst and Hall (2005), *Oxford Desk Reference—Clinical Genetics*, with permission from Oxford University Press.)

Genetic advice (📖 see Figs. 2.13 and 2.14)

- Males carrying the mutation are severely affected; females carrying the mutation are generally either unaffected or more mildly affected than males.
- The degree to which females express the disorder is largely governed by X-inactivation patterns.
- When a carrier female has a pregnancy there are four possible outcomes, each equally likely. These are:
  - a normal daughter
  - a carrier daughter
  - a normal son
  - an affected son
- Another way of expressing this is that in a female pregnancy there is a 50% chance of a carrier daughter; in a male pregnancy there is a 50% chance of an affected son.
- When an affected male fathers a pregnancy, all of his daughters will be carriers and none of his sons will be affected.
- The family tree shows no male-to-male transmission.
- Even if the proband is the only affected member, it is generally more likely that the mother is a carrier than that the proband has the condition as the result of a *de novo* mutation. For XLR conditions where reproductive fitness is zero, there is a two-thirds chance that the mother is a mutation carrier and a one-third chance that the mutation is *de novo* for an apparently sporadic case.
- If the mother of a sporadic case with a presumed *de novo* mutation does not herself carry the mutation in her blood, female siblings of the proband should still be offered carrier testing by mutation detection because of the small possibility of germline mosaicism in the mother.
- Females with unusually severe features of an XLR disorder may have this as a consequence of:
  - Highly unfavourably skewed X-inactivation.
  - Turner syndrome, where the girl has a single X chromosome.
  - X-autosome translocation.

Hence a karyotype is indicated in these circumstances.

X-linked dominant inheritance (XLD) (📖 see Fig. 2.15)

An XLD disorder manifests very severely in males, often leading to spontaneous loss or neonatal death of affected male pregnancies. Hence the disorder appears to affect females exclusively and there is often a history of miscarriage and a predominance of females in the pedigree. XLD disorders are uncommon and examples include the rare genetic disorder Rett syndrome.

Typical family tree
X-linked dominant inheritance

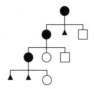

Fig. 2.15 A family tree showing X-linked dominant inheritance. The condition is manifest in female heterozygotes and male hemizygotes. Many of these conditions cause spontaneous loss of affected male pregnancies. (Reproduced from Firth, Hurst and Hall (2005). *Oxford Desk Reference—Clinical Genetics*, with permission from Oxford University Press.)

Genetic investigations

Chromosome basics

- Chromosomes (📖 see Fig. 3.1) are found in a cell's nucleus and derive their name from the Greek for coloured body '*chroma soma*'.
- They carry genes and are composed mainly of **chromatin**, in which the DNA helix is wrapped around core histones (proteins) to form a 'beads on a string' configuration (📖 see Fig. 3.2).
- The human genome is made up of $\sim3.2 \times 10^9$ base pairs, less than 10% of which actually code for proteins (the rest are probably important for maintaining chromosome structure and regulating gene expression).
- A normal human cell has 22 pairs of numbered chromosomes and 2 sex chromosomes (normally XX in a female and XY in a male), i.e. 46 chromosomes in total. This is called a **diploid** complement (2n).
- A single set of chromosomes (e.g. sperm or ovum) is a **haploid** complement (n).
- If there is an abnormal number of chromosomes in a cell, this is termed **aneuploidy**.
- The gain of a single chromosome is referred to as **trisomy**.
- Chromosomes have a **centromere** (where the two chromatin coils appear to join, and where the two coils are pulled apart in meiosis) and two arms ending in **telomeres** (important in maintaining chromosomal stability).
- The shorter arm of the chromosomes is called *p* and the longer arm *q*.

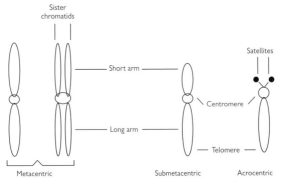

Fig. 3.1 Classification of chromosomes depending on the position of centromeres. (Reproduced from Young (2005), *Medical Genetics*, Fig. 1.5, p. 7, with permission from Oxford University Press.)

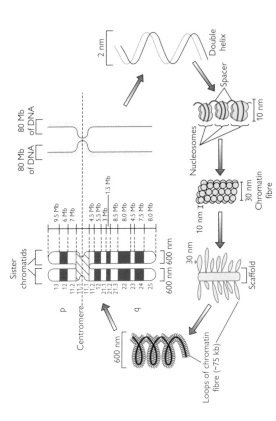

Fig. 3.2 Stages in the packaging of DNA to form chromosome number 17. (Reproduced with permission from Strachan, T. and Read, A.P. (2004) *Human Molecular Genetics 3*. Garland Science, London.)

DNA basics

- Human heredity is encoded by the nucleic acid DNA.
- A nucleic acid is a chain of nucleotides; a nucleotide is a purine or pyrimidine base with attached sugar and phosphate entities.
- In DNA the sugar is deoxyribose (hence deoxyribonucleic acid): in RNA the sugar is ribose (hence ribonucleic acid).
- DNA contains four types of bases—two purines, adenine (A) and guanine (G), and two pyrimidines, cytosine (C) and thymine (T). RNA contains uracil (U) in place of thymine.
- The DNA double helix (structure determined by Watson and Crick in 1953) maintains a constant width and is faithfully replicated, because purines always face pyrimidines in the complementary A–T and G–C base pairs. Thus, DNA:
  - serves as a template for replication that re-establishes the double helix
  - can be 'read' and 'copied' in the process of producing proteins.
- The paired strands of DNA are referred to as the 5′ (five prime) and 3′ (three prime) strands, so named because at the 5′ end a phosphate group is attached to the 5th carbon atom of the sugar component, and at the 3′ end the phosphate group is attached to the 3rd carbon atom of the sugar component.
- The **human genome** (the entire human genetic complement) consists of ~21 000 genes.
- A **gene** is the fundamental unit of heredity and is a sequence of DNA involved in producing a polypeptide chain. It is functionally defined by its protein product. A gene contains:
  - coding segments (**exons**)
  - intervening sequences (**introns**)
  - regulatory elements, e.g. promoter.
- In genetic disorders an individual can be described by their:
  - **Genotype**: their genetic constitution.
  - **Phenotype**: their appearance, or other characteristics, which result from the interaction of their genetic constitution with the environment.
- A **mutation** is a hereditable structural change in the sequence of DNA resulting in a change to an individual's genotype which may, or may not, alter his/her phenotype.

DNA and protein synthesis—the genetic code

Protein synthesis involves transcription of the coding DNA (cDNA) into messenger RNA (mRNA) and then translation of the mRNA into a polypeptide (📖 see Fig 3.3). The 'sense' strand of DNA is read from the 'upstream' 5′ end to the 'downstream' 3′ end and transcribed by RNA polymerase to make mRNA. The non-coding introns are then removed by 'splicing'. mRNA then moves to the cytoplasm where it binds to transfer RNA (tRNA) on the surface of ribosomes. Every tRNA contains 3 nucleotide bases (an anticodon) which complement a set of 3 base pairs on the mRNA (a codon), which specifies a particular amino acid (📖 see Table 3.1) which is then added to the growing protein chain.

Because there are more codons (61 plus 3 STOP codons) than there are amino acids (20), almost all amino acids are represented by more than one codon, i.e. the code is degenerate, particularly at the third base (📖 see Table 3.1). 📖 See Table 3.2 for a list of amino acid abbreviations.

Table 3.1 Triplet codons and their corresponding amino acids and STOP sequences

	T	C	A	G
T	TTT = Phe	TCT = Ser	TAT = Tyr	TGT = Cys
	TTC = Phe	TCC = Ser	TAC = Tyr	TGC = Cys
	TTA = Leu	TCA = Ser	TAA = STOP	TGA = STOP
	TTG = Leu	TCG = Ser	TAG = STOP	TGG = Trp
C	CTT = Leu	CCT = Pro	CAT = His	CGT = Arg
	CTC = Leu	CCC = Pro	CAC = His	CGC = Arg
	CTA = Leu	CCA = Pro	CAA = Gln	CGA = Arg
	CTG = Leu	CCG = Pro	CAG = Gln	CGG = Arg
A	ATT = Ile	ACT = Thr	AAT = Asn	AGT = Ser
	ATC = Ile	ACC = Thr	AAC = Asn	AGC = Ser
	ATA = Ile	ACA = Thr	AAA = Lys	AGA = Arg
	ATG = Met	ACG = Thr	AAG = Lys	AGG = Arg
G	GTT = Val	GCT = Ala	GAT = Asp	GGT = Gly
	GTC = Val	GCC = Ala	GAC = Asp	GGC = Gly
	GTA = Val	GCA = Ala	GAA = Glu	GGA = Gly
	GTG = Val	GCG = Ala	GAG = Glu	GGG = Gly

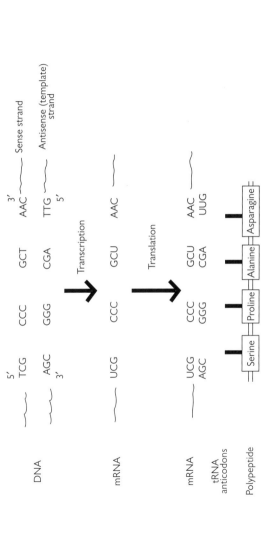

Fig. 3.3 Diagrammatic representation of how information in the sense strand of DNA is converted into a polypeptide chain. For the sake of simplicity, four codons are shown separated by short gaps. (Reproduced from Young (2005). *Medical Genetics*, Fig .1.5 p. 7, with permission from Oxford University Press.

Table 3.2 Amino acid abbreviations and genetic notations

Abbreviation	Amino acid	Genetic notation
Ala	Alanine	A
Arg	Arginine	R
Asn	Asparagine	N
Asp	Aspartic acid	D
Cys	Cysteine	C
Gln	Glutamine	Q
Glu	Glutamic acid	E
Gly	Glycine	G
His	Histidine	H
Ile	Isoleucine	I
Leu	Leucine	L
Lys	Lysine	K
Met	Methionine	M
Phe	Phenylalanine	F
Pro	Proline	P
Ser	Serine	S
Thr	Threonine	T
Trp	Tryptophan	W
Tyr	Tyrosine	Y
Val	Valine	V
STOP	Nonsense	X

DNA sequence variation and mutation

Genetic results are reported according to internationally agreed standards.

c. Refers to a numbered nucleotide in a gene sequence
p. Refers to a numbered amino acid in the protein product

Nucleotide substitutions (point mutations)

These are described by a number representing the nucleotide in the coding DNA (cDNA) sequence, followed by a letter representing the original nucleotide (A, C, G, T) followed by > and the mutated nucleotide, e.g. in the β-globin gene (*HBB*) c.17A>T means that adenine at nucleotide 17 is changed to thymine:

		Codon	
	5	6	7
HbA	CCT	GAG	GAG
	(Pro)	(Glu)	(Glu)
HbS	CCT	G**T**G	GAG
	(Pro)	(**Val**)	(Glu)

If this results in an amino acid substitution, the mutation is termed a **missense mutation**.

In protein annotation this is written with a number representing the amino acid in the translated protein product, the first letter preceding the number being the wild-type amino acid, and the letter after being the altered amino acid, e.g. in sickle cell disease (☐ see Haemoglobinopathies, p. 130), HbS differs structurally from HbA due to a missense mutation in the β-globin gene, denoted by p.E6V (glutamic acid at amino acid 6 is changed to valine). These molecular differences affect the way the protein chain folds, illustrated diagrammatically in ☐ Fig. 3.4.

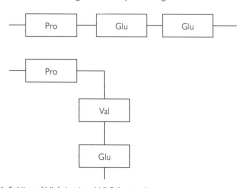

Fig. 3.4 Folding of HbA (top) and HbS (bottom).

If the nucleotide substitution does not alter the genetic code, it is termed a **silent** or **synonymous substitution**, although this could still cause problems by affecting splicing, etc.

Most **splice site mutations** occur in introns. Mutations in introns are referred to by the nearest nucleotide in an exon, e.g. in *CFTR* (the Cystic Fibrosis Transmembrane conductance Regulator gene, 📖 see Chapter 5, Cystic fibrosis, p. 104) c.621+1G>T, the first nucleotide (G) in the intron 3′ to nucleotide 621 in the cDNA is replaced by T and, in c.1717−1G>A, the last nucleotide (G) in the intron 5′ to nucleotide 1717 in the cDNA is replaced by A.

Nucleotide deletions and insertions

The nucleotide number is followed by del/ins and the letter for the relevant nucleotide, e.g. c.394delT means the nucleotide T at position 394 in the cDNA is deleted and c.3905−3906insT means a T is inserted after nucleotide 3905 in the cDNA. Insertions/deletions involving single nucleotides or pairs of nucleotides cause a shift in the reading frame (**frameshift mutation**) and usually result in protein truncation.

In protein annotation, the term delta (or a small triangle) is used to denote a deletion, e.g. in *CFTR*, the ΔF508 mutation means a deletion of phenylalanine at amino acid 508 resulting from a three-nucleotide deletion. Although this particular terminology is not current, it is still in widespread use.

Types of mutation and assessment of their significance

Some mutations, e.g. ΔF508, are well characterized as pathogenic changes (📖 see Table 3.3). On the other hand, interpreting the clinical significance of a newly identified 'private mutation', i.e. a mutation unique to a given individual or family, can sometimes be very difficult.

Missense mutations

A mutation that results in an altered amino acid sequence in the encoded protein is termed a missense mutation. Not all missense mutations are pathogenic as the nature of the amino acid change, and its precise location in the three-dimensional protein structure, will determine whether there is any effect on protein function (📖 see HbS mutation under nucleotide substitution above).

Truncating mutations

Mutations that result in protein truncation are nearly always pathogenic. They include single nucleotide substitutions that encode STOP codons (**nonsense mutations**), **frameshift mutations**, in which the reading frame is lost, and also large **deletions/insertions**.

Splice-site mutations

Splicing is the process by which the introns are removed from the primary transcript, and the exons are joined together. Splice-site mutations disrupt this process.

Some genes have alternative splice variants, where a single gene gives rise to more than one mRNA sequence that may have different tissue distributions. Mutations may abolish a splice acceptor or donor site or impair the efficiency of splicing, resulting in abnormal ratios of splice variants.

Triplet repeat mutations

A mutation caused by an increase in the number of copies of a repeated trinucleotide, e.g. $(CTG)_n$ and $(CAG)_n$. Examples of diseases caused by triplet repeat expansions are myotonic dystrophy (☐ see Chapter 5, Myotonic dystrophy, p. 152), fragile X syndrome (☐ see Chapter 5, Fragile X syndrome, p. 122) and Huntington disease (☐ see Chapter 5, Huntington disease, p. 144).

Triplet repeat mutations are unstable and may increase when transmitted from parent to child. This can cause significant worsening across generations, either causing the disease to appear at an earlier age, or be of worse severity. This phenomenon is called **anticipation**.

Table 3.3 The spectrum of known pathogenic mutations in humans. (Reproduced with permission of Oxford University Press, Young, *Medical Genetics*, Table 1.3, 2005.)

Type of mutation	Proportion of total (expressed as %)
Point mutations	
Missense	47
Nonsense	11
Splice-site	10
Regulatory	1
Deletions and insertions	
Gross deletions	5
Small deletions	16
Gross insertions and duplications	1
Small insertions	6
Other rearrangements	3

Data obtained from the Human Gene Mutation Database (🔗 www.hgmd.org) Sterson, P.D., Ball, E.V., Mort, M. *et al.* The human gene mutation database (HGMD): 2003 update. *Human Mutatation*, **21**, 2003, 577–81. Reprinted with permission of John Wiley & Sons, Inc.

Mechanisms by which mutations exert their effect on phenotype (📖 see Fig. 3.5)

Loss-of-function mutation ('inactivating' mutation)

This term includes nucleotide substitutions that introduce a stop codon, out-of-frame deletions resulting in a truncated protein, or specific mutations that cause loss of function of the protein by disturbing the conformation or charge of a site critical in the interaction of the protein with other molecules. Most mutations in recessively inherited disease are loss-of-function.

Haploinsufficiency arises when the normal phenotype requires the protein product of two alleles, and reduction to 50% of the gene product (as a result of a loss-of-function mutation) results in an abnormal phenotype.

Gain-of-function mutation ('activating' mutation)

These mutations are site-specific and usually result in constitutive activation of a specific protein function. In achondroplasia, *FGFR3* is mutated in a specific position (c.1138G>A or c.1138G>C). As a result, its normal signalling function is constitutively activated (i.e. activated even in the absence of bound fibroblast growth factor (FGF)) resulting in shortening of the long bones.

Dominant-negative mutation

This is a mutation in one copy of a gene resulting in a mutant protein that has not only lost its own function, but also prevents the heterozygously produced wild-type protein of the same gene from functioning normally. It commonly acts by producing an altered polypeptide (subunit) that prevents or impairs the assembly of a multimeric protein (an assembly of two or more protein molecules), e.g. assembly of collagen triple helices in osteogenesis imperfecta (OI) also known as 'brittle bone disease'.

Normal synthesis

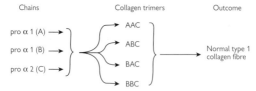

Mutation with a loss-of-function effect

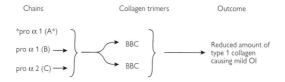

Mutation with a dominant-negative effect

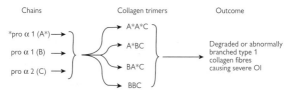

Fig. 3.5 Different mutational mechanisms in osteogenesis imperfecta ('brittle-bone disease'). The normal type I collagen molecule is a trimer made up of two proα1 chains and one proα2 chain. A mutant proα1 that becomes incorporated in the collagen trimers (dominant-negative effect) has more severe consequences than a mutant chain that is not synthesized (haploinsufficiency or loss-of-function effect). (Reproduced with permission from Suri, M. and Young, I.D. (2004). *Genetics for pediatricians*. Remedica, London)

Genetic investigations

Genetic analysis will be described briefly here, moving up through increasing levels of magnification.

Approaches to genetic investigation fall broadly into two groups: (i) genome-wide scans, e.g. chromosome analysis (karyotyping) and genomic microarray analysis ('molecular karyotyping'); and (ii) highly focused analysis of an individual gene. In the latter group, the decision to select one of the ~21 000 genes for mutation analysis is usually made on the basis of a presumptive clinical diagnosis, e.g. Duchenne muscular dystrophy (*DMD* gene), cystic fibrosis (*CFTR* gene).

Karyotyping (chromosome analysis) (📖 see Fig. 3.6)

This requires obtaining living, dividing cells from:
• Lymphocytes from venous blood (usually) or bone marrow pre-cursors
• Fibroblasts (skin)
• Chorionic villi or amniotic cells.

After preparation of these cells, usually by arresting cell division during metaphase when the chromosomes are in their most compact state, they can be stained using a variety of stains, the most common of which is **Giemsa**. After denaturing treatment with trypsin, this dye is added and binds to DNA, giving the characteristic appearance familiar to many of a 'G-banded karyotype'. Analysis is done using light microscopy by a skilled cytogeneticist and is labour intensive (it takes several hours to complete an individual karyotype analysis).

Each of these ~500 bands corresponds to ~ 6–8 Mb (Megabases) of DNA.

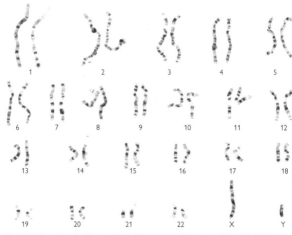

Fig. 3.6 Normal male Giemsa banded karyotype. (Reproduced from Firth, Hurst, and Hall (2005), *Oxford Desk Reference—Clinical Genetics*, with permission.)

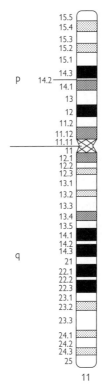

Fig. 3.7 Banding pattern of chromosome 11. (Reproduced from Francke, U. (1994). Digitized and differentially shaded human chromosome ideograms for genomic applications, *Cytogenet. Cell Genet.,* **65**, 206–19, and with the permission of S. Karger, A.G. Basel.)

Given the labelling system of the long and short arms, and the banding appearance, it is then easy to identify, for example, 11p15.5 as being on the short arm 'p' of chromosome 11 in band 15.5 (🕮 see Fig. 3.7).

FISH (fluorescent *in situ* hybridization)

This technique uses a DNA probe to identify a specific chromosomal abnormality that is too small to see with a light microscope, e.g. 22q11 deletion syndrome/DiGeorge syndrome. A DNA probe is made, with a complementary base sequence to a previously identified sequence in a target gene. A fluorescent dye is then attached to the DNA probe. When added to a chromosome spread, the probe hybridizes to the complementary sequence which will then fluoresce under UV light.

Whereas FISH does not give an overall analysis of a chromosome, it can be used in a prenatal setting to give a rapid result for the three common trisomies, i.e. trisomy 21, 18, and 13.

Genomic microarray techniques ('array-CGH')

This is essentially a method for very high-resolution 'chromosome analysis' and is sometimes termed 'molecular karyotyping'. Genomic arrays use competitive genome hybridization (CGH) of a mixture of test DNA from a diagnostic sample (labelled with a green probe) and normal DNA from a control (labelled red) with normal chromosomes. Hence an alteration in the green to red fluorescence ratio between the test sample and the normal sample will demonstrate whether there is more or less DNA from a particular chromosomal region and identify 'duplications' or 'deletions'.

Genomic microarrays vary in terms of their resolution, e.g. some arrays report at a resolution of ~1Mb and others down to resolutions of ~100kb or less. Routine karyotyping by light microscopy has a resolution of ~5–10Mb.

SNP arrays provide a powerful tool for genome-wide genotyping using single nucleotide polymorphisms (SNPs). This approach is commonly used in research studies, e.g. in genome-wide association studies of common diseases, e.g. diabetes, obesity, hypertension. High resolution SNP arrays can also be used for molecular karyotyping.

Genomic array analysis is a relatively new tool and sometimes gives results that, with current levels of knowledge, may be novel and difficult to interpret.

Multiplex ligation-dependent probe amplification (MLPA)

This is a technique for identifying small deletions and duplications. Each MLPA probe consists of two oligonucleotides that are ligated by a thermostable ligase if they bind to the target sequence.

Deletions (or duplications) of exons are an important class of intragenic mutation (e.g. *BRCA1*) that may be missed by conventional sequencing. Unless a strategy such as MLPA is used to detect 'dosage', routine sequencing methods will simply read the sequence from the normal allele, giving a normal result and failing to identify, for example, that an entire exon is deleted from the disease allele.

Chromosomal microdeletions can also be tested for using MLPA kits. e.g. 22q11 deletion syndrome, Williams' syndrome, and telomeric deletions.

Quantitative fluorescence polymerase chain reaction (QFPCR)

Small sections (markers) of DNA from the sample are amplified, labelled with fluorescent tags, and the amounts are measured by electrophoresis. QFPCR is used to test for gene dosage and can be used to test for aneuploidy of whole chromosomes, e.g. chromosomes 13, 18, and 21.

DNA sequencing

Most DNA sequencing methodology in common use is based upon the Sanger dideoxy method, named after its double Nobel prize winning inventor Dr Fred Sanger. The automation of sequencing, using fluorescent labelling of the four nucleotides, has created a faster, cheaper alternative to the original process.

'Next generation' sequencing using new technologies is being developed and is currently being gradually introduced into large-scale research facilities. These machines have a huge sequencing capacity and will enable much faster and cheaper sequencing in the medium to long term, bringing the prospect of the '$1000 genome' ever closer.

Genetic linkage

If two loci are positioned on the same chromosome, the distance between those two loci will affect the chance of there being a crossover, or recombination, during meiosis (gamete formation). This linkage or genetic distance can be measured and is referred to as the recombination fraction, denoted by θ. This is expressed in centiMorgans (cM) where a distance of 1cM between loci means that a crossover will occur between them once per 100 meioses: the greater the value of θ the further apart the two loci are.

Linkage analysis

Prenatal diagnosis

Linkage analysis is occasionally used in the clinical setting for example for prenatal diagnosis of well-characterized monogenic disorders, e.g. cystic fibrosis, where the mutation on only one allele is known and, using linkage, it is possible to 'track' the presumed second mutation on the other allele.

PGH (pre-implantation genetic haplotyping)

Using this method, a series of single nucleotide polymorphisms (SNPs) located in and around the disease gene is used to track a given disease gene. This technique enables PGD for monogenic disorders because the SNP haplotype for a given gene can be analysed, which is technically more straightforward and generalizable than developing customized assays for individual 'private' mutations. The technical challenges are formidable and PGH has limited availability.

Genetic services and the primary care interface

Referral to a genetics service

Who should be referred to Clinical Genetics?

Typical reasons for a referral to a genetics clinic include:

- *Family history of a genetic disorder:* a person with a genetic condition in the family wants to know the risk that he/she will develop the condition or pass it to his/her children.
- *Family history of cancer:* a person worried about a family history of cancer wants to know if he/she is at increased risk and to discuss the options for surveillance and management.
- *Diagnosis:* a child with problems such as developmental delay, learning difficulties, congenital anomalies (e.g. heart defect, deafness) may be referred if there is concern that there may be a genetic basis to the child's condition. If a child has multiple problems, the geneticist may be asked to assess whether there is a unifying genetic diagnosis.
- *Issues related to genetic testing:* a genetic test, e.g. chromosome analysis, arranged by a paediatrician, hospital specialist, or GP has given an abnormal/atypical/unusual result or has diagnosed a genetic disorder.
- *Reproductive advice:* parents of a child with a genetic condition, or a condition that may have a genetic cause, wish advice about the likelihood of similar problems recurring in a future pregnancy.
- *A new diagnosis of a genetic disorder* in the patient or his/her child or a member of their extended family.
- *Teenager/young adult* with a genetic problem that was diagnosed in early childhood may need referral for an explanation about the genetic basis of his/her disorder, and discussion about their reproductive risks and options for prenatal diagnosis.

A family history suggestive of a genetic disorder, i.e. with a problem that affects more than one family member, is the most common reason for PCPs to make a Genetics referral. Familial histories of cancer, particularly breast and bowel, form a significant majority of such referrals.

A recent audit of referrals to a regional genetics service showed that 27% of their referrals came from primary care, with 34% coming from O&G or Paediatrics. Demand for genetic advice is growing, driven mainly by increasing awareness about the importance of genetics in the aetiology of disease. Media interest in genetics is also fuelling patient expectation.

Referral to Clinical Genetics before or during a pregnancy

A referral should be made for:

- Women with a previous pregnancy affected by a genetic disorder.
- Women with a family history of a genetic disorder.
- When the mother or her partner has a genetic disorder.
- When the mother or her partner carries a chromosomal disorder, e.g. translocation.
- Women taking medication or other substances which may have a teratogenic effect.

It is advisable to refer requests for genetic advice in pregnancy as a priority, either by telephone or fax.

The Primary Care—Clinical Genetics interface

A truly *accurate* diagnosis is paramount. Different types of 'muscular dystrophy' have different modes of inheritance, for example autosomal dominant, autosomal recessive, X-linked recessive, and mitochondrial. Advice for offspring and other relatives will depend on the mode of inheritance. For example the X-linked condition, Becker muscular dystrophy (BMD) may be clinically indistinguishable from an autosomal recessive form of limb-girdle muscular dystrophy. The daughter of a man with BMD will be an obligate carrier with a 1 in 2 risk to a future son, whereas the daughter of a man with AR limb-girdle dystrophy will have a very small (<1/200 risk) to her offspring (unless she marries a relative or her partner has a family history of the same type of limb-girdle dystrophy).

- Confirmation of the precise diagnosis is therefore essential before advising on recurrence risks or risks to the extended family, and usually requires obtaining the primary documentation, e.g. mutation reports, pathology reports, etc.
- Regional genetic services will routinely obtain this documentation before providing genetic advice to patients. Hence referral is recommended in order to ensure accurate genetic advice.

✎ Making the referral

Regional genetics services (📖 see Fig. 4.1 and the Directory of UK and Ireland Genetics Centres, p. 415) can be contacted by phone, fax, and, some centres, by email if PCPs have queries about the need for, or the process of, referral. To check catchment areas for the regional services, particularly for the metropolitan districts. (see ✍ www.gig.org.uk.)
Letters should contain (where relevant):
- Name, address, DoB, NHS number
- Contact details for the patient(s) and the surgery
- Current history
- Relevant previous medical/obstetric/birth history
- Family history as given by the patient (📖 see Chapter 2, Taking a family history, p. 52) with:
  - Names of, and relationships between, family members
  - Dates of birth, diagnosis, and death of the affected individuals (where known)
- A précis of your genetic understanding of the patient's condition (e.g. your analysis of a NICE guideline) and an explanation of your expectations of the service.
- A description of what your patient has been told and is expecting from the referral.

Regional genetics services in the UK

There are 23 regional genetics services throughout the UK. They are multi-disciplinary services including clinicians, genetic counsellors, laboratory scientists (molecular geneticists and cytogeneticists) and administrative/secretarial staff. Each regional genetic service serves a population of ~2–3 million people.

Clinical genetics services are provided by teams of consultant clinical geneticists, specialist trainees, and genetic counsellors.

- *Clinical geneticists* are doctors whose main expertise is in the diagnosis of genetic disease and malformation syndromes, and who have undergone specialist training to consultant level following general professional training in medicine or paediatrics. A consultation with a clinical geneticist will usually involve a conventional medical approach, including history (including family history), examination, investigation, diagnosis (or differential diagnosis), genetic advice, and reproductive advice (where relevant).
- *Genetic counsellors* (GC) either have (i) a nursing background, e.g. in midwifery/health visiting, and acquire their knowledge of clinical genetics through working in a regional genetics service and participating in a training/accreditation programme to become registered as a genetic counsellor; or (ii) have an MSc in genetic counselling and acquire their knowledge of health care by working in a regional genetics service and participating in a training/accreditation programme to become registered as a genetic counsellor. Most GCs undertake formal education in counselling as part of their training. They may have their own caseload of patients where the genetic diagnosis is usually established or where further assessment does not require clinical examination. They often have particular expertise in predictive genetic testing, e.g. in familial cancer syndromes.

Genetics clinics

- *General genetics clinics:* the regional genetics services each run regular general genetics clinics in their main centre, which is usually based in a teaching hospital. They also run peripheral clinics in district general hospitals throughout their region (usually on a weekly, fortnightly, or monthly basis).
- *Specialist genetics clinics:* e.g. cardiac genetics, eye genetics, will often be run in the main centre in conjunction with other specialists, e.g. cardiology, ophthalmology, as appropriate.

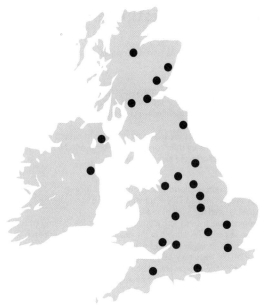

Fig. 4.1 Map showing location of regional genetics services in the UK. (Reproduced with permission from the British Society for Human Genetics.)

Tests—genetic tests in primary care

Samples for genetic tests

Occasionally, PCPs may be asked to obtain samples from patients for genetic testing.

Before samples are obtained, practitioners must check:
- That the appropriate consents are in place.
- Be clear that their patient is aware of the possible implications of the test.
- **Label sample tubes clearly** using three-point patient references, preferably including their name, date of birth, and NHS number on both request form and sample bottles.

Samples of venous blood should be taken as follows:
- **DNA** analysis into an EDTA tube (5ml)—this is usually the same type of tube as used for a full blood count (FBC).
- **Chromosome** analysis into a lithium heparin tube (2–5ml) (this may change to an EDTA sample in the near future as the approach to chromosome analysis changes from light microscopy to genomic array). Occasionally tests may be possible on buccal swabs or mouthwashes. In these cases the equipment will be supplied. Most PCPs will be familiar with the types of kits supplied by private firms who offer paternity testing.

Read the request form carefully and if in doubt, phone the laboratory.

Predictive genetic tests—✍ refer to Clinical Genetics

Predictive genetic testing for significant genetic disease and genetic testing of children should not be undertaken in primary care. Testing should always involve the local genetics service.

Genetic test results—will there be a conclusion?

In brief, often, but not always ... genetic knowledge and interpretation is progressing with ever-increasing speed, but many patients will be left with uncertainty with which they and their family must live. For predictive genetic testing, the variability in gene penetrance, expression, interaction with other genes and/or environmental factors, means that while it may be possible to state with certainty whether an individual has or has not inherited the familial mutation, it may not be possible to accurately predict when the disorder may onset and how severely the individual may be affected. Thus, although individuals testing negative for a familial mutation can be reassured, those testing positive swap one set of uncertainties 'Will I get the disease?' for another 'When will it affect me and how severely?'. They will continue to need long-term support from all involved in their care.

Surveillance of genetic disease

PCPs may be asked to participate in the surveillance of their patients who are either at risk of genetic disease, or getting complications from such diseases.

Disease-specific surveillance is discussed for individual diseases, e.g. neurofibromatosis type 1, myotonic dystrophy, in 📖 Chapter 5, p. 156 and p. 152 respectively.

What happens at a genetics consultation?

There is no standard referral protocol in the UK. The initial response to a new referral may vary, but is likely to include one or both of the following components:

- Contact with the affected individual/family offering a preliminary meeting/telephone consultation with a genetic counsellor.
- A letter to the patient enclosing a family history form which will then be reviewed to determine whether an appointment is required.
- An appointment to see a clinical geneticist/genetic counsellor in outpatients or sometimes in the patients' home or place of residence. In some centres a counsellor may contact the individual/family prior to an appointment to:
- Ascertain the patient(s) understanding of the reason for the referral.
- Take a family history, optimally across three generations or more.
- Initiate specific further enquiries (e.g. establish histologically precise diagnoses of any cancers via a local or national cancer registry).
- Obtain relevant consents for relevant enquiries.
- Explain the need to, and obtain consents from, other family members, and initiate such contact where necessary.
- Discuss the expected next point of contact by the genetics service.

Genetic counselling

Genetic counselling can be defined as: 'The process by which individuals or relatives at risk for a genetic disorder that may be hereditary are advised of the consequences of that disorder, the probability of developing or transmitting it, and the ways in which this may be prevented, avoided, or ameliorated' (Harper 1998).

Most patients coming to a genetics clinic want answers to four simple questions:

1. What is it, i.e. what is the diagnosis?
2. Why did it happen, i.e. what is the genetic basis of the disease?
3. Will it happen again, i.e. what is the recurrence risk or risk to other family members?
4. If so, what can be done to prevent/manage that risk, i.e. surveillance, prenatal diagnosis, etc.?

Genetic advice is 'non-directive', i.e. patients will not be told what course of action to follow. If a patient/couple/family need to make choices about options that are available to them, e.g. for genetic testing or surveillance, they will be given the relevant information to enable them to make an informed choice and offered help and support in reaching a decision.

The genetics consultation

The consultation with the Genetics service may involve a consultant/specialist trainee/genetic counsellor. Appointments with the genetics service will usually last between 30min and 60min. During the consultation, the geneticist will usually:

- **Set an agenda for the consultation** by eliciting the main issues at the outset of the consultation. Is the main issue finding a diagnosis, or determining whether an individual with a family history is themselves at risk of developing the condition, or reviewing the natural history if that is known? If the condition may have implications for future children, they will offer to discuss this. They will try to establish what it is that the family wants to find out.
- **Determine the patient's perception:** what is the patient's interpretation of their problems/their child's problems, or family history?
- **Establish a genetic diagnosis** (where possible) or a differential diagnosis.
- **Explain the genetic basis of the condition** if known, or if unknown, they will advise whether or not it is likely to have a genetic basis.
- **Assess the genetic risk to other family members** and discuss whether or not there is a significant risk to other family members not present at the consultation. If an appreciable risk exists, they will work with the patient/family to agree a strategy for offering genetic advice and investigation to other members of the family.

Further reading

Harper P.S. (1998) *Practical genetic counselling*, 5th edn. Oxford; Boston: Butterworth-Heinemanne.

Common genetic conditions

Introduction

While individual genetic disorders are rare, collectively they are not uncommon. Indeed, since genetic conditions are often life-long disorders they account for a significant burden of disease, especially amongst younger members of the population. Most general practices will have patients and/or families who are affected by some of the conditions outlined in this chapter.

Primary care can play an important role in targeted surveillance for genetic conditions such as myotonic dystrophy or neurofibromatosis type 1. In this chapter we have outlined the surveillance required for individual disorders and indicated when this can be provided in primary care.

If you have additional queries, the following resources may be helpful:

- Regional genetics services, 📖 see Directory of UK and Ireland Genetics Centres, p. 415
- Geneclinics: 🐾 http://www.geneclinics.org/
- OMIM: 🐾 http://www.ncbi.nlm.nih.gov/omim/

Alpha$_1$-antitrypsin deficiency

Introduction

Alpha$_1$-antitrypsin is a proteinase inhibitor that protects the connective tissue of the lungs from the elastase released by leucocytes. Alpha$_1$-antitrypsin deficiency is a common autosomal recessive (AR) disorder (1/1600–1/1800) characterized by a predisposition to emphysema and cirrhosis. Liver damage arises not from deficiency of the protease inhibitor, but from pathological polymerization of the variant alpha$_1$-antitrypsin before its secretion from hepatocytes.

PiM is the normal protein. 10% of the European population are carriers for the S or Z variant (4% (1/25) of northern Europeans carry Z, and 6% (1/17) carry S). Common phenotypes are PiMM, PiMS, PiMZ, PiSS, PiSZ, and PiZZ. Null variants are rare and are only distinguishable from homozygotes by genotyping.

Genetics

Inheritance and recurrence risk

AR inheritance. The possibility that apparently healthy parents of a ZZ or SZ child may themselves be ZZ or SZ should be borne in mind when offering phenotyping. If MZ parents have had a child with a ZZ phenotype and severe neonatal liver disease, there is a 1 in 4 risk for a subsequent ZZ child. However, because of the variable expressivity of the phenotype in alpha$_1$-antitrypsin, the chance that a subsequent ZZ child will also develop severe liver disease is estimated at 20–30%.

Prenatal diagnosis—✍ refer to Clinical Genetics

This is available using chorionic villus sampling (CVS). Parents must have been phenotyped first and subsequently genotyped. In practice, it is rarely requested. Prenatal diagnosis is by genotyping of DNA from CVS.

Other family members

- The most important message for family members is *not to smoke*. Smoking greatly accelerates lung disease in alpha$_1$-antitrypsin deficiency and markedly reduces life expectancy.

Smoking also accelerates smoking-related lung disease in carriers. Offer smoking cessation support.

- Because carrier status is so common in the general population (10% (1/10)) and because so few ZZ individuals experience severe neonatal liver disease, cascade screening of the entire family is rarely appropriate.

Carrier status is common in the general population (1/10) with 4% (1/25) of northern Europeans carrying the Z allele and 6% (1/17) carrying the S allele.

Consultation plan in primary care

History
- May present neonatally with prolonged jaundice.
- May present with chronic recurrent chest infections.
- May present with liver enzyme abnormalities.
- Smoking history.
- Three-generation family tree, with specific enquiry regarding emphysema and liver disease.

Examination
- Jaundice, other signs of liver disease (palmar erythaema, spider naevae, etc.),
- Crackles at lung bases.

Investigations in primary care
- LFTs
- CXR
- Clotted sample (serum) for alpha$_1$-antitrypsin phenotyping could be arranged from primary care after adequate discussion and with appropriate consent, or the patient could be referred for specialist advice and investigation. If interpretation of phenotyping is problematic, it may be necessary to proceed to genotyping (EDTA sample). NB If alpha$_1$-antitrypsin typing is to be attempted on an individual who has had a liver transplant, the alpha$_1$-antitrypsin phenotype will reflect the genotype of the donor liver (since this protein is made in the liver), and mutation analysis (of DNA from lymphocytes) will be needed to determine the genotype of the transplant recipient.

Management in primary care
- Refer patient to paediatrician/adult services as appropriate.
- Consider referring proband and siblings to genetics service.
  NB: Cascade screening the extended family is rarely appropriate.
- Consider influenza and pneumococcal vaccination.
- Agree periodicity of surveillance of liver blood tests (bilirubin/enzymes/clotting) and lung function.
- Aim to minimize pyrexia and acute-phase inflammation by active treatment of incidental infections in ZZ homozygotes, especially in infancy.
- Subsequent affected siblings of an alpha$_1$-antitrypsin deficient proband should receive intramuscular vitamin K at birth to prevent intracranial bleeds.
- Code patient's notes.
- Code notes, with appropriate consents of other family members (see Chapter 1, Confidentiality and consent, p. 8).

Long-term complications
- *Emphysema.* In healthy non-smokers, forced expiratory volume in 1 second (FEV_1) decreases by 35mL/yr, in ZZ non-smokers the average decrease is 45mL/yr, but in ZZ smokers, the rate is doubled at 70mL/yr, reflecting the development of pan-lobar basal emphysema.
- *Cirrhosis.* The risk of cirrhosis in adult life is difficult to quantify, but ZZ individuals are at increased risk for chronic liver disease. Many have subclinical liver disease at post-mortem.

The most important message for family members is **not to smoke**. Smoking greatly accelerates lung disease in alpha$_1$-antitrypsin deficiency and markedly reduces life expectancy. Offer smoking cessation support.

Support groups
UK ✆ www.alpha1.org.uk
USA ✆ www.alpha1.org

Autism and autism spectrum disorders

Introduction
Autism is characterized by qualitative impairments in reciprocal social interaction and communication coupled with restricted and stereotyped patterns of interests and activities. The recurrence risk of autism in siblings is much higher than the rate of the disorder in the general population. The concordance rate in monozygotic (MZ) twins (60–91%) is higher than in dizygotic (DZ) twins (0–6%) suggesting a strong genetic component to autism susceptibility. In addition, the genetic liability to autism confers a risk for a broader range of more subtle impairments in social communication and play development. These variants may be described as atypical autism, Asperger syndrome, or pervasive developmental disorder not otherwise specified. Collectively, these conditions are referred to as **autism spectrum disorders**.

Classical autism
- With a prevalence of 1–2/1000, it is much more common in males with a M:F ratio of approximately 4:1.
- The prevalence of autism spectrum disorders is approximately 6/1000.
- Autistic children fail to use eye contact to regulate social interchanges and are often delayed in their language development, with little babble; some autistic children never acquire speech.
- Although described in terms of social and behavioural abnormalities, autism is also associated with an uneven pattern of cognitive defects. Many autistic individuals have full-scale intelligence quotient (IQ) scores <70, but show greater visuospatial than verbal skills. A small minority have one or more outstanding skill, well above their overall low level of functioning.
- There is evidence for an underlying neurodevelopmental disorder as 25–30% develop epilepsy by adult life (often with onset in teenage years) and 25% have head size >97th centile.
- Only a small percentage of children with autism have a specific genetic diagnosis. Specific identifiable aetiologies include fragile X syndrome (FRAX) (📖 see Fragile X syndrome, p. 122), tuberous sclerosis (TSC) (📖 see Tuberous sclerosis, p. 174), Rett syndrome, and a variety of chromosomal anomalies.
- In 90% the cause is unknown.

Differential diagnosis
- ***Asperger syndrome.*** Asperger syndrome is characterized by higher cognitive abilities and more normal language function. It is much more common in males than females (M:F, 8:1). In one study, there was a high rate of close relatives with autism spectrum problems but also high rates of prenatal and perinatal problems.
- ***Tuberous sclerosis (TSC).*** (📖 See Tuberous sclerosis, p. 174.) Autosomal dominant (AD) neurocutaneous disorder due to mutations in TSC1 and TSC2. TSC is reported in 1% of children with autism. In TSC, autism is seen in 72.5% of individuals. Children who present with seizures, particularly infantile spasms, in the first 2yrs of life are

more likely to have learning disability and autism or autism spectrum disorders than those who develop seizures later or remain seizure-free.
• **Fragile X syndrome.** (☐ See Fragile X syndrome, p. 122.) Autistic features are common in fragile X syndrome.

Genetics

Inheritance and recurrence risk

The rate of autism and other forms of pervasive developmental disorder in siblings of autistic probands is 3–5% (45-fold increase in risk) with an additional 5–7% risk that he/she will have some type of broader social communication disorder of a less seriously handicapping variety (i.e. able to manage in mainstream education with appropriate support). Offspring of unaffected siblings are at a low risk (see below).

Prenatal diagnosis—✍ refer to Clinical Genetics

Not usually possible unless there is a laboratory diagnosis in the affected individual, e.g. a specific monogenic disorder such as TSC or FRAXA or a chromosomal disorder.

Consultation plan in primary care

History
• Pre-, peri-, and postnatal history.
• Detailed developmental history especially of language development.
• Specific enquiry regarding regression/loss of skills.
• Three-generation family tree with specific enquiry about schooling, career, hobbies, and sociability of parents and other close relatives.

Examination
Growth parameters: height, weight, and occipital–frontal circumference (OFC).

Initial management plan in primary care
• Referral for assessment by child psychiatrist/clinical psychologist/ paediatrician.
• Encourage liaison of referral information from SENCO/school, etc.
• Refer to Joint Agency Children's team if available.

Ongoing management in primary care

Traditionally, autism has been considered to be a lifelong and seriously handicapping disorder, but now that subtler forms of autism spectrum disorder are being recognized, it is becoming appreciated that the outcome may not always be so limited.
• Educational and behavioural interventions are the mainstay of management.
• Risperidone shows some promise as a treatment for tantrums, aggression, or self-injurious behaviour in children with these associated features (use if recommended by secondary care).

(Continued)

- Depressive and psychotic disorders may develop and require psychopharmacological treatment.
- Parents require support from health visitors and other primary care members.
- May need extra financial support from care allowances, etc., refer to social services manager.
- Council tax exemption if serious mental handicap.
- Disability living allowance (DLA).
- Code patient's notes.
- Code notes, with appropriate consents, of patient and other family members (📖 see Chapter 1, Confidentiality and consent, p. 8).

Investigations in secondary care
- Chromosome analysis and fragile X.
- Examination of skin with Wood's light for hypopigmented macules (TSC), especially if there is a history of seizures.
- Neuroimaging is not part of routine clinical assessment, but is indicated for specific neurological signs, epileptic focus on electroencephalogram (EEG), or triad of severe learning disability, autism, and epilepsy.

Potential long-term complications
- About 30% will develop seizures by adult life (often with onset in teenage years).
- Most individuals with classical autism will not be able to live independently as adults.

Support group
The National Autistic Society: 🖢 www.nas.org.uk

Autosomal dominant polycystic kidney disease (ADPKD)

Introduction

ADPKD is a common autosomal dominant (AD) disorder with a prevalence of ~1/800 across all ethnic groups. It is caused by mutation in either the *PKD1* gene (85%) or in the *PKD2* gene (15%). It is a systemic disorder characterized by:

- Age-dependent cysts: kidney, liver, pancreas, and spleen.
- Cardiovascular abnormalities: hypertension, mitral valve prolapse, intracranial aneurysms (ICA), and left ventricular hypertrophy (LVH).
- Connective tissue abnormalities: hernias, colonic diverticulae.
- Age at presentation with renal failure is earlier in PKD1 than PKD2, 54yrs vs. 74yrs.

ADPKD is usually regarded as a disease of adult life. However, a small minority may present in childhood with loin pain, etc. A tiny minority (~1%) present *in utero* when multiple intra-renal cysts or 'bright hyperechogenic kidneys' are detected during detailed antenatal USS.

Genetics

Inheritance and recurrence risk

AD with 50% risk to offspring of a mutation carrier. There is usually an extensive family history. *De novo* mutations do occur, but are uncommon. There is marked inter- and intrafamilial phenotypic variability.

Prenatal diagnosis—✍ refer to Clinical Genetics if requested

Technically feasible by chorionic villus sampling (CVS) if the mutation is known, or if the kindred is large enough that clear linkage to chromosome 16 or 4 can be established (Ⓛ see Chapter 3, Genetic linkage, p. 78). In practice, prenatal diagnosis is rarely available.

Predictive testing—✍ refer to Clinical Genetics/Nephrology

Renal USS is the mainstay for predictive testing; mutation analysis is less commonly used. Residual risk of ADPKD following a normal renal USS at 25yrs is <5%; by 30yrs the residual risk has dropped to 2%. Computerized tomography (CT) and magnetic resonance imaging (MRI) are more sensitive than USS, and may be used following a normal USS if an individual is contemplating donating a kidney to a member of the family with end-stage renal failure (ESRF) (living-related transplant). Linkage may also be desirable in clarifying the status of a potential donor, if mutation analysis is not feasible.

Other family members

A cascade approach to diagnosis in adult relatives is appropriate because of the benefits of good control of hypertension and the high morbidity and mortality associated with undiagnosed chronic renal failure.

Differential diagnosis

Includes renal cysts and diabetes (RCAD), von Hippel–Lindau (VHL) and autosomal recessive polycystic kidney disease (ARPKD).

Consultation plan in primary care

History
- History of loin pain, haematuria, or recurrent UTIs.
- Where and by whom was the diagnosis made in a relative?
- Has any family member been seen by a genetics service?
- Three-generation family tree with specific enquiry about affected relatives, age of diagnosis, reason for diagnosis, age of onset of ESRF, history of subarachnoid haemorrhage (SAH)/ICA, cause of death.

Examination
- Blood pressure.
- Heart sounds for mitral valve prolapse.
- Abdomen for palpable kidneys or liver.

Investigations
FBC, RFT, LFT, urine dipstick, and MSU.

Initial management in primary care

- If abnormalities discovered, referral to Nephrology indicated for definitive investigation.
- Consider referral to Clinical Genetics.
- Code patient's notes.
- Code notes, with appropriate consent, of other family members (📖 see Chapter 1, Confidentiality and consent, p. 8).

Ongoing management in primary care

- **Hypertension.** Blood pressure should be monitored annually from teenage years. Aggressive treatment of hypertension is important in reducing the risk of accelerated cardiovascular and cerebrovascular disease seen in ADPKD and in prolonging renal function.
- **Creatinine.** Once a diagnosis of ADPKD is made, plasma creatinine should be monitored annually if normal and, if plasma creatinine is elevated, the patient should be referred to a nephrologist.
- **Pregnancy.** Women with ADPKD usually tolerate pregnancy well but must be under specialist supervision for monitoring of hypertension (which may worsen in pregnancy) and they are at some increased risk for pre-eclampsia (PET). Renal function usually remains stable throughout pregnancy. Fetal anomaly USS may occasionally show renal cysts in an affected fetus.
- **Drugs.** Avoid non-steroidal anti-inflammatory drugs (NSAIDs), e.g. ibuprofen, if renal function is abnormal. Explain about the danger of OTC NSAIDs. Prescribe all drugs with care if renal function is impaired.

Natural history and management

- Many patients with PKD2 will die of another cause.
- Death due to SAH occurs in ~6% of patients with ADPKD, with aneurysmal rupture on average at age 41yrs, a decade earlier than in sporadic cases. Patients with PKD2 as well as PKD1 are at risk of ICA.
- Hypertension is frequent and of early onset.

Potential long-term complications

- *ESRF.* Treated by renal transplantation, haemodialysis, or peritoneal dialysis.
- *UTI.* Prompt treatment of infection is important: if infection becomes established in cysts it can be very difficult to eradicate.
- *ICA.* Asymptomatic 'berry aneurysms' are found in 8% of individuals with ADPKD (population risk is 1–2%). The incidence rises to 16–25% in the presence of a positive family history. Screening by magnetic resonance angiography (MRA) may be considered for adults if there is a strong adverse family history of ICA, and should be arranged in conjunction with neurosurgical colleagues so that a management plan is agreed before imaging is undertaken.

Support group

Polycystic disease charity: ☏ www.pkdcharity.co.uk; ☎ 01388 665004.

Cystic fibrosis (CF)

Introduction

CF is the most common life-limiting autosomal recessive (AR) disorder in the northern European population. Universal neonatal screening is offered in the UK and many other countries. Three clinical phenotypes are associated with mutations in the CF transmembrane conductance regulator gene (*CFTR*) on 7q31–32:

- **Classical CF.** Obstructive lung disease, bronchiectasis, exocrine pancreatic insufficiency, elevation of sweat chloride concentration (>60mM), and infertility in males due to congenital bilateral absence of the vas deferens (CBAVD). Usually presents after neonatal screening but, if not screened, in infancy or early childhood with failure to thrive and recurrent chest infections.
- **Non-classical CF.** Chronic pulmonary disease ± pancreatic exocrine disease ± elevated sweat chloride (>60mM) ± CBAVD.
- **Congenital bilateral absence of the vas deferens** (CBAVD).

More than 1000 mutations in *CFTR* have been identified, of which the most common by far is delta F508 (ΔF508). ΔF508 encodes a three-nucleotide deletion resulting in a CFTR protein lacking phenylalanine (F) at postion 508 in the protein. This causes misfolding of the newly synthesized mutant CFTR ion channel so that it does not integrate into the cell membrane, but remains in the cytoplasm, where it is degraded.

The incidence of CF in people of northern European extraction is 1/2000–1/4000 newborns (1/2500 in the UK). CF is rare in native Africans and Asians. A specific mutation W1282X is common in the Ashkenazi Jewish population. Standard commercial kits for DNA diagnosis usually identify 29 mutations. Using a standard screen, 76% of English patients with CF will have two identifiable *CFTR* mutations, 22% will have a single identifiable CF mutation, and 2% of patients with CF will have no identifiable mutation. For carriers, the detection rate using the same kit is shown in Table 5.1.

Table 5.1 Cystic fibrosis carrier frequency and mutation detection rate

Population	Carrier frequency	Mutation detection rate with panel appropriate to ethnic group (%)
Ashkenazi Jewish	1 in 23	97
Northern European	1 in 23	90
Hispanic	1 in 46	57
African-American	1 in 65	75
Asian	1 in 90	30

Genetics
Inheritance and recurrence risk (📖 see Fig. 5.1)

Autosomal recessive (AR) and so the recurrence risk to parents of an affected child = 1/4. The following recurrence risks are based on pedigree analysis and assume that there is no consanguinity, no family history of CF in a partner, and a CF carrier rate of 1/23 (📖 see Table 5.1 for carrier rates in different ethnic groups).

- Risk to offspring of healthy sib of an affected child is:
  Healthy sib × population carrier rate × AR risk = 1/138

$$2/3 \times 1/23 \times 1/4 = 1/138$$

- Risk to offspring of aunt/uncle or half-sib of an affected child is:
  Carrier rate to second-degree relative × population carrier rate × AR risk = 1/184

$$1/2 \times 1/23 \times 1/4 = 1/184$$

- Risk to offspring of an affected individual is:
  Affected individual × carrier rate in normal population × 1/2 = 1/46

$$1 \times 1/23 \times 1/2 = 1/46$$

These risk estimates based on pedigree analysis can be substantially modified by CF mutation analysis in the relative and his/her partner.

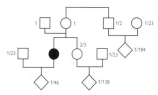

Fig. 5.1 Risk calculations for a family with cystic fibrosis (CF) ● individual with CF 1/23 = population carrier risk, 1 = carrier parent.

Variability and penetrance

Homozygosity for ΔF508 and compound heterozygosity or homozygosity for other non-functional alleles are associated with the classical form of CF. Even in classical CF the age of onset and rate and progression of pulmonary disease are very variable (influenced by modifier genes, infection, nutrition, therapy, smoking, etc.). All classical cases of CF (e.g. ΔF508 homozygotes) have pancreatic insufficiency, but there is considerable variability in pulmonary disease. Decline in lung function in CF is associated with colonization by *Pseudomonas aeruginosa* and *Burkholderia cepacia*.

A partially functional allele in combination with a non-functional allele (e.g. ΔF508) is a typical picture in non-classical CF. However, since the standard screening panel comprises mainly non-functional alleles, many patients with non-classical CF will have only one identifiable CF allele, i.e. those patients in whom clinical diagnosis is most challenging are often those most difficult to diagnose genetically.

Prenatal diagnosis—☞ refer to Clinical Genetics

Possible by chorionic villus sampling (CVS) at 11 weeks' gestation if both mutations are known. If a single or neither mutation is known, diagnosis of CF is secure, and paternity is certain, it is possible to offer linkage studies (📖 see Chapter 3, Genetic linkage, p. 78) to enable prenatal diagnosis. Pre-implantation genetic diagnosis (PGD) using PGH is available in some centres.

Predictive testing—☞ refer to CF paediatrician/Clinical Genetics

This may be applicable in siblings of a child recently diagnosed with CF, in view of the benefits of treatment with prophylactic antibiotics and pancreatic and vitamin supplements.

Other family members—☞ refer to Clinical Genetics

- **Parents:** When an individual is diagnosed with CF, and mutation analysis is performed, it is routine practice to offer carrier testing to both parents. Cascade screening of the extended family for the mutation identified in their relative can then be offered.
- **Partner:** Where an individual is shown to be a CF carrier, population-based screening (📖 see Table 5.1) can be offered to his/her partner to determine the risk to their offspring.
- **Carrier testing of children** is usually deferred until 16yrs when they are of an age to be involved in decision-making and old enough to understand the implications of the result.

Some children are not detected by the neonatal screening programme and may still present with clinical features of CF. This includes children who were born outside the UK, those who were born before the universal neonatal screening programme was introduced, and those whose CF was not detectable by the methods used in neonatal screening.

Consultation plan in primary care

History
- Chronic cough and sputum production.
- Unresolving proven chest infections.
- Neonatal failure to thrive/meconium ileus/rectal prolapse/fetal echogenic bowel in pregnancy.
- Take a family history (three-generation family tree).

Examination
Physical signs from any of the following:

Chronic chest disease
- Chronic cough and sputum production from persistent colonization with typical CF pathogens (*Staphylococcus aureus, Haemophilus influenzae, Pseudomonas aeruginosa, Burkholderia cepacia*).
- Airway obstruction (wheezing and air trapping).
- Sinusitis and nasal obstruction from nasal polyps.
- Clubbing.

Gastrointestinal and nutritional abnormalities
- Meconium ileus (10–20%).
- Rectal prolapse (20%).
- Distal intestinal obstruction.
- Pancreatic insufficiency.
- Recurrent pancreatitis, focal biliary cirrhosis, or multilobular cirrhosis.
- Failure to thrive (protein–calorie malnutrition).
- Hypoproteinaemia and oedema, complications secondary to lack of fat-soluble vitamins.

Salt loss syndromes
- Acute salt depletion.
- Chronic metabolic acidosis.

Male urogenital abnormalities resulting in obstructive azoospermia (CBAVD).

Initial management in primary care

PCPs should refer, on suspicion, to a paediatrician who will liaise with Genetics when appropriate.

Ongoing management in primary care

- Close liaison with hospital and community (e.g. Physiotherapy) services.
- May need extra financial support from care allowances, etc.—refer to social services.
- Support application for council tax exemption if serious physical handicap.
- Support application for disability living allowance.
- Code patient's notes.
- Code, with appropriate consents, notes of other family members (☐ see Chapter 1, Confidentiality and consent, p. 8).

Investigations in secondary care

- Chest X-ray looking for persistent abnormalities (bronchiectasis, atelectasis, infiltrates, hyperinflation).
- X-ray or computerized tomography (CT) abnormalities of paranasal sinuses.
- DNA sample for mutation analysis of *CFTR*.

Potential long-term complications

- ***Respiratory failure.*** Pulmonary disease is the main cause of morbidity and mortality in patients with CF. Heart–lung transplantation may be considered for end-stage disease.
- ***Diabetes.*** 25–50% have an abnormal glucose tolerance test (GTT) by their 20s and 5% require insulin.
- ***Liver disease.*** 5% of adults have cirrhosis and portal hypertension.
- ***Male infertility.*** 97% of males with CF have CBAVD with obstructive azoospermia. Pregnancy may be possible with assisted reproductive technology (ART), in which case mutation analysis will be offered to the partner (📖 see Chapter 9, Assisted reproduction technology, p. 328).

Surveillance

- Management of CF in paediatric and adult CF centres results in a better clinical outcome. Survival to the 30s and 40s is no longer rare.
- Median survival for patients with pancreatic sufficiency (non-classical CF) is 56yrs.
- Primary care team to agree with secondary-care specialist what surveillance they may be involved in, e.g. fasting blood glucose, LFTs, vaccinations.

Pregnancy in women with CF

Fertility in women with CF is impaired, but successful pregnancy is possible. Women with mild to moderate disease may safely go through pregnancy but **specialist input is important** to optimize the outcome for both mother and baby.

Pre-pregnancy counselling

- Consider the drug regimen of your patient and whether any of the drugs have teratogenic potential **BEFORE conception.**
- Discuss and prescribe folic acid supplements, 400 microgram/day.
- Discuss mutation analysis for her partner (they should be offered CVS if partner is a CF carrier).
- *Refer to CF physician for assessment of likely impact of pregnancy on respiratory reserve.*
- Discuss increased risk of gestational diabetes due to pancreatic insufficiency in women with classical CF.
- Pregnancy should be jointly managed by an obstetrician with special expertise in maternal and fetal medicine and a CF specialist.

Neonatal screening (📖 see Fig. 5.2)

Neonatal screening for CF is offered in the UK. The programme combines the assay of immunoreactive trypsinogen (IRT) on a dried blood spot (Guthrie card), with analysis for common CF mutations, e.g. ΔF508. An IRT of 60–70 microgram/L is equivocal and >70 microgram/L is positive. (This approach has been well studied but misses some children with CF and detects more ΔF508 carriers than expected.)

The documents produced by the screening programme give guidance to PCPs about the management of babies with CF and also address the referral of presumed carriers to clinical geneticists for further discussion and family testing.

Support group

Cystic Fibrosis Trust: ℘ www.cftrust.org.uk

Cystic Fibrosis Newborn Screening Flow Chart

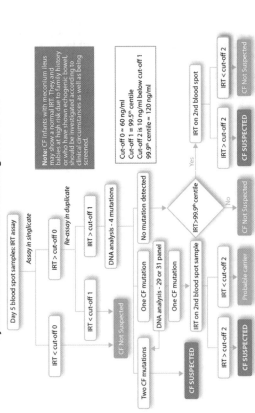

Note: CF infants with meconium ileus may show a normal IRT. They, and babies at high risk due to family history or who have shown echogenic bowel, should be investigated according to clinical circumstances as well as being screened.

Cut-off 0 = 60 ng/ml
Cut-off 1 = 99.5th centile
Cut-off 2 is 10 ng/ml below cut-off 1
99.9th centile = 120 ng/ml

Day 5 blood spot samples: IRT assay
Assay in singlicate

IRT < cut-off 0 → CF Not Suspected

IRT > cut-off 0
Re-assay in duplicate

IRT < cut-off 1 → CF Not Suspected

IRT > cut-off 1
DNA analysis - 4 mutations

Two CF mutations → CF SUSPECTED

One CF mutation
DNA analysis - 29 or 31 panel

No mutation detected

Two CF mutations → CF SUSPECTED

One CF mutation
IRT on 2nd blood spot sample

IRT < cut-off 2 → CF SUSPECTED

IRT > cut-off 2 → Probable carrier

IRT>99.9th centile

No → CF Not Suspected

Yes → IRT on 2nd blood spot

IRT > cut-off 2 → CF SUSPECTED

IRT < cut-off 2 → CF Not Suspected

Fig. 5.2 NSC flowchart for NHS screening for CF on the newborn bloodspot. Figures based on a population sample of 10 000 newborns. (Reproduced with permission of the UK National Screening Committee ℘ www.screening.nhs.uk/an Copyright, 2008.)

Duchenne and Becker muscular dystrophy (DMD and BMD)

Introduction

- *Duchenne muscular dystrophy (DMD)* affects 1 in 3000–4000 male births. It is the most common and severe form of childhood muscular dystrophy, resulting in death by the late teens or early twenties. DMD is an X-linked recessive (XLR) disorder caused by mutations in the dystrophin gene (DMD) on Xp21. In DMD the mutations are 'out-of-frame' resulting in truncation of the gene product.
- *Becker muscular dystrophy (BMD)* is clinically similar to DMD but milder, with a mean age of onset of 11yrs, and survival into middle age and beyond. Cognitive impairment is not a major feature of BMD. BMD is caused by mutation of the same gene as DMD, but in BMD the mutations in dystrophin are 'in-frame', so dystrophin is partially produced and the phenotype is milder.

DMD/BMD are X-linked recessive disorders, so even a distant family history of muscular dystrophy on the maternal side of the family, e.g. a maternal great uncle, may be relevant.

Clinical presentation

- Boys with DMD may present with developmental delay, especially with speech delay and late walking (>18 months). Typically the ability to walk independently is lost between the ages of 7 and 13yrs (mean age 9yrs) and affected boys become wheelchair dependent.
- ~ 30% of boys with DMD have a mild learning disability that is not progressive.
- Cardiomyopathy is almost universal and early detection may allow appropriate treatment; severe symptomatic cardiomyopathy is usually a poor prognostic indicator.
- In BMD loss of the ability to walk may occur late (e.g. middle age or later) with some patients remaining ambulant with aids. In the teens and twenties, muscle weakness becomes evident, causing difficulty in rapid walking, running, and climbing stairs. It may become difficult to lift objects above waist height.
- Some patients present with an intermediate dystrophin phenotype, i.e. a clinical picture intermediate between those of DMD and BMD.

Female carriers

Some female carriers have a mildly elevated creatine kinase (CK), but other female carriers have a CK in the normal range. Hence an elevated CK makes carrier status likely, but a normal CK does **not** exclude carrier status. A small percentage of women are manifesting carriers and have a variable degree of muscle weakness.

Genetics

Inheritance and recurrence risk

- **X-linked recessive (XLR).** In any pregnancy of a carrier female there are four possible outcomes, each equally likely: normal male; normal female; affected male; carrier female.
- **Carrier rate** is similar across different ethnic groups.
- **Penetrance** is complete in males inheriting a pathogenic dystrophin mutation.

Prenatal diagnosis—✎ refer to Clinical Genetics

- Available to carriers of a known dystrophin mutation by chorionic villus sampling (CVS) at 11–12 weeks' gestation.
- Available to mothers of a boy with an apparently *de novo* Duchenne mutation because of the significant risk arising from germline mosaicism.
- Available in families where a mutation has not been found, but where a 'high-risk X' can be identified by linkage studies.
- Testing for fetal sex using free fetal DNA in maternal blood (cffDNA) may have a place in the management of pregnancies at high risk for DMD/BMD, avoiding the need for CVS in female pregnancies.
- Pre-implantation genetic diagnosis (PGD) with selection of female embryos may be an option for women with a high carrier risk in a family where the causative mutation is unknown or those with fundamental objections to TOP.

Predictive testing—✎ refer to Clinical Genetics
Newborn males
Women at risk of being carriers who decline prenatal testing, and who give birth to a son, may wish their infant son to be tested before embarking on another pregnancy. [CK is often mildly elevated in cord blood or in blood samples taken within the first week after delivery in normal infants].

Becker muscular dystrophy
CK levels in BMD can be as high as in DMD but usually are not. CK levels in BMD fall with disease progression and may reach near normal levels in the very elderly.

Other family members: carrier testing and assessment of risk of carrier status in female relatives—✎ refer to Clinical Genetics

The genetics of DMD/BMD is complex and referral to a Clinical Genetics department for expert advice is essential. Even if the mother of an affected boy is shown not to be a carrier, she should still be offered prenatal diagnosis in future pregnancies because the mutation may be present in her ovaries (germline mosaicism).

Similarly sisters of an affected boy should always be referred for genetic advice and carrier testing, even if the mother is shown not to be a mutation carrier.

Consultation plan in primary care

History
- Difficulty rising from the floor, difficulties going upstairs or running.
- Detailed developmental history. Boys with DMD usually have mild delay of motor milestones, e.g. late walking and tip-toe and unsteady gait.
- Difficulties going upstairs (e.g. needing to get both feet on to the step before tackling the next step).
- Three-generation family tree, with careful enquiry for other affected males (e.g. maternal brother, uncles, and great-uncles). Extend the family tree as far as possible on the affected side of the family.

Examination
- Observe the child's gait. You may need more space to observe this than is available in the consulting room. Abnormalities of gait become much more evident when a child tries to hurry (ungainly and slow running).
- Gower's manoeuvre, where the child pushes up on his thighs with his hands to get up off the floor, due to proximal muscle weakness.
- Boys with DMD rarely ever learn to jump with both feet together.
- Calf hypertrophy occurs in most children in the early phase of the disease.
- Tight tendo-achilles.

Investigation
If the diagnosis is suspected, expedite referral to a paediatric neurologist/paediatrician for expert assessment and investigation.

Management of both DMD and BMD in primary care

- Consider flu and pneumococcal vaccines.
- Disabled badge for car.
- Care allowances.
- Code patient's notes.
- Code, with appropriate consents, other family members (◻ see Chapter 1, Confidentiality and consent, p. 8).
- Add patient and carers to Carers' register.

Investigations in secondary care
- CK: usually several thousand. Children with DMD invariably have serum or plasma CK levels >10 times normal.
- DNA for dystrophin deletion/duplication analysis. This analysis is positive in ~75% of boys with DMD and means that a secure diagnosis can be made without the necessity for muscle biopsy. Dystrophin sequencing to look for point mutations in the gene is the next step if deletion/duplication analysis is negative.
- Muscle biopsy to confirm diagnosis, if no dystrophin mutation identified.
- Echocardiogram and electrocardiogram (ECG) at diagnosis.

Management of long-term complications in DMD

Loss of ambulation

- Muscle weakness is progressive and children with DMD will become wheelchair-dependent. This is due to a combination of weakness and contractures affecting the ankles, knees, and hips.
- Ankle splints to prevent contracture of the tendo-achilles are important in maintaining ambulation for as long as possible. Some boys may also find long leg calipers beneficial for the prolongation of ambulation.
- Prednisolone has been shown to preserve ambulation and delay the development of other complications. Side-effects require careful monitoring and may necessitate the introduction of alternative regimes and careful dietary control. Prednisolone does not slow contracture development.

Scoliosis

- More than 90% of boys with DMD will eventually develop a significant scoliosis.
- Bracing may reduce the rate of progression of the scoliosis, but often major surgery is required to stop the progression.
- Surgery is high risk and should be undertaken in specialist centres that have the facility to undertake a comprehensive cardiac assessment prior to intervention.

Nocturnal hypoventilation

- Respiratory muscles are also affected, with respiratory failure from nocturnal hypoventilation.
- Treat with night-time facial or nasal mask ventilation. Without treatment, death often ensues within a few months.

Cardiac problems

- Because of their immobility, patients with DMD rarely develop signs of cardiac failure; however, on investigation signs of cardiomyopathy are almost universal.
- Patients are at significantly increased risk of arrhythmia and other cardiac problems perioperatively.
- Guidelines exist for cardiovascular investigations and management.
- Cardiac investigations (echo and ECG) every 2yrs to age 10yrs and annually thereafter. Echo and ECG should be repeated before any surgery.

Cognitive impairment

- May be a significant part of the condition and may particularly have an effect on verbal rather than performance intelligence quotient (IQ).

Management of long-term complications in BMD

Impaired mobility
- Some men with BMD retain ambulation throughout their lives, but others will become dependent on aids (sticks/walking frames) and eventually become wheelchair-dependent.

Cardiac complications
- Cardiac complications, e.g. dilated cardiomyopathy (DCM), are a major cause of morbidity and mortality in BMD. BMD patients should be under regular review by a cardiologist with regular surveillance from their teens onwards (annual ECG and echocardiogram in the first instance).
- As for DMD, BMD patients are at increased risk perioperatively and an anaesthetist should always be made aware of the diagnosis.

Surveillance

One model of care is for the primary care team and local community paediatric team to share care with a specialist centre with expertise in paediatric neuromuscular disorders.

Gene therapy

This remains a hope for the future. Possibilities currently under development include upregulation of utrophin and targeted exon-skipping to restore the reading frame.

Support groups

Muscular Dystrophy Campaign: ℘ www.muscular-dystrophy.org
Duchenne Family Support Group: ℘ www.dfsg.org.uk
Parent Project UK—Muscular Dystrophy: ℘ www.ppuk.org

Ehlers–Danlos syndrome (EDS)

Introduction
Most forms of EDS cause clinical problems such as easy bruising and scarring, musculoskeletal discomfort, and susceptibility to osteoarthritis (☐ see Table 5.2). However, only the vascular type is associated with an increased risk of death. Approximately 1/5000 people are affected by EDS.

Table 5.2 Villefranche classification of EDS (1997)

Classical (types I and II)	AD up to 50% are due to mutations in *COL5A1* and *COL5A2*
	Soft, hyperextensible skin with easy bruising and thin atrophic scars; joint hypermobility; varicose veins; risk of prematurity in affected fetuses
Hypermobility (type III)	AD
	Common and usually mild disorder. Soft skin with hypermobility of large and small joints (Beighton score 5/9 or greater)
Vascular (type IV)	AD due to mutations in *COL3A1* encoding type III collagen
	Uncommon but serious disorder. Characteristic facies with prominent eyes due to decreased adipose tissue below the eyes and thin, slightly 'pinched' nose, thin lips, and hollow cheeks. Thin translucent skin with visible veins and easy bruising. No significant large joint hypermobility (Beighton score <5/9). Risk of arterial rupture and rupture of bowel, bladder, and uterus leads to reduced life expectancy
Kyphoscoliosis (type VI)	AR due to mutations in *PLOD1* (lysyl hydroxylase deficiency)
	Soft hyperextensible skin, joint hypermobility, muscle hypotonia, scoliosis, and rupture of the optic globe
Arthrochalasia (type VIIA and B)	AD due to exonic deletions in *COL1A1* or *COL1A2*
	Soft skin with or without abnormal scarring, severe joint hypermobility, and congenital hip dislocation
Dermatosporaxis (type VIIC)	AR due to mutations in type I collagen N-peptidase (ADAMTS 2)
	Severe skin fragility with sagging, redundant skin
Other variants	e.g. X-linked (type V) and AD periodontal EDS (type VIII), AR progeroid (*XGPT1* mutation) and AR EDS without scarring (*tenascin-X* deficiency)

EDS hypermobility type (type III)

This is the most common type of EDS, it merges clinically with benign joint hypermobility syndrome (common in gymnasts and ballet dancers) and does not have the skin fragility or easy scarring seen in most types of EDS. EDS hypermobility type follows AD inheritance. It is likely to be genetically heterogeneous and caused by mutations in a variety of genes encoding components of the extracellular matrix.

Vascular EDS (type IV)—✍ refer to Clinical Genetics

Vascular EDS should be suspected in any young person presenting with unexplained arterial rupture or visceral rupture, carotid dissection, or colonic perforation. Diagnosis is based on specific facial features and thin, translucent skin with prominent veins. There may be increased joint mobility of the hands.

Complications are rare in infancy, but occur in up to 25% before 20yrs, and 80% before 40yrs. Median life expectancy is 48yrs, with arterial rupture accounting for most deaths: 80% thoracic or abdominal vessels and <10% from intracranial haemorrhage. Arterial repairs are technically challenging because the vessels are extremely friable. Although no specific therapies delay the onset of complications in patients with vascular EDS, knowledge of the diagnosis may influence the management of surgery, pregnancy, and major complications. Patients should avoid any activity that leads to a sudden increase in blood pressure.

Differential diagnoses

- **Benign joint hypermobility syndrome.** This term is sometimes used synonymously with EDS hypermobility type (see above).
- **Cutis laxa** is a connective tissue disorder characterized by loose skin and variable internal organ involvement, resulting from paucity of elastic fibres.
- **Marfan syndrome.** 📖 See Marfan syndrome, p. 148.

Genetics

Inheritance and recurrence risk

Most are AD with 50% risk to the child of an affected parent. Significant variability is uncommon, but mild phenotypic variability is commonly seen.

Prenatal diagnosis and predictive testing—✍ refer to Clinical Genetics

Technically possible if the familial mutation is known, but rarely indicated (with the possible exception of vascular EDS).

Consultation plan in general practice

History
- Enquire about dislocation/subluxation of joints (especially shoulders, patellae, temperomandibular joints, and digits).
- Three-generation family tree with specific enquiry regarding joint hypermobility, easy bruising, or abnormal scarring.
- For vascular EDS enquire about arterial or intestinal rupture.

Examination
- Ask the patient whether they have any 'party tricks' to demonstrate their joint hypermobility.
- Assess skin. Is it soft and velvety? Is it hyperextensible? (Pick up a small fold of skin over the upper arm and gently draw it away from the underlying muscle.)
- Examine skin over elbows and knees for abnormal scarring (e.g. thin atrophic ('cigarette paper') scars; also examine any scars from surgery for abnormal widening and thinning.
- Examine for bruising.
- Auscultate heart.

Management in primary care
- Code patient's notes.
- Code, with appropriate consents, other family members (📖 see Chapter 1, Confidentiality and consent, p. 8).

Investigations in secondary care
Your patient may undergo the following in a secondary care setting:
- Skin biopsy for electron microscopy for ultrastructural analysis and for fibroblast culture for collagen studies.
- DNA for mutation analysis is generally not performed except for vascular (IV), kyphoscoliosis (VI), and arthrochalasia (VII) types.
- Echocardiogram for mitral valve prolapse (MVP) and aortic root diameter in adults with classical EDS, vascular EDS, and kyphoscoliotic EDS.
- Magnetic resonance imaging (MRI) of thoracic and abdominal aorta and iliac arteries in symptomatic individuals with vascular EDS (whether there is a role for repair of unruptured aneurysms in patients with this syndrome is not clear).

Potential long-term complications
Pregnancy
A woman contemplating pregnancy should be referred to a 'high-risk' unit obstetrician to discuss the risks prior to conception. This applies to all types of EDS except for EDS hypermobility type (type III).
- There is an increased risk for preterm delivery in fetuses affected by classical EDS.
- Overall, postpartum haemorrhage and complicated perineal wounds are more common in women with EDS.
- Women with vascular EDS have a risk of uterine rupture (as well as arterial and bowel rupture).

Since the mortality rate amongst women with vascular EDS who became pregnant was 1 death per 23 pregnancies in a recent US study, the most important topic a GP can raise with affected girls is effective contraception.

Early arthritis
- Joint hypermobility can predispose to premature onset of osteoarthritis in early or mid adult life.
- Refer to physiotherapy and occupational therapists.

Support groups
The Ehlers–Danlos National Foundation: ✆ www.ednf.org
The EDS support group (UK): ✆ www.ehlers-danlos.org

Fragile X syndrome (FRAX)

FMR1, Martin–Bell syndrome

Introduction

Fragile X syndrome is the most common inherited cause of mental retardation, with approximately 1 in 5500 males carrying a full mutation. *FMR1*, at Xq27.3, (📖 see Table 5.3) contains a triplet repeat $(CGG)_n$ in the 5′ untranslated region of the gene. In the presence of a full mutation the *FMR1* gene is methylated ('switched off') and, although mRNA may be produced, no FMR protein (FMRP) is produced. The level of FMRP correlates with the degree of cognitive involvement in both males and females.

Table 5.3 Full, pre-mutation, intermediate, and normal allele sizes in FMR1

Normal individuals	<45 repeats
Intermediate allele (not clinically significant)	45–54 repeats
Pre-mutation carrier females and normal-transmitting males	55–200 repeats
Affected individuals and full-mutation carrier females	>200 repeats

Males with full mutations often show strengths in skills of daily living, relative to their communication and socialization abilities. Nevertheless, a degree of supported living is needed by many.

Clinical presentation

Full mutation in males

- Generally present with developmental delay. Speech and language are delayed and the speech of affected individuals tends to be characterized by the use of many incomplete sentences, repetition, and echolalia.
- Males with a full methylated mutation have an average IQ of 41.
- Behaviour is characterized by overactivity and impulsiveness with marked concentration problems, fidgetiness, and distractibility. Affected individuals are easily overwhelmed by a variety of sensory stimuli. Autistic features are common. Most children with fragile X syndrome are affectionate and have an interest in relating socially, but have notable difficulty in social interaction and tend to be shy and anxious in group situations.

Full mutation in females

- Females are less affected by fragile X than males, because the normal X produces variable amounts of FMRP.
- Up to 50% of females with a full *FMR1* mutation demonstrate learning and behavioural difficulties that are similar to, but usually less severe than, those seen in affected males. 50% have an IQ in the normal range.
- Subtle problems with learning, behavioural and emotional difficulties are common even in females with a full mutation who have a normal IQ.

- As is the case for affected males, verbal abilities tend to be better than performance skills, and special needs in arithmetic, visuospatial abilities, and visual and auditory memory are common.

Pre-mutation alleles

- The vast majority of individuals with a pre-mutation have an IQ in the normal range.
- On rare occasions, males with a pre-mutation (expansion size 55–199 repeats) may be clinically affected with mild learning disabilities or subtle cognitive deficit.
- When a child with learning difficulties is found to have a pre-mutation, this should **not** be assumed to be the cause and other investigations should be considered.

Genetic advice

Inheritance and recurrence risk

Fragile X syndrome is an X-linked condition, although the precise method of inheritance puzzled geneticists for many years. Cloning of the gene *FMR1* confirmed that the gene can be passed from clinically unaffected males (normal transmitting males carrying a pre-mutation) to their daughters, all of whom will inherit a pre-mutation. In contrast, a woman with a pre-mutation is at risk of having an affected child since the repeat may expand in the female germline to a full mutation.

The *Sherman paradox*, named after Stephanie Sherman who observed the worsening of the syndrome with successive generations, and correctly predicted that the responsible gene is mutated in a two-stage process:

- An existing pre-mutation produces no clinical effect and a second event (further expansion) must occur to convert this pre-mutation into a full mutation to exert the clinical effect.
- The pre-mutation must pass through a female in order to convert into a full mutation.

The complex genetic issues surrounding fragile X must be managed by a clinical geneticist.

Females

Women with an FMR1 pre-mutation face the following possible outcomes to each pregnancy, each equally likely: (i) a normal male; (ii) a normal female; (iii) a male with an FMR1 pre-mutation or full mutation; (iv) a female with an FMR1 pre-mutation or full mutation.

Males

- Males with a pre-mutation will pass this on to all of their daughters and none of their sons. The repeat size is likely to remain fairly stable (although small expansions and contractions are possible).
- Males with the full mutation are unlikely to form mature sexual relationships as adults. Several studies have found that adult males who carry a full mutation in their somatic tissues have only pre-mutation size repeats in their sperm/gonadal tissue.

Prenatal diagnosis—✑ refer to Clinical Genetics
Prenatal diagnosis is possible by chorionic villus sampling (CVS) at 11–12 weeks, but note the difficulty of predicting phenotype in females carrying a full mutation (▢ see p. 123).

Other family members—✑ refer to Clinical Genetics
Daughters of mothers carrying a full or pre-mutation
- Testing of sisters of affected boys who have no schooling problems is generally deferred until 16yrs of age or later when they may wish to establish their carrier status before planning a family.
- In sisters who experience mild learning difficulty with no obvious alternative cause, it may be helpful to initiate a referral to a community paediatrician/clinical geneticist to pursue diagnostic testing for Fragile X.

Other family members
Cascade screening of adult family members is indicated. A pre-mutation in a female may have been inherited from her mother or her father, but a full mutation can only be maternally inherited. Remember that, if the familial mutation is maternally inherited, normal brothers may be pre-mutation carriers (normal transmitting males) and should be offered testing because of the potential risk to their daughters' offspring.

Consultation plan in primary care

History
- Pregnancy and perinatal history.
- Developmental milestones, including language development and schooling.
- Behaviour.
- Three-generation family tree, which may need to be extended to further generations in the maternal line to facilitate cascade carrier testing.

Examination
- Height, weight, occipital-frontal circumference (OFC).
- Heart
  - examine for mid-systolic click or murmur (mitral valve prolapse (MVP)).
- Behaviour
  - eye contact, hyperactivity, autism spectrum difficulties.

Management in primary care

- The health visitor is the linchpin for co-ordinating services and supporting the parents.
- Refer to a developmental paediatrician who will arrange pre-school learning support.
- Liaison with community paediatric services.
- Code patient's notes.
- Code, with appropriate consents, other family members (▢ see Chapter 1, Confidentiality and consent, p. 8).

• Individuals with FRAX have special educational needs. Most can manage in mainstream primary school with appropriate support, but others may benefit from a special needs school. Children with FRAX are readily overwhelmed by noisy and busy environments, e.g. supermarkets, leading to tantrums, overactivity, withdrawal, repetitive behaviour, etc. Careful thought needs to be given to this in planning educational support. Children often learn best when auditory and visual distraction is minimized and work is packaged into short (maximum 15min) blocks (📖 see Fragile X Society (details provided in 'Support groups') for further information on educational needs).

Investigations that will be performed in secondary care

• DNA for FRAXA $(CGG)_n$ repeat size.
• Developmental assessment by a paediatrician.

Potential long-term complications in affected individuals

• **Recurrent otitis media** occurs in 60–80%, causing conductive hearing loss. Consider referral to ENT for grommets and/or prophylactic antibiotics if this is troublesome.
• **Seizures** occur in approximately 20%. They usually resolve by adolescence.
• **Mitral valve prolapse (MVP)** is rare in childhood but may occur in 50% of adults.

Potential long-term complications in pre-mutation carriers

Males

• Some adult males with FRAX pre-mutations may develop a late-onset progressive neurological syndrome, *fragile X tremor ataxia syndrome* (FXTAS), with cerebellar tremor/ataxia, cognitive decline, and generalized brain atrophy characterized by intranuclear inclusions. The prevalence of this disorder amongst males with a pre-mutation is not currently known.

Females

• Approximately 24% of female pre-mutation carriers will undergo *premature menopause* (cessation of menses at <40yrs).
• This information may be helpful to carrier women for reproductive planning.

Support groups

Fragile X Society: ☎ 01424 813147; 🖥 www.fragilex.org.uk
National Fragile X Foundation (US): 🖥 www.fragileX.org

Haemochromatosis

Hereditary haemochromatosis (HH), genetic haemochromatosis.

Introduction

HH type 1 is a disorder of iron metabolism causing excessive absorption of dietary iron with progressive iron overload. Eventually, deposition of iron in tissues results in cirrhosis of the liver, diabetes mellitus, skin pigmentation, and testicular failure. It is caused by mutations in the *HFE* gene on chromosome 6.

In evolutionary terms, heterozygotes for mutations in *HFE* may have been at a selective advantage when diets were poor and infestation with gut parasites was common. In Caucasian populations, ~1 in 200 people are homozygous for the common C282Y mutation in the hereditary haemochromatosis (*HFE*) gene. However, this mutation is not fully penetrant and so many of these homozygous individuals will never develop clinically significant disease. Penetrance is influenced by age, alcohol use, other genetic factors, and iron losses.

> Clinically significant disease is ten times more common in men than in pre-menopausal women because menstruation and pregnancy deplete iron stores in women.

There are two common mutations C282Y and H63D. Approximately 90% of patients with HH are homozygous for C282Y; a further 4% are compound heterozygotes for C282Y/H63D. H63D homozygotes do not develop HH. HH due to C282Y is common in populations associated with Celtic migrations, e.g. the UK especially Northern Ireland, Brittany, and Australia. It is rare in Asia, the Middle East, and most of Africa. In *HFE* C282Y homozygotes, it is unusual to get tissue injury from iron overload before 20yrs.

If HH is diagnosed early, before irreversible liver damage, treatment by serial phlebotomy is both straightforward and effective and many of the non-specific symptoms are reversible. It is presumed that iron depletion treatment that is initiated before cirrhosis develops results in a near normal life expectancy.

Genetics

Inheritance and recurrence risk

- HH type 1 is an autosomal recessive (AR) disorder.
- The general population allele frequencies for both mutations are high, e.g. 8% for C282Y and 15.7% for H63D in a survey in north-eastern Scotland—overall an approximate 1/10 risk for carrier status in the general population.
- Genetic risk to sibs is 1 in 4, to offspring is $(1 \times 1/10 \times 1/2) = 1/20$, to grandchildren is $(1 \times 1/10 \times 1/4) = 1/40$, and to nephews/nieces is $(2/3 \times 1/10 \times 1/4) = 1/60$ (see p. 127—'Whom not to screen').

> Penetrance is incomplete and disease expression is variable, so many of those with a genetic predisposition to HH will never manifest serious clinical features.

Prenatal diagnosis

Technically feasible, but rarely requested since this is a treatable condition in which complications are largely preventable and lifespan should be normal with careful monitoring of Fe storage and venesection where indicated.

Predictive testing

Appropriate in adult life to identify whether members of a family, eg. siblings, require regular monitoring of Fe status.

Other family members

Screening in primary care

Adult first-degree relatives of patients with HH should be screened. This is particularly important for siblings, who have a 1 in 4 chance of having inherited an HH genotype and will share more of their remaining genetic factors with the affected individual than will other relatives.

- Siblings of homozygotes should have HFE mutation analysis and iron indices (serum Fe, ferritin, and transferrin saturation) sent.
- Parents should be screened if symptoms suggestive of HH, otherwise likelihood of homozygosity is low.
- Children should not be tested before adulthood although a partner/ spouse may be screened to see if carrier (children only at risk if spouse is carrier = 10% chance).
- If the index case genetics are unknown or where there is uncertainty about counselling. ✎ Refer to Clinical Genetics.

Whom not to screen!

The low penetrance of *HFE* makes cascade screening of extended families inappropriate. Risks to second-degree relatives, e.g. grandchildren, nephews/nieces, and third-degree relatives, e.g. cousins, become sufficiently small that systematic iron studies and genetic testing are not indicated.

Consultation plan in general practice

History

- Obtain a full history of affected relatives where possible, including where and when seen by Genetics.
- For siblings, enquire for symptoms of HH. Late features of the disease are well known, e.g. bronzed skin pigmentation, cirrhosis, and diabetes mellitus, but early features are characteristically non-specific:
  - weakness and lethargy
  - arthralgia, especially interphalangeal (IP) and metacarpophalangeal (MCP) joints of hands (especially digits II and III);
  - ask about impotence or amenorrhoea where appropriate (endocrine failure secondary to Fe deposition in the pituitary);
  - dyspnoea (cardiomyopathy).
- Obtain a three-generation family tree.

Examination

- Hands for arthropathy of small joints.
- Pigmentation (especially shins).
- Cardiac arrythmias.
- Signs of hypogonadism.

(Continued)

Investigations in primary care
- Iron studies including serum Fe, ferritin (reflects total body Fe stores), and transferrin saturation (best screening test).
  - **Ferritin.** In normal subjects, ferritin concentrations of >300mg/L for men and postmenopausal women and >200mg/L for premenopausal women indicate elevated iron stores (levels may vary between different labs). Serum ferritin is an acute-phase reactant and so may be raised in intercurrent illness or inflammation.
  - **Transferrin saturation.** If transferrin saturation >50%, repeat on a fasting morning sample. Fasting transferrin saturation >55% (men) and >50% (women) is abnormal and indicates Fe accumulation. Normal values are 20–40%, carriers may have intermediate levels and genotyping may be helpful in determining significance.
- DNA for *HFE* genotyping after appropriate discussion and with patient consent (alternatively, refer to Clinical Genetics). ✍
- If symptomatic, include measurement of: liver function tests (LFTs), glucose, alpha-fetoprotein (AFP), luteinizing hormone (LH)/follicle-stimulating hormone (FSH) if impotence/amenorrhoea, and ECG.

Management in primary care

Management of those with HH genotypes, e.g. all C282Y homozygotes or C282Y/H63D with abnormal iron studies
For individuals with ferritin >1000mg/L or raised ALT
- ✍ Refer to consultant hepatologist; **and**
- Screen first-degree relatives as below or refer to Medical Genetics, who will arrange this.

For individuals with ferritin <1000mg/L and normal ALT
- Minimal risk of liver fibrosis, but if ferritin >400mg/L will need therapeutic venesection (refer to Hepatology or local venesection service if available, aiming for ferritin of 50mg/L).
  - For those with ferritin 200–400mg/L, reassure that they are unlikely to ever suffer any ill effects and suggest that they donate blood up to 4 times a year via the National Blood Transfusion Service in order to prevent further iron overload. Monitor annually to look for iron accumulation.
  - For those with ferritin <200mg/L fully reassure and monitor 2- to 5-yearly to look for iron accumulation: less frequently if (i) female; (ii) compound heterozygote; (iii) no evidence of accumulation. If ferritin rises, consider blood donation or venesection.

and
- ✍ Screen first-degree relatives as above or refer to Medical Genetics, who will arrange this.
- Code patient's notes.
- Code, with appropriate consents, other family members (📖 see Chapter 1, Confidentiality and consent, p. 8).

Management of those with non-HH genotypes
Refer to hepatologist. NB. Many of these will have alcoholic or non-alcoholic fatty liver disease and with conservative measures (e.g. alcohol reduction, weight loss) ferritin and ALT will improve.

Ongoing management in primary care
- GPs help co-ordinate life-long surveillance and encourage attendance for venesection.
- For individuals with HH who have already accumulated excess Fe, the usual treatment is weekly venesection.
- Once excess Fe has been removed, the transferrin saturation should be maintained below 50% and the serum ferritin at <50mg/L, which can often be achieved on a programme of venesection 2–4 times per year.
- Advise against taking over-the-counter preparations containing Fe, such as multivitamin and mineral supplements, and avoidance of very high dietary intake of Fe (red meat, red wine, etc.).
- Code patient's notes.
- Code, with appropriate consents, other family members (📖 see Chapter 1, Confidentiality and consent, p. 8).

Proven heterozygotes, i.e. those carrying a single copy of C282Y or H63D who are asymptomatic do not require repeated measures of iron status if initial studies are normal.

Investigations in secondary care
- DNA sample for genotype.
- Echocardiogram and ECG.
- Liver biopsy may be considered for any patient with a raised transferrin saturation, a serum ferritin concentration of >1000mg/L, and/or evidence of liver damage (hepatomegaly or raised aspartate transaminase (AST) activity). For patients with a raised transferrin saturation, a ferritin of <1000mg/L, no hepatomegaly, and normal AST activity, biopsy is usually not necessary because the risk of hepatic fibrosis or cirrhosis being present is low.

Potential long-term complications
- **Liver cirrhosis**—with increased risk for hepatocellular carcinoma—irreversible. Hepatoma is responsible for one-third of deaths from HH. The great majority of hepatomata occur in cirrhotic livers, but they have been reported in non-cirrhotic livers.
- **Arthritis**—especially small joints of hands.
- **Congestive cardiomyopathy**. Early cardiac changes on echocardiography may improve with venesection.
- **Diabetes mellitus**. Non-insulin-dependent diabetes or impaired glucose tolerance may be improved in a small proportion of patients by venesection; insulin-dependent diabetics will remain insulin-dependent.
- **Impotence**. Hypogonadotrophic hypogonadism may improve or resolve after iron depletion.

Related illness

Juvenile haemochromatosis (type 2)
A rare AR disorder with clinical onset between 10 and 30yrs of age and caused by homozygous mutation in hemojuvelin (HJV) on 1q21.

Support groups
The Haemochromatosis Society: 🖰 www.ghsoc.org
Hemochromatosis Foundation: 🖰 www.hemochromatosis.org

Haemoglobinopathies

Introduction

Haemoglobinopathies are the most common single-gene disorders in the world population, with ~7% being carriers. The incidence of the various haemoglobinopathies varies enormously in different population groups so that detailed knowledge of your patient's ethnic background is often extremely helpful.

In much of the UK there is universal neonatal screening for sickle cell disease and carrier testing in pregnancy for thalassaemia.

Heterozygotes are often referred to as '**trait**'; homozygotes as '**disease**'.

Hb electrophoresis

Haemoglobin (Hb) is a tetramer composed of two different pairs of globin chains. Adult haemoglobins are HbA ($\alpha_2\beta_2$), HbA$_2$ ($\alpha_2\gamma_2$), HbF ($\alpha_2\delta_2$). The α-globin and β-globin gene clusters are on different chromosomes and so can be inherited independently.

- In *normal* adults ~97% of Hb is HbA, 0–3.5% HbA$_2$, and 0–1% HbF.
- The α-*globin chains* are present in both fetal and adult Hb, so severe homozygous forms of α-thalassaemia cause intrauterine death (IUD) or neonatal death. In α-*thalassaemia*, Hb electrophoresis is normal. DNA analysis is required to make the diagnosis.
- β-*chain* abnormalities do not become clinically significant until Hb synthesis switches from HbF to HbA in early infancy. There are two α-globin genes in tandem array on chromosome 16 (normal genotype: *AA/AA*). The β-like globin cluster is on chromosome 11 and contains one β-, two γ-, and one δ-globin gene (normal β-genotype: β/β). In β-*thalassaemia* trait, HbA$_2$ is >3.5% (usually 4–6%; but not in the presence of Fe deficiency), with a slight elevation of HbF to 1–3% in some.

There are two main types of haemoglobinopathy:

- **Structural** variant haemoglobins, e.g. sickle cell anaemia
- **Reduced rate of production** of one or more of the globin chains, e.g. thalassaemia.

Hereditary persistence of fetal hemoglobin (HPFH)

In this AD condition, expression of the δ-globin gene of HbF persists at high levels in adult erythroid cells. Increased levels of fetal hemoglobin (HbF) ameliorate the clinical course of inherited disorders of β-globin gene expression, such as β-thalassaemia and sickle cell anemia.

Structural variants

Structural variants are named after letters of the alphabet (e.g. S, C, D, E) or places where they were discovered (e.g. Zurich, Constant Spring). More than 750 abnormal Hbs have been characterized.

Most variants have a single amino acid replacement due to a point mutation. For example, HbS (sickle) differs from HbA due to a missense mutation in the β-globin gene E6V (glutamic acid at amino acid 6 is changed to valine). This substitution alters the solubility of the Hb molecule in the deoxygenated state, resulting in aggregation with consequent sickling of the red cell. Sickled red cells have increased fragility and shortened survival, leading to chronic haemolytic anaemia. The sickled red cells can themselves aggregate in the microvasculature, leading to a thrombotic crisis.

Clinical presentation of structural variants

Sickle cell anaemia (genotype β^S/β^S)

The clinical course is extremely variable, ranging from crippling haemo-lytic anaemia with frequent crises to mild disorder. It usually presents in infancy with jaundice and anaemia from about 3 months of age. Hb is typi-cally 6–8g/dL; transfusion is not usually required. Crises due to blockage of vessels by sickled erythrocytes may cause infarction of bone and bone marrow, abdominal pain, chest syndrome (shortness of breath, pleuritic chest pain, and fever), and neurological syndrome (transient ischaemic attacks (TIAs) and strokes). Crises may be precipitated by infection or dehydration but often no precipitant is identified. Repeated splenic infarc-tion in early childhood makes children vulnerable to infection, and pro-phylactic penicillin reduces early mortality. In the long term, avascular necrosis of the hip, renal impairment, and ischaemia of the retinal vascu-lature may occur. A study based on survival of >3000 patients attending a Jamaican clinic estimated median survival for men at 53yrs and for women at 58.5yrs.

Sickle cell trait (β^S/β)

- Asymptomatic, except in conditions of extreme anoxia. It is possible for heterozygotes to suffer vaso-occlusive episodes if they become unusually hypoxic during anaesthesia.
- May have normal FBC. Diagnosed by positive sickling test and Hb electrophoresis demonstrating HbA and HbS (34–40%).
- The co-inheritance of α-thalassaemia causes reduced red cell indices and lowers the %HbS.

Apart from advice about anaesthesia and avoidance of unpressurized air-craft or deep-sea diving, individuals with sickle trait require no treatment. If planning a pregnancy, partners should be offered screening for haemoglobinopathy.

Haemoglobin SC disease (α^S/α^C)

- Relatively common in West Africa, e.g. Ghana.
- Milder anaemia than sickle cell anaemia (SS).
- May be undiagnosed until adult life when patients present with one of the complications, e.g. aseptic necrosis of the femoral head, unexplained haematuria.
- Widespread thrombosis may occur in pregnancy/puerperium or during intercurrent infection.
- Infarction of retinal vasculature may lead to retinitis proliferans with retinal detachment and loss of vision.

Haemoglobin C disease (β^C/β^C)
- Homozygous state for HbC is characterized by mild haemolytic anaemia with splenomegaly.
- Film shows 100% target cells.
- This is a mild disorder for which no treatment is required.

Clinical presentations of thalassaemias

β-thalassaemias
These produce severe anaemia in their homozygous and compound heterozygous states. They occur widely in a broad belt stretching from the Mediterranean and parts of North and West Africa through the Middle East and India to South-East Asia, including the Balkans and southern parts of Russia and southern China. Some mutations are inactivating (β^0) and others cause reduced levels of β-globin synthesis (β^+).

Homozygous β-thalassaemia (β^0/β^0, β^0/β^+, β^+/β^+)—'β-thalassaemia disease'
Most homozygous β^0-thalassaemia presents in the first year with failure to thrive and intermittent bouts of fever. Hb at presentation ranges from 2 to 8g/dL. If regular transfusion is instigated development progresses reasonably normally until puberty when side-effects of secondary haemochromatosis become apparent with lack of secondary sexual characteristics and short stature. With regular transfusion and compliance with optimal iron chelation therapy, life expectancy improves considerably and patients can survive to their third or fourth decade with a good quality of life.

A few β^+-thalassaemia mutations have a milder phenotype than the majority of β^0 and β^+ mutations. Homozygotes for these mutations have a milder condition called thalassaemia intermedia. Patients have a Hb of 6–9g/dL, splenomegaly, and some bone deformities, but are not dependent on regular transfusions for survival.

Heterozygous β⁰-thalassaemia (β/β^0) and heterozygous β⁺-thalassaemia (β/β^+)—'β-thalassaemia trait'
Carriers for β-thalassaemia are usually asymptomatic except in periods of stress such as pregnancy when they may become anaemic. Life expectancy is normal. Hb is 9–11g/dL with hypochromia and microcytosis and low mean corpuscular volume (MCV) and mean corpuscular haemoglobin (MCH). *A heterozygous state for β-thalassaemia may mask a coexistent carrier state for α-thalassaemia* (the latter is usually characterized by microcytosis and reduced MCH, which may be attributed to the β-thalassaemia trait).

α-thalassaemias
These are more common than the β-thalassaemias but pose less of a health problem as the homozygous forms of the severe types (α⁰-thalassaemias) are lethal *in utero*. They occur widely throughout the Mediterranean, parts of West Africa, the Middle East, parts of India, and throughout South-East Asia. The most serious forms of α-thalassaemia are restricted to some of the Mediterranean island populations (e.g. Cyprus) and South-East Asia.

Clinical presentations of thalassaemias with variant haemoglobins

Sickle cell β^o-thalassaemia (β^S/β^o) or sickle cell β^+-thalassaemia (β^S/β^+)—'sickle/thalassaemia disease'

Variable phenotype. In Mediterranean populations where one parent may have β and the other β^S, the picture is one of sickle cell disease. In Africans several mild forms of β^+-thalassaemia are commonly found which, when they interact with β^S, produce a condition with mild anaemia and few sickling crises and normal life expectancy. HbS also interacts with $\delta\beta$-thalassaemia to produce sickle cell disease, in contrast to the interaction of HbS with hereditary persistence of fetal haemoglobin (HPFH) where patients are clinically normal.

Genetics

Inheritance and recurrence risk

Sickle cell disease and other structural variants
Autosomal recessive (AR) with 25% sibling recurrence risk.

Thalassaemias
AR with 25% sibling recurrence risk.
- Beware the possibility of interaction of thalassaemia with variant haemoglobins.
- Beware the possibility that β-thalassaemia trait may mask coexistent α-thalassaemia trait.

Prenatal diagnosis—✎ refer to Clinical Genetics
- Both parents will be tested to define their genotype before embarking on prenatal diagnosis.
- Prenatal diagnosis by chorionic villus sampling (CVS) at 11 weeks' gestation is available if mutations have been identified in both parents.

Carrier testing—✎ refer to Haematology
Carrier testing is appropriate in the following circumstances.
- If there is a significant incidence of haemoglobinopathy in individuals of a given ethnic group.
- If a partner has a known haemoglobinopathy, the other partner should be tested even if they are from a low-risk group (since haemoglobinopathies can occur at very low incidence in most populations).
- In some areas of the UK carrier testing is performed in early pregnancy (📖 see Antenatal screening for genetic disorders, p. 324).

Other family members
Cascade testing of families and of partners should be offered.

Consultation plan in general practice

History

- Three-generation family tree with specific enquiry about ethnic origin and consanguinity. Specific detail about the country of origin of relatives can be very helpful.
- Enquire about previous pregnancies, miscarriages.

Examination

- Height, weight
- Splenomegaly

Investigations

- Full blood count (FBC) with red cell indices.
- Hb electrophoresis.
- Sickle test if indicated by ethnic background.

Management in primary care

- Refer affected individuals to a haematologist.
- Refer affected couples for genetic counselling prior to conception.
- Consider flu and pneumococcal vaccine.
- Code patient's notes.
- Code, with appropriate consents, other family members
  (📖 see Chapter 1, Confidentiality and consent, p. 8).

Investigations in secondary care

- DNA for molecular studies where indicated.
- In the UK samples may be referred to the National Haemoglobinopathy Reference Laboratory, Oxford Haemophilia Centre, Churchill Hospital, Oxford OX3 7LJ; ☎: 01865 225329 after prior discussion with the laboratory.

Neonatal screening

Babies born in England are routinely screened for some haemoglobinopathies, e.g. sickle cell disease, by haemoglobin electrophoresis on the neonatal blood spot test.

Support groups

UK Thalassaemia Society: 🖰 www.ukts.org
The Sickle Cell Society: 🖰 www.sicklecellsociety.org
Advice for carriers is given in the excellent website 🖰 www.chime.ucl.ac.uk/APoGI/menu.htm where it is possible to print off information leaflets about a large range of different haemoglobinopathies.
🖰 www.screening.nhs.uk/sickleandthal/

Haemophilia and other inherited coagulation disorders

Introduction

- Bleeding occurs in haemophilia owing to failure of secondary haemostasis. Primary haemostasis (formation of a platelet plug) occurs normally, but stabilization of the plug by fibrin is defective because inadequate amounts of thrombin are generated. The type and severity of haemophilia run true in families. There is no known family history in approximately one-third of haemophiliacs (📖 see Table 5.4).
- Haemophilia A (*factor VIII deficiency*) and haemophilia B (*factor IX deficiency or Christmas disease*) are clinically indistinguishable. The incidence of haemophilia A is 1 in 5000 male births and that of haemophilia B is 1 in 30 000 male births.

Factor VIII—haemophilia A

The factor VIII gene is located on Xq28 and consists of 26 exons. 45% of patients with severe haemophilia A have an inversion in intron 22 that disrupts the factor VIII gene. Approximately 2% of patients with severe haemophilia A do not have a detectable mutation on sequencing of the factor VIII gene.

Factor IX—haemophilia B

The factor IX gene is located on Xq27 and consists of 8 exons. The vast majority of mutations are point mutations.

Table 5.4 Classification of haemophilia

Severity of haemophilia	Concentration of factor VIII or IX	Clinical features
Mild	5–40% (>0.05–0.40IU/mL)	Spontaneous bleeding does not occur; excessive bleeding after surgery, dental extractions and accidents
Moderate	1–5% (0.01–0.05IU/mL)	Bleeding into joints and muscles after minor injuries; excessive bleeding after surgery and dental extractions
Severe	<1% (<0.01IU/mL)	Spontaneous joint and muscle bleeding; bleeding after injuries, accidents, and surgery

Differential diagnoses

Von Willebrand disease (VWD)

Deficiency or dysfunction of the adhesive glycoprotein Von Willebrand factor (VWF). VWD is common, with incidence figures varying between 0.1

and 1%. There are several different subtypes of VWD, but the phenotype is usually relatively mild. Mucosal bleeding predominates but it is also an important cause of menorrhagia in affected families. VWD does not follow straightforward autosomal dominant inheritance; the inheritance is more variable.

Other coagulation factor deficiencies
Congenital deficiencies can occur in any of the coagulation factors, but all are rare. Inheritance is usually autosomal recessive and they are more common in racial groups where cousin marriages occur. Such disorders should be discussed with a haemophilia specialist.

Babies with a family history of haemophilia or other coagulation problems should not have surgery, e.g. circumcision or tongue tie, until their clotting status has been properly evaluated by a haematologist.

Genetics
X-linked recessive
Females with disadvantageous X-inactivation (see Chapter 2, X-linked inheritance, p. 54) may have mild haemophilia, but severe disease is rare in females unless there is extreme skewing of X-inactivation, or the girl has Turner syndrome or the child has a father who is a haemophiliac and a mother who is a carrier.

Inheritance and recurrence risk
Factor VIII deficiency
Mutations originate far more often in males than in females, such that 80% of mothers of isolated patients are expected to be haemophilia carriers.

Variability and penetrance
Haemophilia is fully penetrant. It runs true in families, so if one relative has 'mild' disease, other affected relatives will also be likely to be mildly affected; similarly for severe disease.

Prenatal diagnosis—refer to Clinical Genetics
- Most patients with mild haemophilia enjoy a normal lifestyle, with appropriate advice about management of trauma or major surgery.
- Prenatal diagnosis is usually only considered for severe haemophilia.
- Offer fetal-sexing by free fetal DNA from 8 weeks gestation.
- Possible by chorionic villus sampling (CVS) at 11–12 weeks' gestation if familial mutation known, or by linkage.
- Pre-implantation genetic diagnosis (PGD) with selection of female embryos may be another option to consider.

Predictive testing—refer to Clinical Genetics/Haemophilia centre
Testing of cord blood of 'at risk' males is indicated to guide future management.

Other family members—✍ refer to Clinical Genetics

> PCPs have an important role to play in referring sisters or other maternal female relatives for carrier testing.

- Carrier testing, or female relative testing, is usually straightforward if the familial mutation is known.
- Mutation testing to determine carrier status is the gold-standard for reliable assignment of carrier status. It is usually deferred until the mid-teens when a girl is able to engage actively in the testing process.
- Only a proportion of carriers have factor levels below the normal range. A reproducibly normal result does not exclude carrier status.
- Some carrier females have low concentrations of factor VIIIC or IXC that can predispose to excessive bleeding, with levels in the mild haemophilia range. Factor concentrations should therefore be measured in girls and women who are definite or possible carriers.

Consultation plan in general practice

Presentation

Bleeding into joints and muscles spontaneously or after minor injuries, excessive bleeding after surgery and dental extractions.

History

- Three-generation family history with specific enquiry re. bleeding disorders; ask about joint bleeding. For milder disorders it is particularly helpful to ask if anyone has bled after surgery, e.g. dental extractions or tonsillectomy. Extend family tree further if other affected relatives are known.
- Try to establish which haemophilia centre affected individuals attend.

Examination

Refer urgently if suspect joint haemarthrosis.

Investigations

When the diagnosis in the proband is uncertain, involve a haematologist:
- Full blood count (FBC) for platelet count.
- Coagulation screen (prothrombin time (PT), activated partial thromboplastin time (APTT). Note that a normal screen does not rule out VWD or some other disorders.

Management in primary care

- Code patient's notes.
- Code notes, with appropriate consents, of other family members (📖 see Chapter 1, Confidentiality and consent, p. 8).

Investigations and management in secondary care

Investigations

- Von Willebrand factor antigen (VWF: Ag).
- Ristocetin cofactor (VWF: RiCof)—a functional assessment of VWF.
- Specific factor levels, e.g. factor VIII or IX.

Management

Management is co-ordinated by the local haemophilia centre. Haemophilia care in the UK is provided by a network of specialist centres and co-ordinated by the UK Haemophilia Centre Doctor's Organization (UKHCDO), who provide relevant protocols and guidelines for management

Your patients may ask you about the following:

- **Recombinant products** are the treatment of choice for people with severe and moderate haemophilia A or B. They have largely replaced plasma-derived factor concentrates in the UK.
- **DDAVP** (desamino-8-D-arginine vasopressin). In mildly affected patients with haemophilia A and mild VWD (some subtypes) it is often possible to use DDAVP instead of factor VIII concentrate. Patients with severe VWD require factor concentrates containing VWF; these are plasma-derived.
- **Plasma-derived factors.** During the 1980s, production of factor concentrates from pooled plasma resulted in a large number of haemophiliacs acquiring one or more of: hepatitis B, hepatitis C, and human immunodeficiency virus (HIV). Virus-inactivation procedures are currently used in product manufacture, but concerns remain about prions (e.g. new-variant Creutzfeldt–Jakob disease (CJD)).
- **Hepatitis B immunization** (vaccinate sexual partner(s) of affected individual too).

Potential long-term complications

Complications of the disorder

- Recurrent joint bleeding with inadequate treatment in severe haemophilia leads to chronic arthropathy, pain, and loss of function, which may lead to crippling.
- Death from bleeding (e.g. intracranial haemorrhage) may occur.

Complications related to treatment

- Transfusion-transmitted infections, e.g. hepatitis B, hepatitis C, HIV (risk is very much reduced with virally inactivated concentrates; risk thought to be eliminated with recombinant products).
- Development of antibodies (inhibitors).

Pregnancy surveillance in carriers

- The whole primary care and obstetric team must be fully aware of the diagnosis.
- Guidelines for the management of pregnancy in carriers for haemophilia are as follows:
  - Baseline factor VIII or IX level to be checked at booking and at 34 weeks' gestation.
  - Fetal sex should be determined by free-fetal DNA and ultrasound scan (USS) and the obstetrician informed prior to delivery.

Support groups

Haemophilia Society (UK): www.haemophilia.org.uk

National Hemophilia Foundation (USA): www.infonhf.org

The Haemophilia Alliance is a national partnership whose aim is to advance and promote high levels of care for people with haemophilia and related disorders. www.haemophiliaalliance.org.uk

Hereditary motor sensory neuropathy (HMSN/CMT)

Charcot–Marie–Tooth disease (CMT), peroneal muscular atrophy

Introduction

Hereditary motor sensory neuropathy (HMSN/CMT) represents a clinically and genetically heterogeneous group of inherited neuropathies. Disorders causing demyelination are usually classified as HMSN1 (CMT1) and those causing axonal loss as HMSN2 (CMT2) (□ see Table 5.5). The mechanisms by which mutations disturb the relationship of the myelin sheath and axon are not fully understood.

There is a wide range of severity: a few gene carriers may be asymptomatic in adult life and a few may have severely impaired mobility and become wheelchair-dependent. For the majority, HMSN causes problems with sporting activities and footwear in childhood and adolescence, and some impairment of mobility by middle life. There are currently >40 genes implicated in CMT. Many of these genes play a role in axonal transport and protein trafficking.

HMSN is not uncommon, with a prevalence of 1/3300.

Table 5.5 Classification of HMSN/CMT

Inheritance	Genetic basis	Clinical features
HMSN1/CMT1 AD ~70–80%	HMSN1A, due to duplication of *PMP22* gene, accounts for 70–80%	Distal muscle weakness and atrophy associated with mild/mod. glove and stocking sensory loss, depressed reflexes and pes cavus
HMSNX/CMTX X-linked semi-dominant (i.e. expressed in females as well as males) ~10–20%	Connexin 32 (also known as *GJB1*)	Affected individuals are clinically very similar to HMSN1, but males are consistently more severely affected than females
HMSN2/CMT2 AD ~10%	Various	Clinically similar to HMSN1 but in general less disabling and with less sensory loss
Complex forms of HMSN/CMT with various modes of inheritance Rare	Various	Neuropathy may be isolated or combined with other features, e.g. deafness, retinitis pigmentosa, etc.

Differential diagnosis

- **Hereditary neuropathy with liability to pressure palsies (HNPP).**
  The history is of recurrent nerve palsies often with an AD history of

similar problems. Caused by deletion of the *PMP22* gene (the same region that is duplicated in HMSN1A/CMT1A).

- **Distal spinal muscular atrophy (SMA).** A heterogeneous group of neuromuscular disorders caused by progressive anterior horn cell degeneration and characterized by progressive motor weakness and muscular atrophy, predominately in the distal parts of the limbs.

- **Friedreich's ataxia (FRDA).**
  - Friedreich's is the most common inherited ataxia, with a carrier frequency in the Caucasian population of ~1:85. Mean onset 15yrs (range 2–51yrs).
  - AR and caused by mutations in frataxin (a nuclear-encoded mitochondrial protein) resulting in a dying back from the periphery of the longest and largest myelinated fibres (e.g. large fibres arising in dorsal root ganglia).
  - The disease is slowly but relentlessly progressive with loss of walking ~15yrs after onset.
  - Mean age of death at ~37.5yrs (usual cause is cardiomyopathy).

Genetic advice

Inheritance and recurrence risk

May be AD inheritance or X-linked or AR. Variability is often displayed within the extended family and gives parents an idea of the range of possible severity. Approximately 10% of affected individuals are asymptomatic and detected either by careful clinical assessment or neurophysiology (e.g. nerve conduction velocity tests (NCVs)) or genetic testing.

Prenatal diagnosis—✎ refer to Clinical Genetics

Prenatal diagnosis is technically possible by CVS if the familial mutation is known, but is seldom desired or requested.

Other family members—✎ refer to Clinical Genetics

Predictive testing is possible for at-risk adult members of the family if the familial mutation has been defined. Genetic testing is usually undertaken in children only if they are symptomatic.

Consultation plan in general practice

History
- Developmental milestones. Difficulty running, walking, participation in sport at school.
- Enquire about difficulty undoing buttons, clumsiness, or frequent falls.
- Document current level of disability.
- Enquire about vision and hearing.
- Three-generation family tree (or more if affected members are known in previous generations) with detailed enquiry for high arches, unusual gait, impaired mobility, e.g. use of sticks, wheelchair.

(Continued)

Examination
- Gait for foot drop with slapping or high-stepping gait. Can they walk on heels (usually difficult due to weakness of foot dorsiflexion)?
- Wasting of calf muscles, high instep, clawing of toes, and enlargement of peripheral nerves.
- Weakness of hands may occur later and is rarely symptomatic before adult life. Wasting of interossei muscles in hands?
- Loss of vibration sense in feet and hands.
- Reflexes: ankle jerks are usually lost early, with progressive loss of other reflexes.

Management in general practice

- Referral to Neurology or Paediatric Neurology to prevent severe foot deformities if possible, and specialist physiotherapy, e.g. ankle–foot orthosis (AFO) for foot drop.
- Consider referral to Clinical Genetics.
- Code patient's notes.
- Code notes, with appropriate consents, of other family members (☐ see Chapter 1, Confidentiality and consent, p. 8).
- Care of feet if sensory deficit, to prevent development of ulcers, etc.
- Monitor adolescents for development of scoliosis.
- Mobility aids, e.g. walking sticks, handrails, wheelchairs, may be required over time.
- If adults are drivers, they should inform the Driver and Vehicle Licensing Agency (DVLA).

Enter a warning on the medical notes to avoid neurotoxic drugs, e.g. vincristine, taxol, cisplatin (chemotherapy), isoniazid (tuberculosis), and nitrofurantoin (antimicrobial used in treatment of urinary tract infections (UTIs).

Investigations in secondary care
- Molecular genetic investigations (DNA).
- Nerve conduction velocities (NCVs).
- Additional investigations will need to be considered for sporadic cases in early childhood.

Potential long-term complications
- **Pes cavus:** Daily stretching exercises to prevent Achilles tendon shortening may be helpful. Careful choice of footwear which has good ankle support. Severe cases may benefit from orthopaedic surgery.
- **Loss of mobility.** With time, some patients may need aids such as walking sticks, but <5% need wheelchairs.
- **Scoliosis** is more common in those with early onset of symptoms. It is rarely severe.

Support group
CMT UK: ℅ www.cmt.org.uk

Huntington disease (HD)

Huntington's chorea

Introduction

HD is a progressive neurological disorder with degeneration of the basal ganglia structures causing involuntary movements, psychiatric disturbance, and dementia. The caudate nucleus is particularly atrophied, although the putamen and globus pallidus are also affected. The brain is generally smaller, especially the frontal lobes.

HD is caused by an increased (CAG) trinucleotide repeat number within the Huntington gene (HD) on 4p16. Epidemiological studies showed evidence for an earlier age of onset through the generations (anticipation) and this was shown to be due to expansion of the (CAG) repeat. Large increases of >70 repeats are almost exclusively seen in the children of affected fathers.

Clinical presentation

- Peak age of onset is between 40 and 45yrs. Chorea may be prominent in the early in stages of the condition (especially with onset >40yrs).
- As the disorder progresses, dystonia, bradykinesia, and decreased voluntary movements are the predominant motor features.
- Psychiatric problems and behavioural problems are common presenting features in young adults.
- Death usually occurs 15–20yrs after the first signs.
- The prevalence of HD in the UK is 4–10 per 100 000.

Juvenile HD

- Is uncommon and in the great majority is paternally inherited.
- Presents with schooling difficulties and paucity of facial movement. Bradykinesia predominates and chorea is not a feature in the early phase of juvenile onset disease.

Differential diagnoses

Conditions associated with chorea

- **Benign familial chorea.** Autosomal dominant (AD). Onset in early childhood with no progression, dementia, or psychiatric features.

Disorders of the basal ganglia

- **Parkinson disease.** Diagnostically there is not usually any confusion except in the juvenile rigid form of HD. Some affected individuals with HD have an erroneous diagnosis of Parkinson disease.
- **Tardive dyskinesia.** Problems arise when an at-risk individual is treated with phenothiazines for psychosis.
- **Spinocerebellar ataxia (SCA).** SCA 3, in particular, has a pronounced movement disorder.

Conditions associated with dementia

- Chorea rather than dementia is the presenting feature in early HD.

Psychiatric conditions
- HD has often been misdiagnosed as schizophrenia or paranoid psychosis.
- It is important to note that both conditions are more common in patients with HD.

Genetics
Inheritance and recurrence risk
- AD, with 50% risk to offspring of an individual carrying an HD mutation.
- Factors influencing the age of onset include: age of onset in other family members and whether the mutation is maternally or paternally inherited.

Prenatal diagnosis—✍ refer to Clinical Genetics
This is possible by CVS at 11–12 weeks' gestation if the diagnosis of HD in the family is molecularly confirmed. Both direct analysis of the triplet repeat expansion and prenatal exclusion testing by tracking grandparental alleles are possible. Couples choosing an exclusion test need to weigh the benefits of ensuring that their offspring will not inherit HD (while choosing not to disclose their own status) against the prospect, in the event of a 'high-risk' result, of terminating a pregnancy that has a 50% chance of never developing HD.

Predictive testing—✍ refer to Clinical Genetics
Predictive testing for HD has been the model upon which much of the predictive testing for other genetic conditions has been based. About 10–15% of first-degree relatives opt for predictive testing. There is usually a series of three or more meetings between the at-risk individual and a genetic counsellor to explore the reasons why they wish to have the test and to discuss possible outcomes and future management.

Follow-up is offered to at-risk relatives to keep them informed of new developments and, if they wish, for clinical assessment for signs of HD.

Other family members—✍ refer to Clinical Genetics
Predictive testing for those at less than 50% risk has a number of difficulties, particularly ethical, that require thought and discussion before testing is offered. If an individual at 25% genetic risk is found to carry the $(CAG)_n$ expansion, a predictive test for the intervening relative has effectively been performed.

Consultation plan in general practice

History
- Age of onset of affected family members and age of death.
- Psychiatric disease, suicide, or dementia in apparently unaffected family members (may actually have been HD).
- Three-generation family tree; extend further if possible to include all known affected family members. Note maiden names of females, addresses of long-term care institutions.

(Continued)

Examination
- Many individuals with early HD have few, if any, signs on examination.
- Observe for choreiform movements (fidgety movements of the legs or facial grimacing may be choreiform but most patients consulting about HD are very anxious, which may manifest as restlessness or facial twitching, so be wary of over-interpretation).

Management in primary care

- For a symptomatic individual requiring initial referral for help with diagnosis, refer to a neurologist, or in the case of possible juvenile disease to a paediatric neurologist.
- For those more concerned about their genetic risk, or that of their children, refer to Clinical Genetics.
- Code patient's notes.
- Code notes, with appropriate consents, of other family members (📖 see Chapter 1, Confidentiality and consent, p. 8).
- Such a slow, and long-term, degenerative condition will need close liaison with all statutory agencies (DWP, etc.) to ensure delivery of appropriate financial and physical care.
- Sensitivity to young people maturing with an HD-affected parent, will be required to enable appropriate support and advice.
- Awareness of the unaffected, but 'at-risk' individual's concerns around their future, e.g. insurance forms, etc.

Investigations in secondary care

An individual with suspected HD but no family history
Diagnostic molecular testing for HD may be undertaken after full discussion about the possible implications of this diagnosis for the individual and their family.

In the case of a clinically unaffected 'at-risk' individual
- Accurate confirmation of diagnosis (preferably with molecular confirmation) is required from an affected member of the family.
- Patients wishing predictive testing will be enrolled in a predictive testing programme which usually runs over several months (📖 see p. 145).
- Written informed consent will be required before predictive testing is undertaken, and your patients may want to discuss this.
- **In juvenile HD** the issues surrounding genetic testing need special consideration.

Management (of at-risk individuals and known gene carriers)

Potential long-term complications
- Onset of signs and symptoms of HD (see above).
- Psychological, social, and family problems that can arise from this knowledge.

Surveillance

- Follow-up is offered to all mutation carriers and those at risk who have declined testing. They may wish to be informed if there are any signs of HD. There is also an obligation for the counsellor to disclose such information to the individual if he/she is considered unsafe to drive a car or to be a danger to themselves or other people as a result of HD.
- Close liaison with HD workers in the community helps ensure that appropriate supportive help is given.

Treatment

- For presymptomatic individuals, new research into treatment offers hope:
  - Experimental work on animals is investigating whether histone deacetylase inhibitors prevent the neuronal damage found in HD.
  - Stem cell and fetal striatal transplantation is another area of research.
- Symptomatic treatment of HD is available for the movement disorder and psychiatric complications.

Families appreciate help and advice in how to talk about the condition in the family and how and when to go about telling the children about HD. This and other issues may be helped by contact with HD support groups.

Support groups

Huntington's Disease Society of America: ✆ http://hdsa.mgh.harvard.edu
Huntington Disease Association, UK: ✆ http://www.hda.org.uk

Marfan syndrome (MFS)

Introduction

Marfan syndrome (MFS) is a multisystem disorder caused in the majority of classically affected individuals by mutations in the fibrillin gene (*FBN1*) on 15q21. Recently three further genes for Marfan syndrome/thoracic ascending aneurysm and dissection have been identified: *TGFBR2*, *ACTA2* and *MYH11*. Fibrillin is a component of microfibrils. The microfibrillar meshwork in the extracellular matrix is important in the integrity of the connective tissue. Various components of the extracellular matrix, such as collagens, elastin, and fibrillin, are present in varying proportions in different tissues and contribute to the elasticity, tensile strength, and durability of various types of connective tissue. Fibrillin is particularly rich in the wall of the proximal aorta and the zonule of the ocular lens.

In clinical terms, there appears to be a continuum between tall, thin patients at the extreme end of the normal population, through patients with mild connective tissue phenotypes, to Marfan syndrome. Diagnosis relies on careful clinical evaluation supported where appropriate by genetic testing.

MFS has an estimated prevalence of 1/3000–1/5000. Cardiovascular involvement is the main cause of major morbidity and mortality in MFS, e.g. aneurysm/dissection of the ascending thoracic aorta (which may present as sudden cardiac death) or mitral and/or aortic valve regurgitation. In untreated MFS, life expectancy is reduced by 30–40%. Death is typically due to rupture or dissection of an aneurysm of the aortic root, or severe aortic regurgitation.

Differential diagnoses

Ehlers–Danlos syndrome

📖 See Ehlers–Danlos syndrome (EDS), p. 118.

Loeys-Dietz syndrome

A newly described and rare condition caused by mutation in the transforming growth factor β genes (*TGFBR1* and *TGFBR2*). It is characterized by generalized arterial tortuosity, young age of aneurysm and dissection of the ascending aorta, with other systemic features. AD inheritance with variable expressivity.

Genetics

Inheritance and recurrence risk

- AD condition with 50% risk to offspring.
- There is a high new mutation rate of ~30%.
- The phenotype can be very variable.
- Cardiovascular involvement tends to be more severe in men than in women. Some families show fairly consistent severe cardiovascular involvement, but others do not.
- Penetrance is age-dependent and this is crucial when determining whether 'at-risk' family members are affected or not.
- Clinical examination combined with genetic testing is the most robust way of determining whether MFS is inherited or sporadic.
- In a sporadic case, if there is no identifiable mutation and both parents are normal on full clinical assessment (including echocardiogram and slit-lamp), the recurrence risk for future pregnancies is low.

Prenatal diagnosis—✍ refer to Clinical Genetics

If an *FBN1* mutation has been identified in the parent, this is possible by chorionic villus sampling (CVS) at 11–12 weeks, but in practice is not often requested unless there is an adverse family history.

Predictive testing—✍ refer to Clinical Genetics

If a pathological *FBN1* mutation has been identified in an affected member, predictive testing is possible and may be offered so that surveillance can be targeted more effectively.

Other family members—✍ refer to Clinical Genetics/Cardiologist with special interest in inherited cardiac disease

- Parents of an individual with MFS should be offered comprehensive evaluation with clinical assessment, echocardiogram, and slit-lamp examination
- Offer evaluation to siblings too, unless genetically proven to be *'de novo'*.
- All children of an affected individual are at 50% risk and should be offered periodic review.
- If the proband has an identifiable, pathological *FBN1* mutation, this greatly facilitates assessment of other family members.

Consultation plan in general practice

History

- **Cardiovascular problems**, e.g. aortic aneurysm (clarify whether thoracic or abdominal), aortic dissection, sudden cardiac death.
- **Skeletal/joint problems,** e.g. unusually tall stature, chest shape (pectus excavatum or carinatum), scoliosis, hypermobility of joints: subluxation, dislocation, discomfort, 'clicky' joints.
- **Eye problems**, e.g. lens dislocation, myopia, and retinal detachment.
- **Other problems** associated with MFS include: dental overcrowding and orthodontic treatment, hernias, easy bruising/abnormal scarring, spontaneous pneumothorax.
- Three-generation family tree with specific enquiry about the above.

Examination

- Height, weight, arm span (arm span/height ratio >1.05).
- Face shape, palate, dental overcrowding.
- Hands for arachnodactyly with wrist and thumb signs, and contractures.
- Joint hypermobility.
- Cardiovascular examination, including BP and auscultation for murmurs.
- Chest shape and back for scoliosis.
- Skin for striae (lumbar region and over shoulders) and unusual scarring.
- Feet for pes planus and medial rotation of medial malleoli on standing.

(Continued)

Management in primary care

- Given the potentially life-threatening nature of MFS, referral should possibly first be made to Cardiology/Paediatric cardiology for early investigation of the aortic root. Then, either Cardiology or a PCP can make a referral to Genetics. Ideally, the patient will be seen in a joint clinic for Inherited Cardiac Conditions where both cardiology and genetics expertise are available.
- Code patient's notes.
- Code notes, with appropriate consents, of other family members (☐ see Chapter 1, Confidentiality and consent, p. 8).

Investigations in secondary care

- Echocardiogram.
- Slit-lamp examination of the eyes.
- Physical assessment for features of Marfan syndrome (Ghent diagnostic criteria).
- DNA for mutation analysis (usually *FBN1*).
- Urine for homocystinuria if sporadic case with lens dislocation or family history consistent with autosomal recessive (AR) inheritance.
- If aortic root enlargement is present, possibly magnetic resonance imaging (MRI) scan of thoracic aorta—a more objective measure of aortic root size and shape.
- MRI scan of lumbosacral spine for dural ectasia may be considered.

Management in secondary care

- *Making the diagnosis:* refer to an Inherited Cardiac Conditions (ICC) clinic for diagnosis if this service exists locally, otherwise refer to Cardiology and/or Clinical Genetics. For patients with one major feature, e.g. aortic root dilatation and/or lens dislocation and/or severe skeletal involvement, who have involvement of a second system, *FBN1* mutation analysis may be very helpful in establishing the diagnosis.
- Patients with MFS need to be under long-term Cardiology/Paediatric cardiology care to monitor for progressive dilatation of the aortic root:
  - β-blockade slows progression of aortic root dilatation by decreasing the stress on the aortic wall. Losartan is currently under evaluation as an alternative or supplementary therapy.

All individuals with MFS should be offered *annual echocardiography*.

  - Individuals with marked aortic root dilatation (>4.5cm) should be reviewed more frequently, as should women in pregnancy and those with a rapidly changing aortic root diameter.
  - Patients with an aortic root diameter at the sinuses of Valsalva of >5.0cm should be referred on for consideration of elective replacement of the aortic root with a composite graft.
- *Paediatric review.* Growth should be monitored in childhood and adolescence with monitoring for scoliosis. If significant scoliosis develops, refer for specialist orthopaedic advice.

- *Periodic ophthalmic review for glaucoma*. Increased risk, particularly in individuals with ectopia lentis and *retinal detachment* (patients with high myopia and increased axial globe length are at increased risk). Contact sports and diving from a board should be avoided.

Lifestyle advice

- *Sports*. Enquire specifically about leisure pursuits. In general, isometric exercise, e.g. weight-lifting, rowing, press-ups, should be avoided (severe cardiovascular stress). Contact sports, such as football, basketball, hockey, volleyball, boxing, and wrestling, may be contraindicated (risk of retinal detachment and deceleration injury to aorta). Regular rhythmic activity such as walking, swimming, and non-competitive cycling is usually fine.
- *The Marfan Association* (℞ www.marfan.org.uk) produces a range of booklets for children, teenagers, and adults, and also for teachers, and can provide help with outlets for clothing and shoes.

Pregnancy

Pregnancy increases the risk of dissection of an aneurysm, the risk increasing with gestational age. ✎ Early referral to Cardiology is important.

- Periodic echocardiographic surveillance is recommended during pregnancy and the puerperium, e.g. echocardiogram in each trimester and a fourth scan 4–8 weeks' postpartum.
- If there is evidence of cardiovascular compromise, e.g. moderate or more severe aortic regurgitation or aortic root diameter >40mm, and/or a family history of early dissection, the risk of dissection in pregnancy is greatly increased.
- If cardiovascular involvement is minor and aortic root diameter <40mm, pregnancy is usually tolerated well with favourable maternal and fetal outcomes, and no evidence of aggravation of aortic root dilatation with time.

Support groups

Marfan Association UK: ℞ www.marfan.org.uk
National Marfan Foundation (US): ℞ www.marfan.org.

Myotonic dystrophy (MD)

Dystrophica myotonica, Steinert disease

Introduction

Myotonia is the continued active contraction of a muscle after voluntary effort has stopped. There is slowness in relaxation of grip.

- MD is the most common heritable neuromuscular disorder. It is caused by a triplet repeat expansion (CTG) in the non-coding region of the myotonin gene at 19q13.3 and occurs with a prevalence of ~1/8000.
- The normal number of (CTG) repeats is 4–37. Affected individuals with MD have an increased number of repeats from 50 to many thousand.

Women carrying an MD expansion who are symptomatic or who have even minimal clinical signs are at risk for a congenitally affected infant. **Congenital myotonic dystrophy** may present in late pregnancy with polyhydramnios (due to poor fetal swallowing) and/or at delivery with a floppy baby who may require prolonged ventilatory support and naso-gastric feeding. There is a 20% neonatal mortality, and most survivors will have significant learning disability and require special educational support.

Table 5.6 demonstrates overlaps between the clinical presentation and the repeat size and the uncertainty of predicting the phenotype on the basis of the molecular results.

Table 5.6 Number of CTG repeats and clinical presentation of MD

Number of CTG repeats	Designation	Clinical features
4–37	Normal allele	None
38–49	Pre-mutation	None
50–80	Proto-mutation	Usually asymptomatic or associated with mild late-onset disease (e.g. cataracts without neuromuscular disease)
200–500	Mutation	Usually associated with onset in 30s to 40s
230–1800	Mutation	Childhood onset but not usually congenital but note overlap with congenital range
>1000	Mutation	May cause congenital MD

Genetics

Inheritance and recurrence risk

- Inheritance is AD with a 50% risk to the offspring of an affected individual.
- Affected families exhibit anticipation in their offspring, with a tendency to increasing severity in successive generations. Older generations may be minimally affected, e.g. by cataract alone with no neuromuscular symptoms.

- Congenital myotonic dystrophy (CMD) occurs if the fetus inherits a greatly expanded CTG repeat from an affected mother. The likelihood of a mutation expanding into the congenital size range depends, in part, on the size of the mutation and particularly on the parent of origin. It is much more common from an affected mother and only very rarely reported from an affected father. ✍ **Refer to Clinical Genetics.**

Prenatal diagnosis—✍ refer to Clinical Genetics

Possible by chorionic villus sampling (CVS) using triplet repeat (CTG) expansion. This will determine whether or not the fetus has inherited the expansion. Predicting prognosis is more difficult, although it is usually possible to offer some guidance as to whether the expansion size is likely to result in adult onset or congenital onset.

Predictive testing—✍ refer to Clinical Genetics

The chance that a sibling/offspring aged 21–40yrs with a normal clinical examination carries a (CTG) expansion is 10%, hence clinical assessment needs to be backed up by genetic testing in order to provide accurate genetic advice.

Other family members—✍ refer to Clinical Genetics

Cascade approach to family screening is appropriate. Even mildly affected women may be at risk of having offspring with CMD.

Consultation plan in primary care

History
- Hands 'locking up', e.g. using can-opener, turning key in lock, holding steering wheel, peeling potatoes. Worse in cold weather.
- Fatigue (tire easily); may have reduced exercise tolerance.
- Choking on food/difficulty swallowing lumps.
- Sleep/sleep pattern. Fall asleep during daytime? Sleep with eyes open? Snoring?
- Gastrointestinal symptoms similar to those of irritable bowel syndrome.
- Three-generation family tree with enquiry for cataracts, diabetes, myotonia, muscle weakness, etc.

Examination
- Facies. Ptosis: long face with reduced ability to wrinkle forehead, bury eyelashes, or clench masseter muscles; frontal balding.
- Sternomastoid muscles. Test muscle power against hand placed on side of chin. Note sternomastoid muscle bulk and power (both often reduced in MD).
- Test power of wrist extension (weakness and wasting of forearm muscles is characteristic).
- Tap thenar eminence to elicit myotonic contraction.
- Ask patient to clench hands into a tight fist, hold, and then quickly release (may elicit myotonia). Alternatively, ask them to grip hold of your index and middle finger and then quickly release (may take many seconds to gradually unfurl hand).

(Continued)

• Deep tendon reflexes may be normal in a mildly affected case, but become difficult to elicit and may be absent in more severely affected individuals.

Investigations
• Electrocardiogram (ECG) looking for heart block.
• Blood glucose (diabetes mellitus).

Management in primary care
• Refer to genetics clinic for genetic testing—mutation analysis of $(CTG)_n$ triplet repeat expansion in myotonin gene and assessment of risk to extended family.
• Refer to Cardiology if ECG changes.
• Ophthalmology referral if suspected cataract. Otherwise recommend regular surveillance by optometrist/optician.
• Consider whether the patient's symptoms could affect driving and advise them to notify the DVLA.
• Code patient's notes.
• Code notes, with appropriate consents, of other family members (📖 see Chapter 1, Confidentiality and consent, p. 8).
• Consider disabled parking badge.
• Consider disability living allowances.
• Consider inclusion of carer in Carers' register.

Unless there is a local specialist clinic offering annual review, the following is recommended:
• Annual cardiac check: ECG with assessment of PR interval (30–80% of patients with MD have some abnormality); for pacemaker consideration.
• Specific enquiry for symptoms suggestive of diabetes, and urine dipstick.
• Annual ophthalmic assessment for cataract.

Potential long-term complications
Anaesthetics
Hazards of anaesthesia in patients with MD include: cardiac dysrhythmias, prolonged recovery, and aspiration pneumonia. There is an increased sensitivity to sedatives and opiates given as premedication and an increased risk for adverse reaction to commonly used anaesthetic agents (e.g. suxamethonium).
• If a general anaesthetic is required, it should be given in a hospital with a high-dependency unit or intensive care facilities for postoperative support and monitoring. Postoperatively, patients with MD are at increased risk for chest infections (weak respiratory muscles + sensitivity to opiate analgesia).
• A pre-operative ECG is advised.
• Consider regional blocks or spinal or epidural anaesthesia where possible.

Discuss the benefits of carrying a Medic-alert card/bracelet with details of the patient's diagnosis. ℘ www.medicalert.org.uk/

Other potential complications
- **Diabetes mellitus:** due to insulin resistance.
- **Cataract:** posterior subcapsular cataract may onset in early or mid adult life.
- **Cardiac involvement.** There is clear evidence of an increased risk of conduction disease, but not of ischaemic heart disease or of impaired myocardial function. Ventricular arrhythmias are likely to explain some cases of sudden death.
  - If annual ECGs show increasing PR interval or other evidence of increased risk of bradycardia, refer to a cardiologist for assessment and a 24-hour tape.
  - Treatment with a pacemaker is indicated when a progressive arrhythmia is detected, even prior to symptoms.
- **Endocrine** disorder, with gonadal atrophy in males and premature menopause in females.
- **Cholelithiasis**
- **Somnolence.** Excessive daytime sleepiness is typical in advanced disease but may also be a consequence of nocturnal sleep apnoea. Consider referral for sleep studies.
- **Apathy** and impaired cognitive processing are features of advanced disease.

Pregnancy
- ✍ Early referral to Clinical Genetics to discuss risk to pregnancy and option of prenatal diagnosis.
- Early referral to obstetrician with expertise in maternal/fetal medicine because of increased risk for:
  - polyhydramnios, 15%
  - prematurity <38/40, 13%
  - failure to progress in labour
  - postpartum haemorrhage (5%) and retained placenta (10%)
  - anaesthetic risks.

Support group
Myotonic dystrophy support group: ℘ www.mdsuk.org

Neurofibromatosis type 1 (NF1)

von Recklinghausen disease

Introduction

NF1 is an autosomal dominant (AD) disorder with a birth incidence of 1 in 2500. The cardinal features are multiple *café-au-lait* spots (CALs), neurofibromas, and Lisch nodules in the iris. NF1 shows hugely variable expressivity and many of the features of NF1 show age-dependent penetrance. The NF1 gene is large, spanning 350 kb of DNA with 59 exons, and has a high new mutation rate. NF1 is caused by mutations within the *NF1* gene in ~90% of patients, or by submicroscopic chromosomal deletions encompassing the *NF1* gene on 17q11.2.

Counselling the parents of a newly diagnosed child, who is fit and well, but nevertheless is affected with NF1, is challenging. It is important to balance the possibility of complications and disfigurement with the likelihood of a lifetime with few difficulties. Parent support groups with their specialist staff can be a great help to families at this time. The PCP's most useful task is to listen and support them through these uncertainties.

Diagnostic criteria for NF1 (NIH 1988)

The patient should have two or more of the following:

- Six or more *café-au-lait* spots: 1.5cm or larger in postpubertal individuals or 0.5cm or larger in prepubertal individuals.
- Two or more *neurofibromas* of any type **or** 1 or more plexiform neurofibromas.
- *Freckling* in the axilla, neck, or groin.
- *Optic glioma* (tumour in the optic pathway).
- Two or more *Lisch nodules* (benign iris hamartomas).
- A distinctive *bony lesion* (usually presenting in infancy), e.g. dysplasia of the sphenoid bone or dysplasia or thinning of the long bone cortex (usually the tibia) ('pseudoarthrosis').
- A first-degree relative with NF-1.

Differential diagnoses

Atypical skin pigmentary changes and unusual disorders of growth can cause diagnostic problems.

- **Segmental NF.** Typical skin changes are only found in one segment of the body. A postzygotic mutation is the cause.
- **SPRED1.** A newly described condition following AD inheritance characterized by *café-au-lait* spots and axillary/groin freckling but without the neurofibromas or tumour risk associated with NF1.
- **Neurofibromatosis type 2 (NF2).** This is less common than NF1 but can cause diagnostic confusion. Some individuals have a few CALs. There is a high incidence of central nervous system (CNS) tumours. Spinal neurofibromata seen in NF1 can appear identical to the spinal Schwannomas seen in NF2. Progressive deafness is a common feature of NF2 due to vestibular Schwannomas, but is rare in NF1. NF2 requires expert specialist management (□ see Chapter 7, Neuro-firbromatosis type 2, p. 272).
- **Constitutional mismatch-repair deficiency syndrome (CMMR-D).** This rare AR condition presents in childhood with CALs, axillary freckling,

subtle generalized increase in skin pigmentation, primitive neuroectodermal tumours (PNETs), non-Hodgkin's lymphoma (NHL), and bowel polyps predisposing to bowel cancer. CMMR-D is caused by biallelic mutation in mismatch-repair genes and has a highly malignant phenotype.

Genetics

Inheritance and recurrence risk

- **Parent affected.** The inheritance is autosomal dominant (AD) with a 50% risk to offspring. The new mutation rate is approximately 50%.
- **Parents unaffected.** If the parents are unaffected (after careful clinical assessment and eye examination), or the proband is known to have a *de novo* mutation, the recurrence risk is less than 1%. A small but significant proportion of parents are gonosomal mosaics, with a higher recurrence risk. Hence referral for specialist assessment and advice is important

NF1 is fully penetrant. Many of the features show age-dependent expression. As NF1 shows highly variable expressivity, it is not possible to predict the manifestations of the condition based on the presence or absence of complications in other family members.

Prenatal diagnosis—✍ refer to Clinical Genetics if requested

Possible by chorionic villus sampling (CVS) at 11–12 weeks' gestation if the familial mutation is known, or by linkage in a family with two or more affected individuals if the markers have been worked up in advance and are informative.

Predictive testing—✍ refer to Clinical Genetics

The children of affected individuals are seen annually, if there are no signs, to age 2yrs and then checked once more at 5yrs. Genetic testing is possible if the familial mutation is known.

Other family members—✍ refer to Clinical Genetics

Clinical evaluation should be offered, together with mutation testing if the familial mutation is known.

Consultation plan in general practice

History

- Detailed family history enquiring specifically for other relatives with CALs, lumps, or bumps on their skin, other tumours/seizures.
- Three-generation family tree.

Examination

- *Skin*
  - *Café-au-lait* patches (CALs)—coffee-coloured macules measuring >0.5 cm. Few or none at birth, increasing in number during infancy and childhood.
  - Axillary, neck, or groin freckling (usually appears at 3–5yrs of age).
  - Most diffuse, disfiguring plexiform neurofibromata are apparent within the first 2yrs of life, or at least evident by a patch of skin with increased pigmentation.

(Continued)

- Dermal neurofibromata appear from late childhood onwards. They are raised and may increase in number and size at puberty and during pregnancy.
- Some patients with NF1 show a subtle generalized increase in skin pigmentation in comparison with unaffected family members.
- *Facial features.* Some coarsening of the features, or Noonan-like features, may be seen (particularly in those with gene deletions).
- *Spine.* Scoliosis is found in 11%.

Investigations possible in primary care

- Measurement of head circumference in a baby to monitor a rapidly expanding head circumference (to exclude aqueduct stenosis).
- Monitor growth.
- Annual BP check (consider further investigation or referral for exclusion of renal artery stenosis and pulmonary stenosis). NB. Small increased risk for phaeochromocytoma (affects ~1%).
- Surveillance of skin lesions.

Management in primary care

- *Children*: refer to a paediatrician who will usually co-ordinate care and make referrals to Clinical Genetics and Ophthalmology (referral for annual ophthalmic surveillance for optic glioma in children <6yrs old). Lisch nodules are not usually present in pre-school children. (NB Slit lamp examination is necessary to distinguish these from iris naevi.)
- Referral to Paediatric neurology/Neurology if symptomatic:
  - Brain imaging, e.g. MRI, is necessary in the presence of: (i) a rapidly expanding head circumference in a baby, to exclude aqueduct stenosis; (ii) focal neurological signs (brain and spinal cord need to be considered); (iii) epilepsy; (iv) visual problems; and (v) precocious puberty or failing growth velocity.
- *Scoliosis*: if there are no neurological symptoms/signs, consider Orthopaedic referral for management of scoliosis.
- Code patient's notes.
- Code notes, with appropriate consents, of other family members (📖 see Chapter 1, Confidentiality and consent, p. 8).
- May require close liaison with Pre-school/SENCO, etc.

Unless there is a local specialist NF clinic: paediatric patients should be under annual paediatric review. Adult patients with NF1 who do not have complex problems may be managed in primary care with:
- Annual BP check
- Annual surveillance of skin lesions
- General systems enquiry
☞ Referral to Genetics as appropriate, e.g. explanation of diagnosis and inheritance to a teenager, adult planning a family.

Natural history
Potential long-term complications

There is an increased incidence of malignant soft tissue tumours, so a low threshold for rapid referral and imaging is required.

Toddler or early childhood: optic nerve gliomas
Approximately 15% of individuals with NF1 have thickening of the optic nerve tracts visible on MRI scan. All merit careful surveillance. Any child with NFI with visual symptoms requires urgent referral to a prediatric ophthalmalogist.

In 20- to 30-yr-olds: malignant peripheral nerve sheath tumours (MPNST)
Median age at diagnosis in NF1 patients is 26yrs. Some originate in existing plexiform tumours, but most arise in deep-seated locations, e.g. brachial plexus or sciatic nerve. Almost all MPNSTs present with pain or rapid growth. Any NF1 patient with these symptoms should have rapid access to specialist advice and imaging.

Support groups
The Neurofibromatosis Association: ℘ www.nfa.zetnet.co.uk
National Neurofibromatosis Foundation (US): ℘ www.nf.org

Noonan syndrome (NS)

Noonan syndrome (NS) is a relatively common autosomal dominant disorder affecting ~1/2500 people. It usually presents after an infant is diagnosed with one of the typical cardiac defects (pulmonary stenosis, atrial septal defect (ASD), cardiomyopathy) and the additional features of Noonan syndrome are recognized. In addition to a cardiac defect, children with typical NS have short stature, ptosis, webbed neck (secondary to prenatal lymphoedema), a pectus deformity of the chest, and coagulation defects.

It may occur 'de novo' as a new mutation, but caution is necessary in ascribing unaffected status to a parent as the typical facial features in childhood become more subtle with time. A family history is reported in 50% of cases. Many individuals with NS probably remain undiagnosed; it is not uncommon to diagnose several members of a family with the condition after the diagnosis is made in the proband.

Other diagnoses/conditions to consider

Noonan syndrome is a member of a family of syndromes with overlapping features caused by mutations in genes that code for proteins in the RAS-MAPK pathway. Since the genetic aetiology of these conditions became known, a number of studies have provided useful clinical information regarding prognosis and surveillance, which are particularly useful when counselling the parents of newly diagnosed infants.

- *LEOPARD syndrome*: **Le**ntigines, **O**cular hypertelorism, **P**ulmonary stenosis, **A**bnormalities of genitalia, **R**etardation of growth, and **D**eafness (sensorineural)
- *Cardiofaciocutaneous syndrome (CFC)*
- *Costello syndrome*

Genetic advice—✍ refer to Genetics

Inheritance and recurrence risk

- AD. If one of the parents is affected, a 50% offspring risk is appropriate. If a mutation is identified and this is not present in either parent, the sibling recurrence risk will be low (small theoretical risk of germline mosaicism).
- Prior to genetic testing, if the NS appeared 'de novo' and both parents had only possible or no signs of Noonan syndrome, an empiric recurrence risk of 5% was given.

Features of Noonan syndrome may be subtle. Parental evaluation should include: (i) clinical examination; (ii) assessment of childhood photographs; and (iii) echocardiogram and ECG.

Prenatal diagnosis—✍ refer to Clinical Genetics

Monitor for nuchal oedema and polyhydramnios. Pulmonary stenosis is difficult to detect by fetal echocardiography. Lymphatic abnormality with increased nuchal oedema is more common in *PTPN11*. Prenatal diagnosis possible by CVS or amniocentesis if the familial mutation has been defined.

Consultation plan in general practice

History—key points
- Detailed pregnancy history with specific enquiry for nuchal thickening/cystic hygroma, or polyhydramnios. Birth weight usually normal or increased because of oedema.
- Was there failure to thrive or poor feeding in infancy?
- Detailed developmental history (developmental milestones may be delayed, e.g. sitting at 10/12, walking at 21/12, simple two-word phrases at 31/12). Schooling.
- History of easy bruising or prolonged bleeding after venepuncture, tooth extraction, surgery.
- Three-generation family tree with specific enquiry regarding short stature, congenital heart disease, learning difficulty.

Examination—key points
- **Growth parameters:** height (mean height follows 3rd centile until puberty), weight, OFC.
- **Facial features:** ptosis, low-set posteriorly rotated ears with thickened helix. Overall, the features may appear coarse, particularly in infancy and childhood.
- Low posterior hairline and short neck with redundant skin/webbing.
- **Chest:** wide-spaced nipples, prominence of sternum superiorly and depression inferiorly.
- **Heart:** 50–80% have a cardiac defect. Most common defect is pulmonary stenosis, but may have an ASD or other structural defects. Hypertrophic cardiomyopathy may occur in 20% and may present at birth, in infancy, or in childhood.
- In males examine for *cryptorchidism* (60%).
- **Skin:** check carefully for CALs, there is some phenotypic overlap with NF-1 and it is important not to miss this diagnosis. Check for lentigines (LEOPARD syndrome).

Management in primary care

- **Heart:** refer for specialist cardiological follow-up if a heart defect is identified.
- **Growth:** short stature is a very common manifestation of Noonan syndrome (NS) and most children should be under the care of a paediatric endocrinologist for monitoring growth and consideration of growth hormone therapy.

Investigation in secondary care

- DNA for mutation analysis.
- Karyotype in all sporadic females (phenotypic overlap with Turner syndrome) and in all patients with developmental delay.
- Echocardiogram and ECG, if not already done.
- PT, APTT, platelet count—thrombocytopenia, platelet dysfunction, and varied coagulation factor defects may occur alone or in combination in ~50% of patients with NS.
- Eye exam.

Natural history

- **Fertility:** normal in females, but may be reduced in males who have had cryptorchidism.
- **Hearing:** approx. 30% have chronic serous otitis media in infancy and childhood—increased parental awareness for hearing impairment and low threshold for referral to ENT are appropriate.
- **Vision:** >50% have strabismus and/or a refractive error, so orthoptic referral is appropriate in children at the time of diagnosis.
- **Bleeding:** two-thirds of individuals with Noonan syndrome give a history of abnormal bleeding or mild to severe bruising. The coagulopathy is variable and may be subclinical, cause easy bruising or severe surgical haemorrhage.
- **Development and education:** early milestones may be delayed. IQ usually falls in normal range (30% have mild learning disability) and most are educated in normal school, but 10–15% require special education. Verbal IQ is frequently < non-verbal IQ.

Support group

⅍ www.noonansyndrome.org

Retinitis pigmentosa (RP)

RP is the most common inherited retinal dystrophy, affecting about 1 in 4000. In RP there is early loss of rod photoreceptor function (causing progressive night blindness 'nyctalopia') followed by impaired peripheral cone function (causing field loss); foveal cones (central vision) are affected late in the disease. Examination of the fundus shows pigmentary changes in the mid-peripheral retina. Specialist assessment, including an electroretinogram (ERG), may be required to detect early changes.

RP may be isolated or occur as part of systemic disease or syndrome. It is genetically heterogeneous, and where known, inheritance follows:

- Autosomal dominant (AD) inheritance in 20% of cases.
- Autosomal recessive (AR) inheritance in 20% of cases.
- X-linked recessive (XLR) inheritance in 15% of cases.
- It is also a frequent manifestation of mitochondrial disease.

X-linked retinitis pigmentosa (XLRP) is a severe form, consistently symptomatic in early childhood (📖 see Chapter 2, X-linked inheritance, p. 54).

This section deals only with isolated RP.

Very many genes have been implicated in non-syndromic RP. Many of these can be grouped by function, giving insights into the disease process. These include components of the phototransduction cascade, proteins involved in retinol metabolism and cell–cell interaction, photoreceptors, cilia, structural proteins and transcription factors, intracellular transport proteins, and splicing factors.

Differential diagnoses

- **Usher syndrome:** AR condition characterized by sensorineural hearing loss and progressive retinitis pigmentosa.
- **Multisystem disorders:** A variety of inherited disorders, particularly those affecting function of the cilia, e.g. Bardet–Biedl syndrome, or cellular energy metabolism, e.g. mitochondrial and peroxisomal disorders may have RP as a feature.

Genetic advice

Inheritance and recurrence risk

All forms of autosomal inheritance have been found. In 50% of cases there is no family history. Many of these individuals may have AR disease, but some will represent de novo AD mutations, AD disease with incomplete penetrance, or X-linked disease. The AR and XL types are associated with more severe disease with an earlier age of onset.

Prenatal diagnosis—✎ refer to Clinical Genetics

Is feasible only for families with a known mutation.

Predictive testing of apparently unaffected individuals, other family members—✎ refer to Clinical Genetics

- Carrier risk may be determined from the pedigree, and female carriers of XLRP can often be detected clinically.

- Female carriers of XLRP display a broad spectrum of fundus appearance from normal to extensive retinal degeneration. 90% of female carriers have fundus and/or ERG abnormalities.
- May be possible by genetic testing in large families and/or those with a known mutation.

Consultation plan in general practice

History
- History of night blindness.
- Age of onset and rate of progression.
- Registered as totally or partially sighted?
- Other medical problems, e.g. deafness?
- Three-generation family tree, or more if there is a suggestion of X-linkage.

Examination
Visual fields and fundal examination (or report from ophthalmic optician).

Management in primary care
- Arrange for ophthalmological assessment of at-risk individuals. ERG and other investigations are required to detect the early stages of the disease.
- Help and support with disability allowances.
- Liaison with DVLA.
- Code patient's notes.
- Code notes, with appropriate consents, of other family members (📖 see Chapter 1, Confidentiality and consent, p. 8).

Investigations done in secondary care
- Full opthalmological evaluation of affected individuals, including testing of visual fields and electroretinography (ERG).
- DNA testing/storage—mutation analysis is available for the main types of XLRP which are caused by mutations in the *RP2* gene (~15%) or the *RPGR* gene (~75%).
- More extensive investigations are required in sporadically affected individuals and children to exclude syndromes and systemic conditions.

Support groups

British Retinitis Pigmentosa Society: ☎ 01280 860363; 🖰 www.brps.org.uk
Foundation Fighting Blindness (US): 🖰 www.blindness.org

Spinal muscular atrophy (SMA)

SMA is an AR disorder characterized by symmetrical proximal muscle weakness as a consequence of degeneration of the anterior horn cells of the spinal cord. Three classical types are recognized (see below) but these are somewhat arbitrary and there is, in fact, a continuum of clinical severity. Intelligence is unaffected.

- *Type I SMA—severe (Werdnig–Hoffmann)*: onset of severe muscle weakness and hypotonia in the first few months of life, never able to sit or walk. Fatal respiratory failure usually occurs by age 2yr and often before 6/12. Nearly all present by 6/12 and in one-third abnormal fetal movements are reported.
- *Type II SMA—intermediate*: onset before 18/12 (median age 8/12), ability to sit but not to walk unaided, survival into adult life is usual.
- *Type III SMA—mild (Kugelberg–Welander)*: onset of proximal muscle weakness after 2yr, ability to walk independently initially, survival into adult life.

The combined birth incidence or early childhood prevalence of all types of SMA is ~1/10 000. All three types are associated with deletions and small intragenic mutations in the survival motor neuron gene *SMN1* on 5q13. Carrier rate is estimated at 1/50. Most carriers have only one copy of *SMN1*.

> Carrier testing is not straightforward and requires specialist clinical and laboratory input— refer to Genetics.

Natural history and management

Type I SMA

Conventionally, infants with a confirmed diagnosis of SMA type I are offered palliative and terminal care via hospital and community paediatric teams.

Type II SMA

- *Impaired mobility*. Patients require specialized physiotherapy and seating input appropriate to the level of disability. Although type II SMA is said to be a non-progressive disease, many patients do notice a deterioration of mobility with time.
- *Feeding difficulty*. Patients with type II SMA are at risk of feeding difficulties, e.g. aspiration, which may manifest as recurrent chest infections, and some may require gastrostomy feeding.
- *Respiratory insufficiency*. Some may experience progressive respiratory failure (a severe scoliosis may exacerbate this) and ultimately may require assisted nocturnal ventilation.
- *Scoliosis*: Monitoring of scoliosis and appropriate intervention is important in preserving respiratory function in patients with type II SMA, all of whom have pronounced weakness of trunk muscles.
- *Cognitive function* is normal.
- *Pregnancy*. Successful pregnancy has been reported in women with SMA type II. Pulmonary function may remain stable throughout pregnancy, although it may deteriorate temporarily after delivery.

Type III SMA
The complications listed under type II SMA are much less common in type III.

Genetic advice
A result showing that an individual with clinically typical SMA is homozygously deleted for *SMN1* confirms the diagnosis.

Inheritance and recurrence risk
- AR for all except for rare types of SMA.
- A '*de novo*' deletion occurs in ~1.7% of individuals with SMA. Carrier testing of parents is important as this will have an important effect on recurrence risk and on the counselling and testing of other family members.

Variability and penetrance
Usually the type of SMA will be consistent within sibships, but with some variability.

> Within wider families, any type of SMA may occur, i.e. if counselling the uncle of a child who died from SMA type I, the risk that he will have a child with SMA of any type will be ($1/2 \times 1/50 \times 1/4 = 1/400$) assuming no consanguinity and no family history in his partner.

Prenatal diagnosis—⮠ refer to Genetics
Possible by CVS at 11/40 if mutational basis of the SMA in the family is known. Need to genotype both parents prior to CVS.

Carrier testing—⮠ refer to Genetics
If an individual at population risk (i.e. with a negative family history) has two copies of *SMN1* on carrier testing, the residual probability that he/she is a carrier is 1/820.

    If an unaffected sibling of an individual with a homozygous *SMN* deletion has two copies, the chance that he/she is a carrier reduces from 2/3 to 1/13 (but could be reduced to negligible if it were known that both parents were single-copy carriers).

Other family members
Cascade carrier testing can be offered and is especially important if there is consanguinity.

Consultation plan in primary care

History
- History of progressive muscular weakness and motor delay.
- Three-generation family tree.

Examination
- Floppy baby.
- Hypotonia.
- Normal intellectual development.

Management in primary care
- Referral to paediatric neurologist.
- Refer to clinical geneticist for prenatal and carrier testing.
- Ongoing role in co-ordination between several specialties.
- Code patient's notes.
- Code notes, with appropriate consents, of other family members (📕 see Chapter 1, Confidentiality and consent, p. 8).
- If severely affected child, involve Children's Disability Team.

Support group

The Jennifer Trust: ℘ www.jtsma.org.uk

Stickler syndrome

Stickler syndrome is a dominantly inherited disorder of collagen, causing eye problems (myopia and predisposition to retinal detachment), deafness, and joint problems. Affected individuals may have characteristic facial features, such as a flat midface with a depressed nasal bridge, small chin, and sometimes a cleft palate. The facial features are more obvious in infancy and childhood.

Most affected individuals have joint laxity with joint hypermobility in infancy and childhood, but develop early joint pain from degenerative arthritis (especially hips, knees, and lumbar spine) in their 3rd or 4th decade. Individuals with Stickler syndrome frequently have early onset or congenital myopia (short sightedness) and this, in conjunction with the congenital vitreous anomaly, which is a cardinal feature of Stickler syndrome, predisposes to retinal detachment, which may occur at any age. The sensorineural high-tone deafness seen in Stickler syndrome is usually mild and may be asymptomatic in some individuals.

> When retinal detachment occurs in childhood, young, or mid-adult life, it should prompt consideration of Stickler syndrome.

Proposed diagnostic criteria for Stickler syndrome (after Snead and Yates 1999)

Congenital vitreous anomaly plus any of:
- Myopia with onset before 6yrs.
- Rhegmatogenous retinal detachment or paravascular pigmented lattice degeration.
- Joint hypermobility with abnormal Beighton score ± radiological evidence of joint degeneration.
- Audiometric confirmation of sensorineural hearing defect.
- Midline clefting.
- First-degree relative with a diagnosis of Stickler syndrome (i.e. meeting the above diagnostic criteria).

The majority of patients have Stickler syndrome type 1, which is caused by mutations in the gene *COL2A1*. Type II collagen fibrils are formed by triple helices of polypeptides, each encoded by the *COL2A1* gene. Most mutations result in a reduction of the normal quantity of type II collagen present in both cartilage and the vitreous gel of the eye (haploinsufficiency). The gene is alternatively spliced (expressed), so that certain types of mutation may result in minimal systemic involvement, but all patients with type 1 Stickler syndrome have ocular involvement with a high risk of retinal detachment.

Differential diagnoses
- ***Perthes disease***. Perthes disease of the hip can occur in families, segregating in an apparently AD fashion with incomplete and variable penetrance. Exclude other causes for a dysplastic femoral head, such as multiple epiphyseal dysplasia.

- **OSMED**. 'Non-ocular Stickler syndrome' is caused by mutations in the type XI collagen gene *COL11A2*, which is not expressed in the eye. The other features of the condition affecting joints, hearing, and facial appearance overlap with those seen in Stickler syndrome.
- **Pierre–Robin sequence**. Pierre–Robin sequence (PRS) is the congenital combination of a U-shaped cleft palate and small jaw (microganathia). Stickler syndrome is a common cause of Pierre–Robin sequence. All children diagnosed with PRS in whom a more specific diagnosis has not been made should have an ophthalmic assessment to rule out Stickler syndrome.

Genetic advice

Inheritance and recurrence risk

AD—50% risk to offspring of affected individuals. Wide inter- and intrafamilial variability of systemic features. Ocular involvement and abnormalities of vitreous development are pathognomonic and are a consistent finding.

Prenatal diagnosis—✍ refer to Clinical Genetics

Technically feasible in families with a known mutation, but rarely requested.

Predictive testing—✍ refer to Clinical Genetics

Prophylactic retinopexy is appropriate to reduce the risk of retinal detachment in type 1 Stickler syndrome. Predictive testing could be used in families with a known mutation to target this intervention more effectively.

Other family members

All first-degree relatives should be examined and offered an expert eye assessment.

Consultation plan in primary care

History

- Three-generation family tree asking about congenital or early childhood short-sightedness, retinal detachment, deafness, joint laxity in youth with premature arthritis in 3rd–4th decade, hip and knee problems, and cleft palate.

Examination

- Assess for subtle facial features—flat mid-face, small chin (see above).

Management in primary care

- Referral to ophthalmologist with expertise in vitreoretinal surgery or paediatric ophthalmologist for diagnosis and management.
- Referral to other specialties, e.g. Orthopaedics, as indicated.
- Code patient's notes.
- Code notes, with appropriate consents, of other family members (📖 see Chapter 1, Confidentiality and consent, p. 8).

Investigation in secondary care

Careful assessment of the vitreous gel by an ophthalmologist familiar with Stickler syndrome.

Natural history and management

Potential long-term complications

- **Eye**. Moderate/severe myopia (>−5 D) is common and, in combination with the abnormal vitreous, can result in retinal detachment. Prophylactic retinopexy should be considered in type 1 and 2 Stickler syndrome. There is also an increased risk for cataract and glaucoma.
- **Ear**. Conductive loss due to glue-ear is common in young children with Stickler, particularly those with cleft palate. Some sensorineural hearing loss is found in 60% of adult patients with Stickler. It is milder in type 1 Stickler than in type 2, and generally no more progressive than age-related loss.
- **Joint**. Joint discomfort from degenerative joint disease is a problem for many Stickler patients in adult life. In one study 80% of adults had chronic hip pain. 16% had a history of femoral head failure in youth.

Surveillance

Periodic (at least annual) ophthalmological review from infancy.

Support group

The Stickler syndrome support group: ℡ www.sticklers.org

Tuberous sclerosis (TSC)

Tuberous sclerosis complex (TSC), epiloia, Bourneville disease, Pringle disease

TSC is a multisystem disorder characterized by hamartomas (tumour-like lesions) in the brain, skin, and other organs, and often associated with seizures and mental retardation. The prevalence of TSC is 1/10 000. It can present at any age from fetal to late adult life and is characterized by highly variable expressivity.

TSC follows autosomal dominant (AD) inheritance with a high proportion of cases caused by new mutations (~60%). It is caused by mutations in the genes *TSC1* (hamartin) or *TSC2* (tuberin). Tuberin and hamartin act in a pathway playing a critical role in the regulation of cell growth and proliferation.

The most common presentation is with infantile spasms or seizures in early childhood. After a young child is diagnosed, it is not uncommon to discover that one of the apparently healthy parents is mildly affected.

Natural history

- **Life expectancy** is usually normal, even in those with severe learning difficulties. However, early death may result from epilepsy, cardiac arrhythmias, renal involvement, pulmonary lymphangiomyomatosis (LAM), or complications of giant cell astrocytoma.
- **Learning disability**. 50% of individuals with TSC have normal intelligence quotient (IQ). The majority of people who are seizure-free have normal intelligence. Severe learning disability is not thought to occur in the absence of seizures. Two-thirds of individuals with TSC who have epilepsy also have learning disability. Children who present with seizures, particularly infantile spasms, in the first 2yrs of life are more likely to have learning disability.
- **Behavioural problems** are common. Learning disabilities frequently occur in conjunction with behavioural problems, but this need not always be so. Autism is seen in ~25–61% and more broadly defined pervasive developmental disorders in ~50–86%. Sleep disturbance is very common, especially if a child's epilepsy is poorly controlled.
- **Seizures** occur in 80% of individuals with TSC. Most respond at least to some extent to anticonvulsants, but a small minority have epilepsy that is refractory to anticonvulsant therapy.

Genetic advice

Inheritance and recurrence risk—✑ refer to Clinical Genetics
AD inheritance, with 50% risk to the offspring of an affected individual. 60% of cases arise 'de novo' (i.e. with no family history) as a result of a new mutation.

Affected parent
If one parent is affected, the risk of inheriting TSC is 50% to each offspring. In view of the variation in disease severity (expressivity), the overall risk of having a child with mental retardation is likely to be 25% or less (since 50% or less of individuals with TSC are mentally retarded).

Unless the causative mutation is known, parents of an apparently sporadic case will be evaluated by a geneticist by: (i) detailed family tree; (ii) detailed skin examination including Wood's light exam; (iii) expert ophthalmological assessment of the fundi; (iv) consideration of cranial imaging (CT or MRI); and (v) consideration of renal USS.

Parents unaffected
If neither parent is affected with TSC the recurrence risk is 2% due to germline mosaicism (this has been reported for both *TSC1* and *TSC2* and can be either maternal or paternal).

Apparently unaffected siblings
Should be offered a similar evaluation before they plan a family of their own (unless the causative mutation is known, in which case genetic testing should be offered).

TSC is highly penetrant by adult life; true non-penetrance is extremely rare. TSC is highly variable; hence the need for comprehensive clinical assessment of apparently unaffected relatives (or molecular testing if the familial mutation is defined).

Prenatal diagnosis—✍ refer to Clinical Genetics
Possible by chorionic villus sampling (CVS) where a mutation is known.

Consultation plan in primary care

History
- Developmental and behavioural history.
- Three-generation family tree asking about TSC, infantile spasms, epilepsy, learning disability, facial angiofibromata.

Examination
- **Angiofibromata** ('adenoma sebaceum') are rarely obvious at <2 yrs of age and may not appear until middle age. They occur in 85% of affected individuals in 'butterfly' distribution over nose, nasolabial folds, and cheeks—also chin.
- **Hypomelanotic macules** ('ash-leaf' spots) occur in 95% of affected individuals by the age of 5 yrs, and are usually the earliest skin feature. They may be present from birth or develop in infancy. 0.8% of normal neonates have similar macules, but rarely >3. Typically oval. May need Wood's light to visualize them (UV light).
- **Other skin features of TSC** include forehead fibrous plaque, shagreen patches, and subungual fibromata.

(Continued)

Management in primary care
- Referral to neurologist/paediatric neurologist or clinical geneticist, depending on whether the individual is symptomatic or whether concerns have arisen based on the family history.
- Ongoing role in co-ordination between several specialties.
- Code patient's notes.
- Code notes, with appropriate consents, of other family members (📖 see Chapter 1, Confidentiality and consent, p. 8).
- If severely affected child, involve Children's Disability Team, SENCO, etc.
- If severely affected individual, consider inclusion of carer in Carers' register.
- DSS benefits.

Investigation in secondary care
- **Cranial imaging** by computerized tomography (CT) will often show subependymal nodules (SENs) along the lateral walls of the lateral ventricles, and may demonstrate cortical tubers (seen in 66% of cases), but these are better visualized by magnetic resonance imaging (MRI), when they are seen in 95% of cases.
- Onward referral for **ophthalmology assessment**. Retinal hamartomas are found in 40–50% and are almost always asymptomatic and only interfere with vision if overlying the macula (rare).
- **Renal ultrasound scan** (USS). Angiomyolipomata (AMLs) are the most common renal manifestation of TSC. Renal cysts occur in 17–47% of patients with TSC and are often present from early childhood. They are usually multiple and bilateral.
- In infants consider an **echocardiogram** as cardiac rhabdomyomas are common at this age in children with TSC and may be very helpful in making the diagnosis.
- *Genetic testing:* mutation analysis of *TSC1/2*.

Potential long-term complications
- **Giant cell astrocytomas** occur in 10–15%. Peak incidence is late childhood through adolescence. Cases present with symptoms of raised intracranial pressure (headaches, vomiting) due to obstruction of foramina of Munro.
- **AMLs** of the kidney are common and usually multiple and bilateral, increasing in size and number with age. They are readily identified on renal USS. Usually asymptomatic, but can cause renal pain, haematuria, and even intrarenal or retroperitoneal haemorrhage.
- **Renal cysts** are often present from early childhood. They are usually multiple and bilateral.
- Symptomatic **LAM** is uncommon and occurs almost exclusively in adult females. Prognosis can be poor if lung involvement is extensive. It usually presents in adult life, but can present earlier. Can cause progressive respiratory impairment with emphysematous change, loss of lung volume, and risk of pneumothorax. If symptomatic, refer to chest physician.

- ***Cardiac rhabdomyomas*** may be identified on USS in fetal life or cause outflow obstruction or arrhythmias in the neonatal period. They usually regress in number and size with age.
- ***Hepatic hamartomas*** are present in 25% and are usually of no clinical significance.

Current research is focused on drugs such as rapamycin that may be helpful in inhibiting the uncontrolled cell proliferation seen in TSC.

Support groups

UK Tuberous Sclerosis Association: ☎ 01527 871898; ✆ www.tuberous-sclerosis.org
Tuberous Sclerosis Alliance (US): ✆ www.tsalliance.org

Common consultations in primary care

Introduction

One of the main discoveries of recent genetic research is the emerging importance of genetic factors in common disorders. Technological developments such as genome-wide scans are enabling large-scale research studies to identify specific regions of the genome that appear to have a role in susceptibility to certain common disorders.

In the long-term, it is hoped that this will enable a clearer biological understanding of the genetic factors and the gene–environment interactions underlying common disorders. Armed with this knowledge, it may then become possible to define genetic subtypes and tailor advice and therapies accordingly. At the present time this is very rarely possible and, despite media hype, current clinical practice is yet to reap significant benefits from these promising developments.

Atopy

Asthma, eczema, and allergic rhinitis are allergic or atopic disorders with a complex genetic aetiology but well-recognized environmental triggers. The genetic background of an individual influences the response to allergens. The prevalence in the adult population is 5–8%.

PCPs are aware that atopy clearly clusters in families. Most atopic families do not just present with asthma or eczema but an increased risk for all allergic disorders.

These conditions were poorly documented prior to the Industrial Revolution which has led to the hypothesis that both 21st century 'cleanliness' in the home and pollution may be implicated in the increasing prevalence of allergy.

Genetics

- Research studies of atopic families have identified gene loci that may either increase the risk or have a protective effect. It is hoped that research into identifying the genetic cause may offer therapeutic benefits as we begin to understand the way in which the genes interact with the environmental trigger.
- Genetic predictive testing is not yet possible within families.

Clinical implications for primary care

- Promotion of breastfeeding.
- Stop smoking.
- Advice on avoidance of obvious environmental triggers.
- Appropriate medical management of atopic disorder.

Autoimmune disease

Autoimmune disorders are diseases caused by the body producing an immune response (antibodies) against its own tissues, which then leads to tissue and organ damage.

These conditions show familial clustering but do not follow a regular Mendelian pattern of inheritance.

Large-scale research projects looking at affected sib-pairs, or families with a high incidence of autoimmune disorders, recently showed that certain chromosomal loci and SNPs had associations with different autoimmune disorders.

In addition, studies have looked at gene expression in selected tissues from patients with autoimmune disorders. These have shown the activation of specific pathways in these diseases. In the future, combining this gene and protein expression together with SNP data should help our understanding of the pathogenesis of autoimmunity.

There have always been interesting differences in the sex ratios of affected individuals. For example, females more frequently develop rheumatoid arthritis and scleroderma, whereas males more commonly develop ankylosing spondylitis (AS). It has been thought that this could be explained partially by the presence of fetal cells in mothers or conversely the mother's cells persisting in the affected individual, triggering the immune response.

Autoimmune disorders fall into two general types: those that damage many organs ('systemic'), and those where only a single organ or tissue is directly damaged by the autoimmune process ('localized').

Major histocompatability complex (MHC)

These are a series of genes that are subdivided into three groups, of which the Class I and II make up the human leucocyte antigen (HLA) genes, which encode for cell surface proteins designed to produce an immune response when they bind to an antigenic protein. Such a reaction is appropriate when that antigen is foreign, e.g. invading pneumococci, but, clearly, destructive if the antigen recognized is an individual's own tissue.

There are clear disease associations with the MHC, such as AS and other joint diseases, e.g. psoriatic arthritis. The complex also contains the tumour necrosis factor (TNF) gene, which produces a protein product that is the target of the new anti-TNF drugs being used for rheumatoid arthritis.

Transplantation of human organs necessitates elimination of antigenic dissimilarity between donor and recipient, which explains why the risk of rejection is least when the two have identical HLA genes—they are *histocompatible*.

Ankylosing spondylitis (AS)

This condition is well known as a cause of sacro-iliitis and progressive spinal damage and has an incidence of ~1:1000. It is best known as one of the first diseases to have a link to a cluster of genes on chromosome 6, known as the major histocompatability complex (MHC).

Genetics

Genetic factors contribute ~90% of an individual's susceptibility to AS, with about half of that being from HLA-B27 and other major histocompatability genes and some non-major histocompatability genes, e.g. interleukin-1 (IL-1), with other links to chromosomes 3, 10, 16, and 19.

Although a positive HLA-B27 may predict more severe disease and systemic involvement in an individual, the test needs to be used carefully.

Clinical implications for primary care

90+% of individuals with AS are HLA-B27 positive, but so are 10% of the general population. Given the incidence above, in a population of 1000, 1 will have AS but 100 (10% of 1000) will be HLA-B27 positive. This is therefore a test of *minimal predictive value* which may cause unnecessary concern in the 99% of the HLA-B27+ population who will never develop AS. However, it may be a useful investigation in those with a probable clinical diagnosis of AS.

Coeliac disease

Introduction

Coeliac disease (CD) is a complex, inflammatory disorder of the small intestine induced by gluten. The clinical presentation can be very variable from severe 'failure to thrive' as a baby to mild abdominal symptoms or unexplained anaemia as an adult.

It is common and has a prevalence of approximately 1:200 in Western populations, with a sibling relative risk of 30. Monozygotic twin studies have shown a concordance of 70%. The highest prevalence is in the west of Ireland.

Genetics

- Coeliac disease has a strong genetic component, higher than for many other common complex diseases. Possession of the HLA-DQ2 variant is required for presentation of disease-causing dietary antigens to T cells, although this is also common in the healthy population.
- However, the genetic contribution of this region is limited to approximately 40%, so non-HLA genes must also be involved in the disease aetiology.
- Genetic studies have so far identified multiple loci that may potentially be involved in disease aetiology, although the majority of these loci are expected to point to genes with a small effect.
- A major CD locus on chromosome 19 was recently identified in the Dutch population.
- There is some marked overlap when comparing genetic linkage studies conducted in different autoimmune disorders, suggesting that common pathways contribute to these diseases.
- Coeliac disease is more prevalent among patients with type 1 (insulin-dependent) diabetes mellitus, and coeliac disease-related antibodies have been reported to increase in frequency in their first-degree relatives.

It is very useful for the PCP to be aware of a family history of coeliac disease, leading to a high index of suspicion for checking endomysial antibodies (EMA) on a first-degree relative who becomes symptomatic.

Clinical implications for primary care

- Routine screening of first-degree relatives of a patient with coeliac disease should be discussed by the gastroenterology clinic that made the diagnosis.
- Patients with coeliac disease are at risk of osteoporosis. This is often forgotten by the gastroenterologists and can be discussed in primary care.
- The increased prevalence of coeliac disease (CD) among children with type 1 diabetes mellitus (T1D) implies that there is more than a simple association. A link between the gut immune system and T1D has been suggested, both in animal models and in humans. GPs should be aware of this.
- Prevalence of coeliac disease among siblings of children with type 1 diabetes appears to be correlated with the prevalence of coeliac disease associated HLA-DQB1 alleles. However, routine screening for coeliac disease among all first-degree relatives of patients with type 1 diabetes is not warranted.
- The two major complications of coeliac disease are T-cell lymphoma and ulcerative jejunoileitis. Any previously well coeliac who presents with abdominal pain, diarrhoea, weight loss, and anaemia needs urgent referral.

Support groups

Coeliac Society: ℘ http://www.coeliac.org.uk
Coeliac UK: ☎ 01494 437 278; ☎ 01494 474 349

Deafness of congenital or childhood onset

Severe or profound deafness affects approx 1/1000 infants at birth or during early childhood (pre-lingual phase). Acquisition of speech is a major difficulty for these children, and some may be considered for cochlear implantation. A further 2–3/1000 children have moderate/progressive deafness requiring aids. In developed countries, deafness has an important genetic origin and at least 60% of cases are inherited. The pattern of inheritance can be AD, AR, XLR or mitochondrial. The most common genetic cause of severe to profound deafness in infants is recessive mutations of *GJB2* (connexin 26).

> Mutations in connexin 26 *Cx26* (*GJB2*) may account for up to 50% of all cases of pre-lingual AR non-syndromic hearing loss and 10–40% of sporadic cases.

Genetics—✎ refer to Clinical Genetics

- If the child is the only affected individual and no environmental or genetic diagnosis can be made, recurrence risk for future pregnancies is 10% (empiric figure; in reality some families will have 25% recurrence risk, and others much lower risks, but it is not possible to discriminate without a more precise diagnosis of the cause).
- If two affected sibs or consanguinity, the cause will be assumed to be AR with a 25% risk in future pregnancies.
- If affected parent and child, the cause will be assumed to be AD with a 50% risk in future pregnancies.
- If one parent has severe congenital hearing loss, and environmental and genetic forms have been excluded as far as possible, empiric risk to offspring is 5%.
- If both parents have severe congenital hearing loss (neither with environmental or genetic form) and there is no consanguinity or likelihood of consanguinity, empiric risk to offspring is 10%.
- PCPs should be aware that some deaf couples would not wish to pursue genetic testing and may have a preference for a deaf child.

Carrier detection

- Audiograms will be done in all parents, with sibling audiograms if there is any clinical suspicion of hearing loss.
- For connexin 26 deafness and other types where the mutations are defined, it is possible to offer accurate carrier detection to family members.

Neonatal screening

In the UK there is a national newborn hearing screening programme (NHSP) to detect bilateral hearing loss of greater than 40dB (🖰 http://hearing.screening.nhs.uk/surveillance).

Best practice guidelines have been produced and babies who are detected with hearing loss have a wide range of investigations both to understand the aetiology and to plan management. These are performed in secondary care by the paediatrician and audiologist.

Clinical implications for primary care

PCPs *may* be the first to detect hearing problems at the neonate's 8-week check, if the child has missed the neonatal screening.

Natural history and further management (preventative measures)

- *Hearing aids.* Skilled assessment by an audiologist is required to ensure good results. In young children the ear moulds need to be changed periodically as the ear canal grows.
- *Cochlear implants.* These represent an exciting advance in the management of very young children with profound hearing loss. They are best suited to children in the pre-school years who, with optimal hearing aid correction, still have a loss >65dB.
- *Education.* Provision needs to be carefully matched to the child's level of hearing loss.

Support groups

National Deaf Children's Society (NDCS): 🖰 www.ndcs.org.uk
Royal National Institute for the Deaf: 🖰 www.rnid.org.uk
🖰 www.deafplus.org

Deafness of adult onset

As in childhood, the aetiology is an interplay of genetic and environmental factors. Environmental influences include

- Noise
- Infections
- Drugs such as aminoglycosides.

Deafness of adult onset is usually progressive. Although all patterns of inheritance can be found, recessive and syndromic causes are less likely, AD is the most likely mode of inheritance. The family history may suggest AD inheritance with incomplete penetrance. The pattern of hearing loss combined with knowledge of the rate of loss is documented.

Adults who have hearing loss may present for counselling and it is possible to follow a similar investigation protocol to that used to assess infants.

Initial investigations in secondary care may include:

- Hearing assessment of first-degree relatives.
- Ophthalmology referral for syndromic associations.
- CT/MRI of temporal bone.
- Renal USS.
- Urine dipstick.
- ECG (🕮 see Long QT, Sudden cardiac death: cardiac channelopathies, p. 224).
- Connexin 26 and 30 (*GJB6*) mutation analysis.
- Maternal family history of hearing loss, or hearing loss following exposure to aminoglycosides, will indicate the need to test for A1555G mitochondrial DNA (mtDNA) mutation.
- Chromosome analysis if developmental delay or dysmorphic features.

These give additional information that may help delineate both the cause and probable inheritance.

Clinical implications for primary care

- Developmental delay (mild delay in motor milestones is common in deaf children who are otherwise neurologically normal, probably due to involvement of the vestibular system).
- Vestibular symptoms may coexist.
- Referral to Audiology for investigation.
- ✍ Referral to Clinical Genetics for:
  - children and adults with syndromic forms of deafness;
  - families with defined mutations (including carriers of *GJB2*);
  - families in whom no definitive cause for severe deafness has been established.

Support group

Royal National Institute for the Deaf: ℘ www.rnid.org.uk

Dementia

The Royal College of Physicians Committee on Geriatrics (1981) defined dementia as 'The global impairment of higher cortical functions including learned perceptuomotor skills, the correct use of social skills, and the control of emotional reactions in the absence of gross clouding of consciousness. The condition is often irreversible and progressive.'

Clinically, dementia affects memory, speech, perception, and mood. The risk of developing dementia increases with age. Alzheimer disease is the most common neurodegenerative condition affecting older people.

> Alzheimer disease has a prevalence of 1–2% among those aged 65–69yrs increasing to 40–50% among persons 95yrs of age and over.

Dementia is a feature of many progressive disorders affecting the central nervous system (CNS) but the most common dementia over the age of 40yrs is Alzheimer disease. Other common causes include vascular dementia, Lewy body dementia, frontotemporal dementia, and Parkinson disease.

Pathologically, Alzheimer disease and many other neurodegenerative disorders are characterized by neuronal loss and intracellular and/or extracellular aggregates of proteinaceous fibrils. In Alzheimer disease these are intracytoplasmic neurofibrillary tangles (hyperphosphorylated forms of the microtubular protein tau) and extracellular amyloid or senile plaques.

Early-onset Alzheimer disease can be defined as onset at age <65yrs. A prevalence study based on the population of Rouen, using a very strict definition of early-onset Alzheimer disease with age of onset <61yrs, found a prevalence of early-onset Alzheimer disease of ~40/100 000 persons at risk.

Causes of dementia

- *Alzheimer disease* (📖 see p. 191).
- *AD frontotemporal dementia with parkinsonism (including Pick disease).* The second most common pre-senile dementia after Alzheimer disease.
- *Lewy body dementia.* Clinical presentation is typically with fluctuating cognitive impairment, visuo-spatial dysfunction, marked attentional deficits, psychiatric symptoms (especially complex visual hallucinations), and mild extrapyramidal features.
- *CADASIL* Cerebral Autosomal Dominant Arteriopathy with Subcortical Infarcts and Leukoencephalopathy.
- *Huntington disease* (📖 see Chapter 5, Huntington disease, p. 144).
- *Prion diseases* (Gerstmann–Straussler–Shencker syndrome and Creutzfeldt–Jakob disease (CJD)). AD, and caused by mutations in the *PRNP* gene on 20p. Prion diseases may also be sporadic or have infectious aetiologies (e.g. new-variant CJD).
- *Late-onset metabolic disorders.*

- *Other (non-genetic) causes*
  - AIDS-related: the most prevalent dementing disease in the USA among those aged <40yrs
  - Treatable conditions such as drug toxicity in the elderly, nutritional deficiency, hypothyroidism
  - Alcohol-related
  - Tumour
  - Vasculitis
  - Head injury
  - Transmitted CJD

Genetic advice—Alzheimer disease

- Alzheimer disease may be caused by monogenic, high-penetrance mutations, but Alzheimer disease risk can also be influenced by complex predisposition alleles, e.g. apolipoprotein E (APOE).

> There is no clinical or pathological way of distinguishing genetic from sporadic Alzheimer disease in an individual. Family history and age of onset are used initially to determine the likelihood of an inherited form of Alzheimer disease.

- Three genes have been identified, β-amyloid precursor protein on chromosome 21, presenilin 1 and presenilin 2, that cause early-onset Alzheimer disease and show AD inheritance.
- The inheritance of different APOE genotypes affects the age of onset and apparent risk of Alzheimer disease. The usefulness of APOE testing is controversial—50% of those with a pathological diagnosis of Alzheimer made at post-mortem do not carry an *APOE´4* allele. APOE testing is generally not indicated in a clinical setting, e.g. for clinical diagnosis/prediction. However, it may be useful in research contexts.

Inheritance and recurrence risk

- *Early-onset dementia.* For families with a known mutation, or clearly dominant family history, autosomal dominant risks may be used.
- *Later-onset dementia.* For most families empiric risks are all that can be given. Risks are higher when both parents have had dementia and when there is a younger age of onset. There is a three- to fourfold risk of developing Alzheimer disease in the first-degree relatives of individuals with Alzheimer disease compared to controls (19% against 5%). Risks for second-degree relatives are about twice that for controls (i.e. about 10%).

Predictive testing—✍ refer to Clinical Genetics

This is possible in families with known Alzheimer disease mutations using a protocol similar to that used in HD.

Natural history and management

Individuals affected by early-onset dementia should be referred to a neurologist or psychiatrist with special expertise in dementia for comprehensive evaluation, investigation, and care. Cholinesterase inhibitors, e.g. Donepezil, may be of limited benefit. Drug therapy for vascular dementia is under development.

Potential long-term complications

Progressive loss of higher mental functions with loss of independence.

Surveillance

At-risk individuals are advised to avoid deleterious environmental factors such as alcohol excess. Folic acid supplementation may have some protective value.

Clinical implications for primary care

- Affected individuals need a full systems interview, examination, including Mini-Mental State Examination (MMSE), and diagnostic evaluation by an appropriate specialist (e.g. neurologist or old-age psychiatrist) in order to identify potentially treatable causes of cognitive impairment or dementia.
- There are no clinical differences between sporadic Alzheimer disease and early-onset AD types, other than the age of onset.
- A depression questionnaire may aid diagnosis of depression vs. dementia.
- Onward referral to appropriate local screening resource (Integrated Team for Older People, old-age psychiatrist, Clinical Psychology, Neurology) for diagnosis and assessment.
- Discuss Social Service input re. personal services, day care, etc.
- Elderly Care community psychiatric nurse (CPN).
- DSS benefits.
- Code patient's notes.
- Code notes, with appropriate consents, of other family members' (☐ see Chapter 1, Confidentiality and consent, p. 8).
- May need to discuss driving/DVLA contact.
- Manage relatives with sensitivity with respect to possible familial disease.
- Refer to Genetics under advice from, or in conjunction with, specialist if genetic disease suspected.
- Consider DNA storage on affected individuals when a genetic aetiology is possible, after obtaining appropriate consent.

Support group

Alzheimer's Society: ℬ www.alzheimers.org.uk

Diabetes mellitus

Diabetes mellitus is a common and rapidly increasing medical problem arising from a combination of environmental and genetic risk factors. The condition is divided into two types:
- Type 1 diabetes mellitus (T1D) formerly known as insulin-dependent diabetes mellitus (IDDM).
- Type 2 diabetes mellitus (T2D) formerly known as non-insulin-dependent diabetes mellitus (NIDDM), although ~50% of T2D subjects require insulin within 6yrs of diagnosis. This condition becomes more common as a population ages and obesity levels rise.

Individuals with all types of diabetes require regular medical and nursing supervision to ensure accurate control of the disease in order to help prevent long-term complications. Assessment of cardiovascular risk is probably the most important part of management of T2D in terms of prognosis, due to the constellation of associated metabolic risk factors for atherosclerosis.

It is important to remind patients of the risks in pregnancy to the fetus if the diabetes is poorly controlled (📖 see Chapter 9, Maternal diabetes mellitus and diabetic embryopathy, p. 382).

Clinical implications for primary care

See Chapter 11 in *Oxford Handbook of Endocrinology and Diabetes* for a full description of the management and surveillance of diabetes. If investigating/ seeing an 'at-risk' family member, consider:
- A fasting blood glucose >7mmol/L on two occasions = diabetes mellitus (American Diabetic Association diagnostic criteria); a fasting blood glucose 5.6–6.9mmol/L = impaired fasting glucose (i.e. needs follow-up by GP/physician).
- NB. Individuals with mutations in glucokinase (see Maturity-onset diabetes of the young, below) have stable hyperglycaemia throughout life.

  PCPs will be well aware of diabetes as the greatest exemplar of multi-disciplinary team (MDT) working: primary care doctors/nurses, specialist diabetic nurses, consultant physicians, dieticians, medical photographers, chiropodists, etc.

  Diabetic research, including genetics, is very active across the UK. Since much care is shared with hospital departments, they will usually identify the small proportion of patients for whom genetic mutation testing is both appropriate and possible.
- Code patient's notes.
- Code notes, with appropriate consents, of other family members (📖 see Chapter 1, Confidentiality and consent, p. 8).
- May need to discuss driving/DVLA contact.
- For paediatric patients liaison with school nurses is important.

  Manage patient and relatives with sensitivity at the time of diagnosis, as, for many, the spectre of previous generations' problems associated with diabetes (e.g. persistent ulcers, amputations) may immediately appear.

Type 1 diabetes

Affects about 0.3% of Caucasians, with the highest rates in northern Europe. Treatment of T1D is insulin replacement therapy by percutaneous injection.

The HLA (human leucocyte antigen) or MHC (major histocompatability complex) region (🕮 see Autoimmune disease, p. 182) and the insulin gene region are thought to contain the main susceptibility genes for IDDM, although at least 20 regions have been linked to IDDM.

Most studies have been on European and US families and there may be ethnic differences. Risks follow a multifactorial mode. Genetic factors can be seen in the difference in concordance between monozygous twins and siblings.

> The aetiology is complex and the condition arises from the action of many genes and environmental factors. There is rarely evidence for monogenic inheritance.

Genetic advice

Inheritance and recurrence risk

- 30–50% concordance in monozygous twins.
- Sibling risk 6%, with HLA identical sibs having a greatly increased risk of developing T1D.
- Offspring risks show some differences between affected fathers and mothers; a greater proportion of fathers (approximately 4%) than mothers (approximately 2%) of children with IDDM have the disease themselves.

Predictive testing

HLA testing of sibs has been used but half of HLA-compatible sibs will never develop the condition. There is currently no pre-symptomatic treatment to alter the disease process. Consideration must be given to the ethical position and issues of informed consent. Autoantibodies (anti-islet cell, anti-glutamic acid decarboxylase (GAD), etc.) have been used predictively to assess risk in sibs in research, but not in routine clinical practice.

Other family members

Individuals who are at high genetic risk should know the symptoms of diabetes mellitus and attend for prompt assessment if they develop these features.

Type 2 diabetes

Type 2 diabetes is becoming more common as the population becomes older and fatter. It is estimated that 1 in 10 European and US individuals will develop T2D.

T2D is pathologically heterogeneous, but is most commonly the result of defects in the action of insulin (insulin resistance) with a secondary failure of the β-cells to compensate with increased insulin production.

Treatment is by dietary and lifestyle manipulation and oral hypoglycaemic medication in the early stages, with many progressing to insulin therapy within a few years.

> Although the environmental factors are more apparent than in T1D, there has been more success in identifying monogenic forms of T2D.

Maturity-onset diabetes of the young (MODY)

MODY is a form of T2D with autosomal dominant (AD) inheritance, non-obese body habitus, and an age of onset before 25yrs. It accounts for 1–2% of people with diabetes. Five genes account for 87% of UK MODY.

> Asymptomatic family members at high genetic risk require biochemical investigation for diabetes.

Predictive testing—✍ refer to Clinical Genetics

Possible in those with a known familial mutation. Mutation testing is recommended for other affected family members in order to confirm the aetiology of their diabetes. Consider predictive testing for MODY in children of affected parents, together with appropriate dietary and lifestyle advice.

Other types of diabetes

- **Mitochondrial disorders.** The most common symptom, other than the diabetes, is *deafness* and this usually precedes the diabetes.
- **Insulin receptor mutation.** AD inheritance of a single dominant-negative mutation may cause type A insulin resistance ± diabetes mellitus.

Support group

Diabetes UK: 🖰 www.diabetes.org.uk

Epilepsy

Introduction

Epilepsy is a disorder of the brain. It may occur as part of an acute or acquired process affecting the central nervous system (CNS). Genetic factors and genetically determined syndromes contribute in many patients. Epilepsy and seizures are common medical problems—in the general population the cumulative incidence for developing epilepsy to the age of 40yrs is just under 2%.

One epidemiological survey of >10 000 patients with epilepsy found that the prevalence of epilepsy in first-degree relatives of patients with idiopathic generalized epilepsies was 5.3%. Probands with idiopathic generalized epilepsies were highly concordant with respect to their relative's type of epilepsy. Risks to relatives were higher when the epilepsy in the proband began at <14yrs of age. Concordance has been found to be higher in monozygotic (MZ) twin pairs than in dizygotic (DZ) twin pairs. In 94% of concordant MZ pairs and 71% of concordant DZ pairs, both twins had the same major epilepsy syndrome. *This strongly suggests the presence of syndrome-specific genetic determinants rather than a broad genetic predisposition to seizures.*

Most genetic epilepsies have a complex mode of inheritance and genes identified so far account only for a minority of families and sporadic cases. Many of the genes associated with idiopathic generalized epilepsy are within the ion-channel family and show autosomal dominant inheritance. Other genes are implicated in AD lateral temporal lobe epilepsy, malformations of cortical development and X-linked mental retardation syndromes in which seizures are a component.

The following definitions may be helpful:

- **Epileptic seizure.** A transient episode of abnormal cortical neuronal activity. This may manifest as a motor, sensory, cognitive, or psychic disturbance.
- **Epilepsy.** A disorder of the brain characterized by recurrent (two or more) unprovoked seizures.

Other diagnoses/conditions to consider

- Long QT syndromes, 📖 see Sudden cardiac death: cardiac channelopathies, p. 224.
- Non-epileptic causes, e.g. syncope, pseudoseizures, Münchausen syndrome (by proxy in children). These diagnoses should be evaluated by a neurologist.

Genetic advice (📖 see Table 6.1)

Idiopathic epilepsy

In practice, genetic testing is rarely available but there are some specific forms of epilepsy that have a known genetic cause that can be identified by the patient's neurologist.

Inheritance and recurrence risk

For isolated/idiopathic epilepsy with no clear familial inheritance, multifactorial inheritance is assumed and empiric risk figures used. The offspring risk for epilepsy is between 1.5% and 7.5%.

Table 6.1 Genetic risks in idiopathic epilepsy

Individual affected	Cumulative risk of clinical epilepsy to age 20yrs (%)*
Monozygotic twins	~60
Dizygotic twins	~10
Sibling with onset <10 yr	6
Sibling with onset >25 yrs	1–2
Overall sibling risk	2.5
Parent	4 (1.5–7.5)
Parent and sibling	~10
Both parents	~15
General population	~1

*Excluding febrile convulsions.

Variability and penetrance
Most of the familial epilepsy syndromes show intra- and interfamilial variability.

Prenatal diagnosis
Only available in conditions with a known mutation or cytogenetic abnormality.

> Be alert to the teratogenic effects of anti-epileptic medications as seizure disorders are one of the most common neurological problems affecting women of childbearing age (📖 see Drugs in Pregnancy, p. 336 and Fetal anticonvulsant syndrome, p. 360).

Approximately 0.4% of pregnant women take anticonvulsant medication. Overall, there is a fairly solid consensus that treatment with anticonvulsants in pregnancy, for whatever reason, i.e. epilepsy or mood disorder, is associated with an overall two- to threefold increased risk of congenital malformation, compared to the risk in the general population (📖 see Chapter 9, Drugs in Pregnancy, p. 336).

Potential long-term complications
- Fetal anti-epileptic drug effects and increased risk of neural tube defects. Possible neurodevelopmental consequences for fetus of frequent maternal tonic–clonic seizures in pregnancy.
- Increased risk of sudden death in patients with epilepsy (mainly attributable to the underlying disease, accidents, or suicide), especially in certain groups (e.g. young people and those with frequent generalized seizures and mental retardation).
- Restrictions on driving; possible discrimination; long-term effects of the epilepsy, seizures, and medication.

Surveillance
- By a neurologist, unless fit-free and stable, in which case PCPs can manage.
- Refer back to secondary care if nature, or frequency, of fits change, or for prenatal counselling.
- Seek neurology advice if a patient wishes to stop medication.

Clinical implications for primary care

- Refer to neurologist if a first fit occurs, or *on suspicion* that the patient may have had an epileptic event.
- ECG if hint of cardiac problems (e.g. long QT).
- Contact Neurology if there is a change in nature/frequency of fits.
- Liaison with school re. care of epileptic fits and general effects on education.
- Discuss fears and anxieties.
- Patient to notify diagnosis (when confirmed) to DVLA.
- Code patient's notes and add to epilepsy register.
- Annual epilepsy check (fit frequency, medication review, etc.) as in Quality and outcomes Framework (QoF).

Support groups

Epilepsy Action: ℅ www.epilepsy.org.uk
The National Society for Epilepsy: ℅ www.epilepsynse.org.uk
Epilepsy Foundation of America: ℅ www.efa.org

Family history of a possible genetic disorder

One of the most frequent referrals from PCPs to Clinical Genetics is of the patient who is worried about the implications of a medical problem within a family.

The most common times for individuals to present are immediately after a diagnosis has been made, in early pregnancy, at the time a child leaves home/school, at the start of a serious relationship, or after the death/funeral of the affected individual. These are all times of heightened emotion and the added input of a potentially serious genetic problem means that the PCP often has to deal with a very anxious and apparently demanding patient/family.

Even if the diagnosis has been apparent for some time, this second event brings it to attention and the family suddenly want answers.

The PCP not only needs to support the family's emotional need, but also to assess whether the diagnosis is known and, if so, is whether it is possible to confirm the diagnosis (see Chapter 7, Confirmation of diagnosis of cancer, p. 254).

Clinical implications for primary care

- Draw the family tree, highlighting affected individuals. This may show the likely pattern of inheritance.
Assess urgency of need for referral. Pregnancies require urgent referral and assessment.
- Find out more about the diagnosis: the family may be able to provide a death certificate or have copies of hospital letters and discharge summaries.
- See appropriate section of this handbook for more clinical information.
- Families may get support from relevant patient support groups for the familial condition.

Support groups

Genetics lutent group ♫ www.gig.ork.uk
 See also Chapter 11, p. 421 and p. 422.

Glaucoma

Introduction

Glaucoma is an optic neuropathy with characteristic field loss that may or may not be associated with increased intraocular pressure. It is classified, according to the mechanism causing the glaucoma, into the following:

- Primary open-angle glaucoma (POAG) is due to an intrinsic disorder of the trabecular meshwork.
- Closed-angle glaucoma (acute and chronic).
- Secondary glaucomas arise as a consequence of disease or abnormality, either elsewhere in the eye or in other systems, e.g. Marfan syndrome, ectopia lentis, and homocystinuria, where acute glaucoma secondary to lens dislocation may develop.

Most adult-onset glaucoma is a complex disease showing multifactorial inheritance, and family history is an important risk factor.

Glaucoma in infancy and childhood may form part of a wider condition. Primary congenital glaucoma is rare and is also known as buphthalmos.

Glaucoma is usually a purely ocular condition but associated non-ocular features may suggest a syndrome diagnosis.

Potential long-term complications

Untreated glaucoma can lead to irreversible constriction of the visual fields and, eventually, blindness.

Surveillance

Ensure ophthalmological surveillance for affected individuals and arrange ophthalmological follow-up for 'at-risk' family members.

Genetic advice

Inheritance and recurrence risk

Juvenile and adult primary glaucoma. If inherited, it is mainly AD but most *adult glaucoma* is a complex (multifactorial) disease.

Other family members

First-degree relatives need screening, the age at which to begin screening depending on the family history, but screening is free for those >40yrs of age with a positive family history. Seek guidance from your ophthalmological colleagues if there is an unusual history.

Clinical implications for primary care

Identify first-degree relatives who require ophthalmological screening.
For affected individuals:
- Onward referral, enclosing GOS18 form from optician (UK) to ophthalmologist.
- Regular repeat prescriptions for ophthalmologist-recommended eye drops.
- Code patient's notes.
- Code notes, with appropriate consents, of other family members (☐ see Chapter 1, Confidentiality and consent, p. 8) as they are eligible for free glaucoma screening >40yrs.
- Recommend local services for those with low visual acuity.

Support group

International Glaucoma Association: ☎ 020 7737 3265; ⌨ www.iga.org.uk

Hyperlipidaemia

Introduction

The level of serum cholesterol increases in an individual with advancing age, and is the result of the interplay between a number of genetic and environmental factors; hypercholesterolaemia in the population has a multifactorial basis. Hydroxymethylglutaryl coenzyme (HMG-CoA) reductase inhibitors ('statins') have revolutionized the treatment of hypercholesterolaemia.

The most common genetic cause of hyperlipidaemia is familial hypercholesterolaemia (FH).

There are other rare causes of hyperlipaemia that may be diagnosed by the lipid clinic.

Familial hypercholesterolaemia (FH)

Approximately 1/500 of the population in Europe and North America are heterozygous for mutations in the low-density lipoprotein (LDL) receptor (*LDLR*). There is a much higher incidence of FH in certain populations, such as the Afrikaaners (1/80), Christian Lebanese, Finns, and French-Canadians, due to founder effects.

Guidelines for a diagnosis of FH (Scientific Steering Committee on behalf of the Simon Broome Register Group 1999) are a serum cholesterol >6.7mmol/L in children <16yrs, or >7.5mmol/L in adults plus tendon xanthomata in the patient or in a first- or second-degree relative of the patient.

- Homozygotes and compound heterozygotes have very severe hypercholesterolaemia, and develop xanthomata in childhood over tendons, the skin of the popliteal and antecubital fossae, buttocks, and in the webs between the fingers. Most die by the age of 20yrs due to supravalvular aortic stenosis and coronary heart disease.
- Heterozygotes develop xanthomata over tendons, especially the Achilles tendons and the tendons overlying the knuckles of the hand. Corneal arcus and xanthelasma also tend to develop at a younger age than in the general population.

Heterozygotes are at high risk of coronary heart disease, and without treatment the elevated serum cholesterol concentrations lead to a more than 50% risk of fatal or non-fatal coronary heart disease by age 50yrs in men and of at least 30% in women aged 60yrs.

- The clinical diagnosis of FH is based on a family history of hypercholesterolaemia and premature coronary atherosclerosis, the lipid profile, and the presence of xanthomata.
- Treatment is with statins, which are usually started in the late teens in men and later, perhaps after completion of childbearing, in women. Lifestyle modifications such as a healthy diet, and especially avoidance of smoking, are important adjuncts to drug therapy.
- The prognosis for patients with heterozygous FH has improved with the introduction of more effective treatment, with recent studies showing a decline in the relative risk of coronary mortality in patients aged 20–59yrs from an eightfold risk prior to 1992 and the introduction of statin therapy to 3.7-fold thereafter.

Genetic advice—FH

Mutations are currently only detected in 30–50% of patients with a clinical diagnosis of FH. Some families with FH are more susceptible to coronary heart disease than others and, in a few, coronary heart disease occurs at a strikingly young age, e.g. affecting men in their 20s.

Prenatal diagnosis

May be considered for the homozygous form of FH, but is not generally indicated for the heterozygous form for which treatment is available.

Predictive testing

This is possible by analysis of lipid profiles or, more definitively, by molecular genetic analysis if the familial mutation has been defined.

Cascade screening of family members is indicated, but in FH, since treatment is not usually initiated until the late teens, it may be appropriate to defer genetic testing until individuals are in their mid-teens and able to participate in the testing process.

Clinical implications for primary care

History

- Three-generation family tree, with enquiry about relatives with hypercholesterolaemia, heart attacks (document age), angina (document age of onset), and cause of death (document age).
- History of Achilles 'tenosynovitis'.

Examination

- Examine carefully for tendon xanthomata over the Achilles tendons (often there is fibrous swelling overlying cholesterol accumulation deep within the tendon, so the xanthoma may feel hard) and over the tendons overlying the knuckles with the fingers outstretched.
- Check blood pressure (BP).

(Continued)

Investigation
- Fasting lipid profile including triglycerides.
- LFTs.

Management in primary care

- Affected patients should either be under the care of a lipid clinic, or, with clear surveillance guidelines, primary care.
- Referral to appropriate secondary care expert (e.g. biochemist with an expertise in lipid management).
- Prescribe initial statins (where advised) and manage long term with advice about side-effects and drugs, etc. to avoid (e.g. macrolides, grapefruit, etc.), yearly monitoring of lipid profile, LFTs.
- Advice on healthy lifestyle (smoking cessation, exercise).
- Code patient's notes.
- Code notes, with appropriate consents, of other family members (☐ see Chapter 1, Confidentiality and consent, p. 8).

Support group

Heart UK: ☎ 01628 628638; ✍ www.heartuk.org.uk

Osteoporosis

Introduction

Osteoporosis is a skeletal disorder of compromised bone strength leading to an increased risk of bone fracture. It affects postmenopausal women, if they live long enough (virtually all >85yrs) and 1 in 12 men.

A fragility fracture (sustained as the result of a fall from standing height or less) is the clinically apparent and relevant outcome of osteoporosis. In the absence of fracture, osteoporosis is asymptomatic and often remains undiagnosed. Indeed, women may develop a 'dowager's hump' from asymptomatic osteoporotic vertebral fractures without presenting to their GPs at all. Osteoporotic fragility fractures occur most commonly in the vertebrae, hip, and wrist, and are associated with substantial disability, pain, and reduced quality of life.

Osteoporosis is defined by the World Health Organization (WHO) as a T-score of –2.5 standard deviations (SD) or lower on dual-energy X-ray absorptiometry (DXA) scanning.

'Case finding' indicators of a low bone mineral density are:
- A low body mass index (BMI < 22kg/m^2).
- Medical conditions such as ankylosing spondylitis and rheumatoid arthritis.
- Any malabsorption (Crohn's disease, ulcerative colitis, coeliac disease, pancreatic insufficiency).
- Conditions that result in prolonged immobility (stroke, paralysis).
- Untreated premature menopause (<45yrs old).
- Oral glucocorticoid usage is a special risk factor.
- A first-degree relative with a fractured hip.
- Smoking.
- High (>3units/day) alcohol consumption.
- Chronic obstructive airways disease has a very high risk as these patients often smoke, are relatively immobile, often thin, and have intermittent courses of oral glucocorticoids.
- Women on anastrozole for breast cancer are at increased risk for osteoporosis and local guidelines for DXA scans and management should be followed.
- Thyroid disease.

The diagnosis may be assumed in women aged 75yrs or older sustaining a fragility fracture, if the responsible clinician considers a DXA scan to be clinically inappropriate or unfeasible (NICE guidelines).

Treatment

Standard pharmacological therapy for the prevention and/or treatment of osteoporosis includes bisphosphonates (alendronic acid 70 mg once weekly), selective oestrogen receptor modulators (SERMS), or second-line alternative regulators of bone turnover, such as calcitonin, strontium ranelate, and teriparatide: all with appropriate supplementation with adequate levels of calcium and vitamin D. (See NICE guidelines.)

Genetic advice

Inheritance and recurrence risk

- There is an increased risk if a first-degree relative has osteoporosis (RR 2.3) but the disease is so multifactorial that general bone health advice should be given to all (see National Osteoporosis Society (NOS) website)
- RR of other indicators of low bone mineral density are:
  - glucocorticoids, 2.3
  - alcohol excess, 1.7
  - smoking, 1.6
  - previous fracture, 1.6
  - low BMI, 1.4.

Clinical implications for primary care

- History to determine any indicators of a low bone mineral density.
- Height (how much shrinkage?), weight, BMI.
- Referral for DXA scan.
- Referral, if locally available, to specific osteoporosis classes/physio.
- Encourage smoking cessation, increased physical activity.
- Refer for alcohol counselling if appropriate.
- Use WHO Fracture Risk Assessment tool (see Medical resources, below)
- Code patient's notes.
- Code notes, with appropriate consents, of other family members (see Chapter 1, Confidentiality and consent, p. 8).
- At present surveillance is controversial, with some clinical services offering follow-up DXA scans at intervals which vary from 1 to 3yrs. Other bone metabolic units follow up patients with bone markers such as P1NP on a blood test, which gives some idea of bone turnover.
- Refer patient to osteoporosis specialist if further advice is required, or if male.

Medical resources

NICE guidelines (see website for latest iteration): ✆ www.nice.org.uk
WHO Fracture Risk Assessment (FRAX) calculator: ✆ www.shef.ac.uk/FRAX

Support group

The National Osteoporosis Society (NOS): ✆ www.nos.org.uk

Parkinson disease

Introduction

Parkinson disease is a neurodegenerative disease characterized by tremor, slowness of movement and difficulty initiating movement, rigidity, and poor postural reflexes. This disturbance of motor function is due to the loss of neurons in the substantia nigra and elsewhere, in association with the presence of Lewy bodies (cytoplasmic protein deposits containing aggregates of A-synuclein) and thread-like proteinaceous inclusions within neurites, also containing A-synuclein (Lewy neurites).

It is the second most common neurodegenerative condition after Alzheimer disease, with a prevalence of 0.5–1% at age 65–69yrs and 1–3% amongst persons of 80yrs and older.

Most cases are sporadic, but there are occasional families with dominant or recessive inheritance. There are few patients with clear Mendelian inheritance compared with the number of sporadic cases.

Monozygotic (MZ) twins with early-onset disease have a very high rate of concordance (much higher than for dizygotic (DZ) twins) suggesting a significant genetic component, at least in early-onset disease.

Other similar diagnoses/conditions

- **Parkinsonism** may be post-encephalitic, drug-induced (antipsychotic agents) or arteriosclerotic, and these may all cause confusion with the idiopathic or familial forms of Parkinson disease.
- **Huntington disease** in previous generations is not infrequently mistaken for PD.
- **FXTAS (fragile X tremor ataxia syndrome),** 📖 see Chapter 5, Fragile X syndrome, p. 122.
- **AD Parkinson disease,** see below.
- **Demetia variants**, 📖 see Dementia, p. 190.
- **Benign essential tremor.** A common disorder inherited as a late-onset -AD condition. May be mistaken for PD.

Genetic advice

Inheritance and recurrence risk

- There are a few families with a clearly Mendelian pattern of inheritance (AR or AD) or a defined disease-causing mutation.
- For the remainder, advice is based on empirical data. A threefold increase in risk for first-degree relatives of patients with classical Parkinson disease seems appropriate. Given the fairly low prevalence of Parkinson disease in the population, i.e. 0.5–1% at age 65–69yrs and 1–3% amongst persons of 80yrs and older, the absolute risks remain fairly low.
- A 7.75-fold increase in risk may be appropriate in first-degree relatives of patients with onset of Parkinson disease before the age of 50yrs.
- Storage of a DNA sample from an affected member of the family may be considered, although relevant mutations are rare—mutation analysis for parkin and A-synuclein being usually only available as part of a research programme.

Post-mortem reports are very helpful as the diagnosis is not always accurate in life.

Natural history and management

The early treatment of Parkinson disease involves education for the patient and family, access to support groups, regular exercise, and good nutrition. Dopamine agonists rather than levodopa should be the initial symptomatic therapy. There is active research into disease-modifying therapies that will provide neurorescue or neuroprotection.

Clinical implications for primary care

- Does the consultee have any symptoms of Parkinson disease (tremor, cogwheel rigidity, posture/balance problems)?
- Are there neurological features in the affected individual or other family members?
- Examine for clinical features of Parkinson disease.
- Mini-Mental State examination (MMSE).
- Depression questionnaire may aid diagnosis of depression vs. dementia.
- Three-generation family tree with careful enquiry about who in the family is/was affected, the age at onset of symptoms, treatment given, and age and cause of death.

Management in primary care

- Referral to a neurologist for evaluation.
- Liaise with available local services (e.g. specialist Parkinson nurse).
- Consider DLA, invalidity benefit where appropriate.
- Discussion on driving (🖰 www.dvla.gov.uk).
- Remain aware of an increased incidence of both depression and dementia.
- Code patient's notes.
- Code notes, with appropriate consents, of other family members (📖 see Chapter 1, Confidentiality and consent, p. 8).
- Add patient to Carers' register.
- Add family carers to Carers' register.

Support group

Parkinson's Disease Society: ☎ 0808 800 0303; 🖰 www.parkinsons.org.uk

Psychiatric disorders

- These are common and well represented in GP consultations.
- There has long been debate about the relative contribution of nature and nurture in the aetiology of these conditions.
- Family, twin, and adoption studies have shown a clear genetic contribution to schizophrenia and bipolar disorders but only recently has research begun to tease out the underlying genetic mechanisms.

Schizophrenia

- Schizophrenia is has a population prevalence of about 1%. The condition is diagnosed by the presence of hallucinations, delusions, and other cognitive abnormalities.

> Twin studies have shown a high concordance between identical twins and the risk of schizophrenia, in the children of parent(s) with the condition, is not reduced if they are adopted, and heritability has been estimated at 70–90%.

- For many years genetic studies looking for susceptibility genes have given inconsistent results, but recent work looking at rare variants and small chromosome deletions and duplications has shown these changes to be more frequent in patients with schizoprenia.
- Geneticists are most commonly asked to advise about genetic risks by the normal siblings of affected individuals, or by adoption agencies that are placing children born to affected parents. Despite new promising research, at present empirical risk data are still used.
- The cumulative risk of schizophrenia in the offspring of an affected individual is 10–15%. The risk to nephews and nieces is much lower at about 3.5%.

Major affective disorder (bipolar disease, manic depression)

- 1–2% prevalence.
- Like schizophrenia, there are strong genetic risk factors with concordance in monozygotic and dizygotic twins, respectively, of 40–70% and about 10%. There have been many genes reported as possible candidates for increasing susceptibility, but none are currently of use clinically to help predict at-risk individuals in the population.
- Clinical geneticists still use empirical data if family members wish to be informed of their genetic risk. A first-degree relative has a lifetime risk of 5–10%.

Depression

Depression is very common, with lifetime prevalence for major depressive disorder in the community estimated at 15–17% (DSM4 1994). It occurs twice as frequently in women as in men. Depression can begin at any age, but usually has its onset in the mid-20s. Genetic factors have an important role in the aetiology of depression. Heritability has been estimated from twin studies as 31–42%.

Clinical implications for primary care

- Consider genetic advice if children of parents with a major psychiatric problem are to be adopted.
- Support the family appropriately through liaison with community psychiatric services.

Support group

The Royal College of Psychiatrists has information leaflets for patients and families on all mental health issues: ℜ http://www.rcpsych.ac.uk/mentalhealthinformation.aspx

Sensitivity to anaesthetic agents

Introduction

There are two main types of inherited sensitivity to anaesthetic agents: suxamethonium sensitivity and malignant hyperthermia/hyperpyrexia. Patients with myotonic dystrophy may also be sensitive to anaesthetic agents (📖 see Chapter 5, Myotonic Dystrophy, p. 152).

Suxamethonium sensitivity

Pseudocholinesterase deficiency, butyrylcholinesterase deficiency.

Suxamethonium (succinylcholine) is a drug used in general anaesthesia to induce neuromuscular blockade to facilitate tracheal intubation. It is metabolized in the plasma by the non-specific esterase pseudocholinesterase. Normally this happens quickly and the neuromuscular blockade lasts less than 5 min. Patients who are homozygous or compound heterozygotes for some pseudocholinesterase (BChE) variants produce pseudocholinesterase of abnormal affinity and reduced amount and metabolize the suxamethonium only slowly, resulting in markedly prolonged neuromuscular blockade and paralysis. Artificial ventilation is used to support the patient until the neuromuscular blockade wears off (usually ~90 min after succinylcholine and ~5h after mivacurium). Apnoea after suxamethonium can last for up to 3 days in a highly sensitive individual.

- Affected individuals are otherwise entirely asymptomatic (although they may be sensitive to cocaine).
- The gene encoding pseudocholinesterase is *CHE1* on 3q26.1. 'Silent' alleles are also found, due to nonsense mutations/deletions in the *CHE1* gene.
- Using biochemical assays, the patient's phenotype can be defined. It is often not possible to ascribe a *definitive* genotype without performing family studies and therefore usually only the phenotype is reported. Molecular genetic studies may be available in some centres.
- The frequency of the atypical variant (A) is 0.017 in Caucasians, giving a homozygous frequency of ~1/3500.
- Cholinesterase levels can also be reduced in pregnancy, liver disease, and by other drugs. However, any clinical prolongation of effect is small.

Malignant hyperthermia (MH)

MH is a dangerous hypermetabolic state after anaesthesia with suxamethonium and/or volatile halogenated anaesthetic agents such as halothane and methoxyflurane. It affects ~1/20 000 anaesthetized patients. MH may also be triggered in susceptible individuals by severe exercise in hot conditions, infections, neuroleptic drugs, and overheating in infants, and the overall prevalence is estimated at 1/10 000. The body temperature rises acutely to 40 or 41°C with muscle stiffness, tachycardia, sweating, cyanosis, and tachypnoea. Hyperkalaemia, acidosis, and hypercapnia, as well as the fever, alert the anaesthetist. Dantrolene, which decreases the amount of calcium released from the sarcoplasmic reticulum, is an effective treatment that has reduced case fatality from 70% to 5%.

The inherited abnormalities in MH-susceptible individuals lie in the regulation of myoplasmic calcium (Ca).

Genetic advice

Inheritance and recurrence risk

- ***Suxamethonium sensitivity.*** The condition follows autosomal recessive (AR) inheritance and therefore siblings are at 1 in 4 risk.
- ***MH*** is inherited in an autosomal dominant (AD) manner, giving a 50% risk to offspring of an affected individual.

Other family members

- ***Suxamethonium sensitivity.*** All siblings should be tested biochemically (and molecularly if available). Parents should also be tested, both to help define the phenotypes and also because the relatively high carrier rate in Caucasians means there is a small chance that they, too, could be affected.
- ***MH.*** Parents and offspring should be offered *in vitro* muscle testing if an *RYR1* mutation that would enable predictive genetic testing is not identified within a short time.

Clinical implications for primary care

- Three-generation family tree with specific enquiry about anaesthesia.
- Detailed history from the proband regarding experience following anaesthesia.
- For MH, enquire specifically about muscle pains after exercise or episodes of rhabdomyolysis (myoglobinuria).
- Most cases will have received, or begun, the appropriate investigation pathway after a general anaesthetic in hospital.
- Code patient's notes.
- Code notes, with appropriate consents, of other family members (📖 see Chapter 1, Confidentiality and consent, p. 8).
- Refer to the condition when making any referral to secondary care.
- May be asked to take relevant bloods on other family members.

Reinforce the advice that patients with suxamethonium sensitivity or susceptibility to MH should carry a laminated warning card and consider wearing a Medic-Alert bracelet.

Sudden cardiac death (SCD)

- The major risk factor for sudden cardiac death in adults is the presence of **ischaemic heart disease**. The sudden death of a young adult aged <35yrs from coronary artery disease may be a presentation of Familial hypercholesterolaemia (□ see Hyperlipidaemia, p. 206).
- Inherited cardiomyopathies and channelopathies are of particular importance in sudden cardiac death in young adults.
- In children undiagnosed congenital cardiac anomalies may be detected at post-mortem.

- *Structural cardiac abnormalities* evident at autopsy may include hypertrophic and dilated cardiomyopathy, and arrhythmogenic right ventricular cardiomyopathy.
- *Cardiac channelopathies* may account for one-third of autopsy-negative sudden unexplained deaths (SUDs) during childhood and adolescence. They are a heterogeneous group of conditions and include: long QT syndrome, catecholaminergic polymorphic ventricular tachycardia, Brugada syndrome and short QT syndrome. Sometimes sudden death due to one of these conditions is misdiagnosed as death due to epilepsy.
- *Thoracic ascending aortic aneurysm and dissection* is seen in Marfan syndrome and related disorders (□ see Chapter 5, Marfan syndrome, p. 148). There should be other clinical and autopsy features to suggest the diagnosis.

It is important to try to store a DNA sample (with consent) following the sudden cardiac death of a young person. This can be from blood (~5mls in an EDTA tube) within a short time of death or from a skin biopsy (placed into tissue culture medium up to 48hrs after death).

Because of the diagnostic difficulties even after a full post-mortem, genetic testing (which may be at a later date) can clarify the diagnosis and DNA should be stored. This post-mortem genetic analysis is sometimes called a molecular autopsy.

Management of these families requires specialist cardiac and genetic input and most regional centres will have an inherited cardiac conditions (ICC) clinic.

Clinical implications in primary care

- Three-generation family history with specific enquiry about the following:
  - deaths attributed to heart problems
  - sudden unexplained deaths
  - shortness of breath, chest pain/discomfort, palpitation, light-headedness, and black-outs
  - history of fainting, 'epilepsy', sudden death, and congenital deafness.
- 12-lead electrocardiogram (ECG) looking for LVH, rhythm disturbance, long QT.
- Try to obtain death certificate/post-mortem report/copy of echocardiogram report to verify diagnosis in an affected family member.
- At-risk family members should be reviewed by a specialist cardiologist who will refer where appropriate to genetics or preferably be seen in an ICC clinic.
- Code patient's notes.
- Code notes, with appropriate consents, of other family members (📖 see Chapter 1, Confidentiality and consent, p. 8).

Support groups

British Heart Foundation (BHF): Genetic Information Service ☎ 0300 456 8383 🖰 www.bhf.org.uk
SADS UK The Sudden Arrhythnic Death Syndrome Foundation UK 🖰 www.sadsuk.org
Cardiac Risk in the Young 🖰 www.c-r-y.org.uk

SCD: ischaemic heart disease

Ischaemic heart disease (IHD) remains the most significant cause of death in those living Western lifestyles and is characterized by angina (chest pain on exercise) or myocardial infarction, with possible adverse effects on cardiac rhythm, cardiac efficiency, etc.

Genetics

- Single-gene defects account for a very small number of cases, and IHD is therefore a frequent expression of polygenic disease combined with environmental factors.
- PCPs should manage the obvious, primary or secondary, preventative measures (lipid control, weight reduction, smoking cessation, aspirin, β-blockade, etc.) with which they are currently familiar.
- It would be helpful to record a 'family history of IHD' in patients with such, using the relevant code, as the pace of genetic advancement may allow improved, effective screening and preventative measures in the future.

Clinical implications for primary care

(📖 see p. 219)

Support group

British Heart Foundation (BHF): 🕸 www.bhf.org.uk Heart helpline ☎ 0300 330 3311

SCD: structural cardiac abnormalities

Hypertrophic cardiomyopathy (HCM)

- Previously hypertrophic obstructive cardiomyopathy (HOCM), this is a disease of the myocardium characterized by ventricular hypertrophy. Individuals with HCM are at risk for arrhythmia (which may cause sudden death), myocardial ischaemia, and heart failure. Cardiac hypertrophy can also be secondary to hypertension and valvular or supravalvular aortic stenosis. In the absence of a family history, these need to be excluded before a diagnosis of HCM is made. HCM can also occur in Noonan and LEOPARD syndrome (🕮 see Chapter 5, Noonan syndrome, p. 160), Friedreich's ataxia (FRDA), and some mitochondrial disorders.
- Familial HCM affects up to 1/500 young adults. It follows an autosomal dominant (AD) mode of inheritance and many of the identified genes encode cardiac sarcomere proteins.
- Overall, mutations are found in 60–70% of families with HCM.
- Progression of symptoms due to left ventricular (LV) dysfunction is usually slow, but about 10% of patients develop a dilated end-stage cardiomyopathy. β-blockers, calcium-channel antagonists, and disopyramide may improve symptoms. Surgery or catheter intervention is an option for patients with obstruction that has not responded to medical therapy. LV outflow tract obstruction at rest is a predictor of progression to severe symptoms of heart failure and of death.

Potential long-term complications

- **Sudden death.** Annual cardiovascular mortality is 0.7–1.4%. The greatest risk is in young patients with recurrent syncope or with a strong family history of sudden death. Intense physical exertion may trigger sudden death and should be avoided in high-risk patients. Amiodarone reduces risk of sudden death, and implantable cardioverter-defibrillators have a role in some high-risk patients.
- **Arrhythmia.**
- **Subacute bacterial endocarditis (SBE).** Patients with outflow obstruction and/or mitral regurgitation may need antibiotic prophylaxis, e.g. for dental work (see NICE guidelines).

Affected individuals will be under regular long-term surveillance by a cardiologist. Variable expression of disease is common even amongst family members carrying the same mutation. Where the familial mutation is known, definitive genetic testing may be possible to determine who needs surveillance.

Dilated cardiomyopathy and left ventricular non-compaction

This may be familial and follow a variety of patterns of inheritance. There are also many non-genetic causes.

Arrhythmogenic right ventricular dysplasia (ARVD) or cardiomyopathy (ARVC)

This is an AD heart muscle disorder that causes arrhythmia, heart failure, and sudden death. It is characterized by replacement of the right ventricular myocardium by adipose and fibrous tissue. This disorder may be as prevalent as 6 in 10 000. This disorder is difficult to diagnose and cardiac MRI rather than echocardiography may be needed for full evaluation.

Genetic advice—HCM

Inheritance and recurrence risk
AD with 50% risk to offspring of affected individuals.

Prenatal diagnosis
In a family with a known mutation this is technically possible. It is usually only considered by families with mutations carrying a high risk of sudden death.

Predictive testing
In a family with a known mutation this could be offered so that cardiac surveillance could be targeted more appropriately. Otherwise, screening of at-risk relatives should be offered (📖 see Chapter 1, Genetic testing of children, p. 24, for a discussion of the issues related to genetic testing in children).

Clinical implications for primary care
(📖 See Sudden cardiac death, p. 219)

Support group
Cardiomyopathy Association: ⅓ www.cardiomyopathy.org

SCD: cardiac channelopathies

A number of genetic disorders can predispose to cardiac arrhythmia, these include: long QT syndrome, Brugada syndrome, catecholaminergic poly-morphic ventricular tachycardia, and short QT syndrome.

Long QT syndromes

- These are characterized by prolonged ventricular repolarization that predisposes carriers to life-threatening arrhythmia, most characteristically *torsade de pointes*, a type of ventricular tachycardia that causes syncope but may degenerate to ventricular fibrillation and cause cardiac arrest.
- AD mutations in the potassium and sodium channel genes are the most common causes of long QT syndrome. A recessive type, Jervell–Lange–Nielsen syndrome, is distinguished by profound congenital deafness.
- Birth incidence is unknown but has been estimated at 1/5000–1/7000.
- Typically, syncope occurring during physical activity or emotional upset begins in pre-teen to teenage years and usually continues into the 20s, but may present at any age. First cardiac events are uncommon after 30–40yrs.
- Importantly, it is estimated that in excess of 30–50% of carriers of mutations associated with this syndrome never have symptoms. Most others have one or many episodes of syncope but do not die suddenly. Sudden cardiac death occurs in only about 4% of affected individuals. Syncope typically occurs without warning, as distinct from vasovagal syncope, for example, in which patients feel dizzy or faint prior to collapse.
- Long QT syndrome is often misdiagnosed as epilepsy, especially in children, and this needs careful attention.

Diagnosis of long QT syndrome

- This is often a difficult diagnosis, relying on careful evaluation of the patient's history, his/her non-invasive test results especially the 12-lead ECG, his/her family history, and, ideally, genetic analysis.
- Known triggers for long QT-related arrhythmias include:
  - swimming, running
  - startle: alarm clock, loud horn, ringing phone
  - emotions: anger, crying, test taking, or other stressful situations.
- NB. Sudden death may also occur during sleep.
- Patients should be advised to avoid activities associated with intense physical activity and/or emotional stress, e.g. competitive sports, amusement park rides, scary movies, jumping into cold water, etc.

Long term β-blockers

The first-choice therapy in patients with long QT. Effective in ~70% of patients; cardiac events continue in the remaining 30%.

Implantable cardioverter defibrillator (ICD)
ICD may be necessary for those with symptoms despite β-blockade or for those with a history of cardiac arrest.

Annotate patient's notes with (exhaustive) list of prescribable drugs that are contraindicated. ✒ See www.qtdrugs.org for list.

Clinical implications for primary care
(📖 see p. 219)

Support groups
SADS UK (The Sudden Arrhythmic Death Syndrome Foundation UK): ✒ www.sadsuk.org
The Cardiac Arrhythmia Research and Education Foundation: ✒ www.longqt.org
Cardiac Risk in the Young: ✒ www.c-r-y.org.uk/

Thrombophilia

Introduction

Individuals with thrombophilia have blood that clots more easily than normal. In the normal state there is a balance between the natural clotting and anticoagulant systems. Both of these systems may be affected by either inherited or acquired (including both intrinsic and environmental) influences. The most common manifestation of thrombophilia is venous thrombosis. The incidence of venous thrombosis is about 1 per 1000 person-years. In the USA this leads to 50 000 deaths annually. Venous thromboembolism (VTE) is a multifactorial disorder, with well-characterized examples of gene–gene and gene–environment interactions underlying its pathogenesis. Genetic causes are present in approximately 25% of unselected venous thrombosis cases and up to 63% of familial cases.

Genetic causes

Genetic causes of inherited thrombophilias (hypercoagulabilities) include the following.
- *Factor V Leiden* (R506Q mutation), causing activated protein C (APC) resistance is the most common genetic risk factor for venous thrombosis. 20% of individuals with an idiopathic first venous thrombosis have this mutation, and 60% of pregnant women with a venous thrombosis have this mutation. 4.4% of Europeans and white Americans carry the factor V Leiden mutation.
- *Prothrombin 20210A* mutation (factor II Leiden) is carried by 1–2% of Europeans and white Americans.
- *Antithrombin III deficiency*.
- *Deficiency of protein C.* Purified human activated protein C selectively destroys factors Va and VIII:C in human plasma and thus has an important anticoagulant role.
- *Deficiency of protein S.* Protein S is a vitamin K-dependent plasma protein that inhibits blood clotting by serving as a cofactor for APC.
- Elevation of homocysteine is another potential risk factor in those found to be positive for factor V Leiden, as are anti-phospholipid antibodies which can cause APC resistance.

Acquired or environmental causes

Include the following.
- *Surgery.* Only major surgery is associated with a risk, e.g. abdominal surgery under general anaesthetic or an orthopaedic operation.
- *Pregnancy* (high factor VIII levels).
- *Oestrogens,* e.g. oral contraceptives, hormone replacement therapy (HRT).
- *Malignancy.*
- *Immobility,* e.g. plaster casts, long-haul flights, stroke with limb weakness.

- Patients with *postoperative* VTE have a very low risk of recurrence and a low incidence of thrombophilic defects. Patients with an *unprecipitated* VTE have a 20% cumulative recurrence rate at 2yrs; however, despite 27% of such patients having heritable thrombophilic defects, thrombophilia testing does not allow prediction of a high risk of recurrence.
- Testing in patients from thrombosis-prone families may be warranted in order to identify individuals who might benefit from thromboprophylaxis during risk periods.

If a PCP is considering the need for such testing, they should consult with colleagues in Haematology.

The American College of Medical Genetics (ACMG) guidelines on testing for factor V Leiden currently suggest that testing should be performed in the following circumstance:
- Age <50yrs, any venous thrombosis.
- Venous thrombosis in unusual sites, e.g. mesenteric, hepatic, and cerebral veins.
- Recurrent venous thrombosis.
- Venous thrombosis and a strong family history of thrombotic disease.
- Venous thrombosis in pregnant women or those taking the contraceptive pill.
- Relatives of individuals who have had a venous thrombosis at <50yrs.
- Myocardial infarction in female smokers <50yrs.

Random screening of the general population for Factor V Leiden is NOT recommended.

Potential long-term complications
- **Pregnancy.** Heterozygosity for factor V Leiden has been linked to 2–3× increased risk of late pregnancy loss and has been associated with a higher risk of pre-eclampsia, abruption, intrauterine growth retardation (IUGR), and stillbirth. Individual assessment is required to assess whether the risk of thromboembolism, fetal loss, and pre-eclampsia is greater than the risks related to anticoagulation. Warfarin is a known teratogen with a recognizable embryopathy. Heparin prophylaxis is preferred for those at high risk.
- **Homozygotes for factor V Leiden** have a higher overall risk of recurrence of VTE than heterozygotes. The thrombophilia team will make an assessment about treatment, balancing the risk of recurrence against the risk of major bleeding from oral anticoagulation therapy.

Genetic advice
Inheritance and recurrence risk
The genetic thrombophilias are usually inherited as an autosomal dominant (AD) trait. If both parents are carriers for the same disorder, then there is a 1 in 4 risk of a homozygous affected child.

Variability and penetrance

Although the relative risk of venous thrombosis is increased between four- and eightfold for factor V Leiden heterozygotes, the majority of heterozygous individuals never have a thrombotic event.

Predictive testing and testing of other family members

- Routine testing of at-risk family members is not recommended for factor V Leiden or prothrombin *20210A* as there is only a mildly increased risk for the individual and testing does not decrease morbidity or mortality.
- As a general rule, young children should not be tested. Children have special defences against forming blood clots and it is not until they reach puberty that their risk of blood clots due to thrombophilia begins to increase.
- Teenage daughters of patients with thrombophilia can be considered for testing if the results would influence decisions relating to contraceptive use.
- For some individuals there is an indication to test, such as management of a pregnancy or avoidance of hormonal medication (oral contraceptive pill, HRT), and predictive testing can be offered to adults within families with known mutations after appropriate consent is obtained.

Clinical implications for primary care

- Patients on anticoagulants require regular surveillance of their INRs.
- Advice should be given on ways to modify environmental risks and to report signs or symptoms of thrombosis.
- Surgery, e.g. postoperative or associated with trauma. Minor surgery, such as dental surgery or biopsies under local anaesthetic, are not high-risk situations.
- Pregnancy (high factor VIII levels).
- Oestrogens. Consider alternative forms of contraception or progesterone-only preparations if oral contraceptive use is desired. HRT generally confers a two- to threefold increased risk for VTE. Early evidence suggests an interaction of HRT with thrombophilic states such as the factor V Leiden mutation, resulting in a synergistic increase in the risk of VTE.
- Immobility, e.g. long-haul flights (ensure adequate hydration, relevant exercise, and the use of venous compression stockings).
- Code patient's notes.
- Code notes, with appropriate consents, of other family members (📖 see Chapter 1, Genetic testing of children, p. 8).

Support groups

Thrombophilia: information for patients and their relatives: 🖰 www.bcshguidelines.com
Thrombophilia support: 🖰 www.fvleiden.org

Cancer

Introduction

Cancer is a common condition that affects ~1 in 3 of the population during their lifetime. The great majority of cancers are sporadic occurrences related to the gradual accumulation of somatic mutations with age and exposure to carcinogenic factors in the environment, such as cigarette smoke, UV radiation, X-rays, etc. Genetic variation in (i) cellular repair mechanisms which affect the efficacy with which mutations in DNA are recognized and repaired, together with (ii) genetic variation affecting the likelihood of such cells surviving or undergoing apoptosis (programmed cell death), and (iii) genetic variation in the metabolism of carcinogens, will all affect an individual's likelihood of developing cancer.

A small but important minority of cancers are caused by the inheritance of a mutation in a cancer susceptibility gene. Such cases are exemplified by:

- **Young age at diagnosis.**
- **Family history.** Multiple affected members on the same side of the family.
- **Patterns of cancer.** Recognizable tumour types occurring together in the same family, e.g. colorectal cancer and endometrial cancer in HNPCC or breast and ovarian cancer in *BRCA1*.
- **Multiple primary tumours** in a single individual.
- **Rare tumours.** Rare and unusual tumour types, e.g. small bowel carcinoma in HNPCC.

This chapter outlines some of the common familial cancer syndromes. Predictive testing and effective surveillance are available for many of these conditions. Effective care relies on accurate diagnosis which, in turn, relies upon the clinical acumen of PCPs and oncologists, recognizing when their patient is a member of a family affected by a familial cancer syndrome and referring to Clinical Genetics for risk assessment and discussion of genetic testing and advice on surveillance and risk-reducing options (where applicable).

Obtaining a DNA sample from an affected member of such a family along with appropriate consent for genetic testing is crucial in order to define the genetic basis of the disease (e.g. *BRCA1* or *BRCA2*) and identify the causative mutation, thus enabling predictive testing for other members of the family.

If an affected member of a family likely to have a familial cancer syndrome is terminally ill, contact the local genetics service promptly to discuss obtaining a blood sample with consent for DNA storage and, where appropriate, genetic testing.

Breast cancer in women

Breast cancer is the most common form of cancer affecting women. The cumulative incidence of breast cancer in developed countries is 6.3 per 100 women by age 70yrs, with a lifetime risk of approximately 9–11%. The Western diet is associated both with earlier menarche and with postmenopausal obesity, which, combined with low parity, later first childbirth, and shorter breastfeeding, may account for the much higher incidence of breast cancer in the developed world than in many developing countries.

Much of breast cancer is caused by the interaction of weak susceptibility alleles with environmental or hormonal factors and ageing. The combined contribution of *BRCA1* and *BRCA2* to overall breast cancer is 2–3%.

Factors proven to affect breast cancer risk in the general population

- *Pregnancy and parity.* Breast cancer incidence is transiently increased by pregnancy but is permanently lowered by high parity. The relative risk of breast cancer decreases by 7% for each birth. Breast cancer incidence is reduced by early first childbirth. Women having their first child at >30yrs have double the risk of women having their first child at <20yrs.
- *Breastfeeding.* The longer women breastfeed, the more they are protected against breast cancer. The lack of, or short duration of, breastfeeding typical of women in developed countries makes a major contribution to the high incidence of breast cancer in these countries. The relative risk of breast cancer decreases by 4.3% for every 12 months of breastfeeding. This is in addition to a decrease of 7.0% for each birth. This protective effect is more marked in women having a later first pregnancy.
- *Menarche and menopause.* Cumulative breast cancer incidence is permanently lowered by late menarche and early menopause.
- *Obesity.* Obesity is associated with an increased risk for postmenopausal breast cancer. Regular exercise probably reduces the risk of breast cancer although the quantitative effect is uncertain and the evidence is weak.
- *Alcohol.* Compared with non-drinkers, the relative risk of breast cancer amongst women drinking 35–44g alcohol/day was 1.32, and for ≥45g alcohol/day was 1.46. The relative risk increased by 7% for each additional 10g/day (i.e. for each unit or drink of alcohol consumed on a daily basis). The data suggest that 4% of breast cancer in developed countries may be attributed to alcohol. The effect of alcohol needs to be interpreted in the context of its beneficial effects in moderation on cardiovascular disease.
- *Oral contraceptive pill (OCP).* For both for current users and up to 10yrs post-use, there may be a 24% increase (relative risk (RR), 1.24) in risk of breast cancer. Overall use of OCPs by women with a family history of breast cancer (affected mother, sister, or daughter) was *not* associated with an increased risk of breast cancer (odds ratio (OR), 0.8). Women who are *BRCA1* mutation carriers who have ever used

the OCP or who used the OCP for ≥5yrs may have an increased risk of early-onset breast cancer (RR 1.2 and 1.33, respectively), but a reduced risk of ovarian cancer.

- *Hormone replacement therapy (HRT).* For women in the general population postmenopausal combined oestrogen and progestin replacement therapy results in an increased risk of breast cancer of 5% per year of use. The risk is substantially higher than for oestrogen replacement therapy alone and does not appear to be influenced by a family history of breast cancer in a first-degree relative (mother, sister, daughter) The added risk disappears within 5yrs of cessation of use.

Close to 10% of women diagnosed with breast cancer at less than 40yrs are likely to carry a germline mutation in one of the known high-risk genes, but most of these will have a positive family history.

Factors suggesting a familial susceptibility gene

- Large number of individuals with breast/ovarian/prostate cancer in the family (on one side of the family).
- Multiple generations affected.
- Young average age at which the breast cancers were diagnosed (>25% of breast cancers diagnosed at <30yrs are due to a mutation in a dominant gene; 50% of all breast cancers in the general population are diagnosed after 65yrs of age).
- Pattern of different types of cancers occurring within the family.
- Multiple primary cancers in one individual with early age of onset (usually first primary at <50yrs).
- The combined contribution of *BRCA1* on 17q and *BRCA2* on 13q to overall breast cancer is 2–3%. The vast majority (>90%) of families with a clearly dominant predisposition to breast and ovarian cancer are known to harbour germline mutations in either *BRCA1* or *BRCA2* but, for breast cancer-only families with three or more affected individuals, <50% have mutations in these known genes (☐ see *BRCA1* and *BRCA2*, p. 238).

A family history on the paternal side of the family can be just as significant as one on the maternal side. Men can inherit a *BRCA1/2* mutation and transmit it to their daughters who may then be at risk for breast/ovarian cancer.

Genetic advice

Averaged across all ages, the risk of breast cancer to the sister, mother, or daughter of an isolated case is increased about twofold (1.5– to threefold). The risk then increases with increasing numbers of affected relatives, and also with young age at diagnosis of affected relatives.

Reassurance is currently the appropriate management for women where:
- There has been one family member diagnosed with breast cancer at age >40yrs.
- There have been two family members diagnosed with breast cancer at age >60yrs; provided that there has been no bilateral breast cancer, no male breast cancer, and no ovarian cancer.

Risk assessment

Breast cancer is a common disease amongst women in late middle-age and old age in the developed world.
- The risk that women in the general population will be diagnosed with breast cancer is 1 in 11 (9%) to age 80yrs. This provides a benchmark against which to evaluate the additional (and sometimes larger) risk attributable to the family history.
- Generally, for women seeking advice about a family history of breast cancer, risk estimates will vary between the population risk of 9% (e.g. third-degree relative is only family member affected) and 40% (50% probability of inheriting an 80% penetrant gene mutation, e.g. *BRCA1/2*).

Penetrance

Will be discussed by the clinical geneticist.

Predictive testing—⚎ refer to Clinical Genetics

Possible if there is a known familial mutation. Only offered to adults and often deferred until a time at which surveillance may be initiated or intervention such as prophylactic oophorectomy may be considered.

Diagnostic testing—⚎ refer to Clinical Genetics

Guidelines for consideration of *BRCA1* and *BRCA2* testing in an affected family member are as follows.
- High and high/moderate risk where a DNA sample from an informed affected relative is available.
- For Ashkenazi Jewish individuals, one or more relative with breast or ovarian cancer at any age can be offered testing for the Ashkenazi mutations only.

Consultation plan in primary care

History
- Detailed three-generation family tree, noting affected blood relatives, the types of cancer, age at diagnosis of cancer, and, when relevant, age at death. Extend the family tree back as far as possible on the relevant side(s) of the family. Reported cases of ovarian cancer, even in close relatives, are often wrong (e.g. cervical, endometrial).
- Check ethnicity. Three mutations in *BRCA1/2* in the Ashkenazi Jewish population (*BRCA1* 185delAG, 5382insC, and *BRCA2*, 6174delT) occur with a combined frequency of 2.5% and may account for >90% of highly penetrant families in that population.

Examination

Important for a woman presenting with symptoms, but for women presenting to discuss a family history, examination rarely gives diagnostic information.

Management in primary care

- Refer to a specialist clinic for diagnosis if breast cancer suspected in an individual. Surgical teams will then refer to Genetics as appropriate.
- Use NICE referral algorithm (📖 see Fig. 7.1) to identify correct management regarding referral, or not, of currently unaffected individuals to Genetics.
- Code patient's notes.
- Code, with appropriate consents, notes of other family members. (📖 see Chapter 1, Confidentiality and consent, p. 8.

✐ Use NICE referral algorithm (📖 see Fig. 7.1) to identify patients whose family history indicates referral to Clinical Genetics.

Management in secondary care

- DNA testing for *BRCA1* and *BRCA2* mutation analysis will be done in an affected member of a family meeting the appropriate criteria.
- Clinical Genetics will consider DNA storage from a key affected individual if she/he has advanced cancer.

Risk management and surveillance (📖 see Fig. 7.2)

- Patients may be given written information from the genetics clinic that they might wish to go through with you.
- Risk information about population-level and family history levels of risk.
- Breast awareness information.
- Lifestyle advice about breast cancer risk, including information about HRT, OCPs, breastfeeding, lifestyle, including diet and alcohol, etc.

Breast awareness

- 'Breast awareness' should be encouraged so that women understand the importance of seeking prompt advice if they notice any unusual changes in their breasts.

Mammographic surveillance

A widely adopted pragmatic approach has been to offer mammography where the risk due to the family history for a woman <50yrs of age is at least equivalent to the risk for a woman >50yrs of age in the general population. This roughly equates to a threefold increased risk of breast cancer by the age of 50yrs compared with the general population.

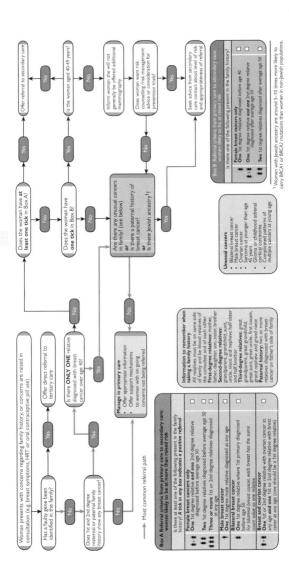

Fig. 7.1 Primary-care management algorithm. From National Institute for Health and Clinical Excellence (2006). CG 41 Familial breast cancer: the classification and care of women at risk of familial breast cancer in primary, secondary, and tertiary care. NICE, London. Available from ⌖ www.nice.org.uk/GG41. (Reproduced with permission from NICE.)

Update family history

Emphasize the importance of notifying the Genetics department of any new diagnoses in the family, as these may significantly change the risk assessment.

	Mammography	MRI
20–29 years	Should not be available for women younger than age 30.	Should be available only for those at exceptionally high risk (that is, annual risk greater or equal to 1%), for example TP53 carriers.

30–39 years	Should be available to women satisfying referral criteria for secondary or specialist care:
	• only as part of a research study (ethically approved) or nationally approved and audited service.
	Individualized strategies should be developed for exceptional cases, such as:
	• women from families with BRCA1, BRCA2 or TP53 mutations (or women with equivalent high risk).
		+/− Should be available annually to:
		• women with a 10-year risk of greater than 8%
		• TP53, BRCA1 and BRCA2 mutation carriers
		• women who have not been tested but have a high chance of carrying a BRCA1 or TP53 mutation, specifically:
		  – those at a 50% risk of carrying a BRCA1 or TP53 mutation in a tested family
		  those at 50% risk of carrying a BRCA1 or TP53 mutation from untested or inconclusively tested families with at least a 60% risk of a BRCA1 or TP53 mutation (that is, a 30% chance of carrying a mutation themselves).

40–49 years	Should be available annually to:
	• women at raised and high risk satisfying referral criteria for secondary or specialist care.
		+/− Should be available annually to:
		• women with a 10-year risk of greater than 20%
		• women with a 10-year risk of greater than 12% whose mammography has shown a dense breast pattern†
		• TP53, BRCA1 and BRCA2 mutation carriers
		• women who have not been tested but have a high chance of carrying a BRCA1 or TP53 mutation, specifically:
		  – those at a 50% risk of carrying a BRCA1 or TP53 mutation in a tested family
		  – those at 50% risk of carrying a BRCA1 or TP53 mutation from untested or inconclusively tested families with at least a 60% risk of a BRCA1 or TP53 mutation (that is, a 30% chance of carrying a mutation themselves).

Aged 50 and over	Should be available every 3 years as part of the NHS Breast Screening Programme. • more frequent mammographic surveillance should take place only as part of a research study (ethically approved) or nationally approved and audited service. Individualized strategies should be developed for exceptional cases, such as: • women from families with BRCA1, BRCA2 or TP53 mutations (or women with equivalent high risk).	Should not be available for women older than age 50.

†As defined by the 3-point mammographic classification used by UK breast radiologists (Breast Group of the Royal College of Radiologists 1989)

Supporting information

An 8% risk aged 30–39 and a 12% risk aged 40–49 years would be fulfilled by women with the following family histories:
• 2 close relatives diagnosed with average age < 30 years*
• 3 close relatives diagnosed with average age < 40 years*
• 4 close relatives diagnosed with average age < 50 years*.
*All relatives must be on the same side of the family and one must be a mother or sister of the consultee. A genetic test would usually be required to determine a 10-year risk of 20% or greater in women aged 40–49 years.

For the purposes of these calculations, a women's age should be assumed to be 30 years of age for a women in her thirties and 40 years of age for a women in her forties. A 10-year risk should then be calculated for the period 30–39 and 40–49, respectively.

Fig. 7.2 Breast cancer surveillance. (Reproduced from NICE guidelines.) NICE professional guidelines. From National Institute for Health and Clinical Excellence (2006). *CG 41 Familial breast cancer: the classification and care of women at risk of familial breast cancer in primary, secondary, and tertiary care.* NICE, London. Available from ℘ www.nice.org.uk/GG41. (Reproduced with permission from NICE.) (🕮 See also p. 414.)

Support groups

Breakthrough breast cancer ℘ www.breastcancergenetics.org.uk
Cancerline UK ℘ www.cancerlineuk. net/index.asp
NICE familial breast cancer guideline has written info for patients ℘ www.nice.org.uk

BRCA1 and *BRCA2*

The majority of families with a clearly dominant predisposition to breast and/or ovarian cancer are known to harbour inherited mutations in either *BRCA1* or *BRCA2*. However, the combined contribution of *BRCA1* and *BRCA2* to overall breast cancer is <2%.

- ***BRCA1*** is a large gene with 22 exons at 17q21. The BRCA1 protein is involved in many important cellular pathways including DNA repair and regulation of transcription. Several founder mutations are common in specific populations: 1% of Ashkenazi Jewish women carry the 185delAG mutation which accounts for 20% of early-onset breast cancer in these women.
- ***BRCA2*** at 13q12.3 is also a large gene. The BRCA2 protein is involved in DNA repair. The mutation 6174delT is found in 1–1.5% of Ashkenazi Jews and accounts for ~8% of early-onset breast cancer in that ethnic group.

Cancer risks associated with *BRCA1*

Female carriers with a mutation in *BRCA1* have an increased risk of breast and ovarian cancer (📖 see Fig. 7.3). The risk for any individual is affected by both genetic modifiers and environmental exposures, but approximate averages are as follows:

- 65% risk of breast cancer to age 70. *BRCA1*-related breast cancers are usually 'triple-negative' high-grade aneuploid carcinomas. They do not express oestrogen receptor, progesterone receptor or HER2. This phenotype is called 'basal-like breast cancer'.
- 39% risk of ovarian cancer (including the Fallopian tubes) to age 70.
- The relative risk of breast cancer in *BRCA1* carriers, relative to the general population, declines with age from >30-fold below age 40yrs to 14-fold above age 60yrs.
- The incidence in *BRCA1* carriers rises to a plateau of ~3–4% per annum in the 40–49yr age group.
- There is a high risk of contralateral breast cancer in affected carriers.
- Ovarian cancer risks in *BRCA1* carriers below age 40yrs are low (in absolute terms); thereafter the incidences are 1% per annum between 40 and 59yrs and 2% after age 60.

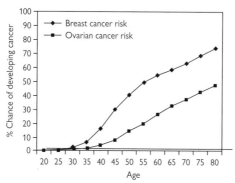

Fig. 7.3 Risk of breast and ovarian cancer by age in female BRCA1 mutation carriers. (Reproduced from Firth, Hurst and Hall (2005). *Oxford Desk Reference—Clinical Genetics*, with permission from Oxford University Press.)

- *Male* **BRCA1** mutation carriers are at modest increased risk of prostate cancer.
- Male and female **BRCA1** mutation carriers are also at modest increased risk of pancreatic cancer.

Men carrying a *BRCA1* mutation have a modestly increased cancer risk whereas men carrying a *BRCA2* mutation have a much higher risk, particularly for prostate cancer.

Cancer risks associated with BRCA2

Female carriers with a mutation in *BRCA2* have an increased risk of breast and ovarian cancer (💷 see Fig. 7.4). The risk for any individual is affected by both genetic modifiers and environmental exposures, but approximate averages are as follows:
- 45% risk of breast cancer to age 70yrs.
- 11% risk for ovarian cancer (including the Fallopian tubes and peritoneum).
- The relative risk of breast cancer in *BRCA2* carriers is 11-fold in all age groups above 40yrs, and is not significantly higher at younger ages.
- The incidences in *BRCA2* carriers show a pattern parallel to that in the general population, rising steeply up to age 50yrs and more slowly thereafter.
- There is a high risk of contralateral breast cancer in affected carriers.
- Ovarian cancer risks in *BRCA2* carriers are, in contrast, very low below age 50yrs but then increase sharply in the 50–59yr age group, perhaps declining somewhat thereafter.
- *Male* **BRCA2** mutation carriers are at greatly increased risk for prostate cancer (>fivefold). Their relative risk is particularly increased at younger ages and the pathology is often more aggressive.

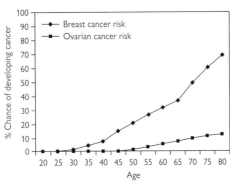

Fig. 7.4 Risk of breast and ovarian cancer by age in female *BRCA2* mutation carriers. (Reproduced from Firth, Hurst and Hall (2005). *Oxford Desk Reference—Clinical Genetics*, with permission from Oxford University Press.)

- Male and female *BRCA2* mutation carriers are also at significant increased risk of pancreatic cancer (three- to fivefold) and increased risk for melanoma (skin and eye).

Consultation plan in primary care

History

Three-generation family tree with specific enquiry for breast, ovarian, prostate, and other associated cancers.

Examination

Usually not necessary for evaluation purposes.

Management in primary care

- 🖎 Referral to Genetics as indicated by the NICE breast cancer protocol either if there is a clear history or if there is doubt about the family history which requires full evaluation by searching medical records of affected family members.
- Code patient's notes if BRCA1/2 mutation found.
- Code, with appropriate consents, other family members' notes. 📖 See Chapter 1, Confidentiality and consent, p. 8.
- The role of the GP after referral to the clinical genetics clinic is to support the BRCA1/2 carrier regarding risks to his/her own health and arrange appropriate screening and/or prophylactic surgery.
- Identify other 'at risk' members of the family and ensure that the offer of genetic advice, screening, and/or predictive testing is made available to all at-risk relatives from an appropriate age in early adult life.
- Women who are contemplating prophylactic surgery may appreciate an individualized assessment of their risk by a clinical geneticist.

Genetics

Risk assessment

See section on cancer risks associated with *BRCA1* and 🕮 Fig. 7.3, p. 239 or section of cancer risks associated with *BRCA2* and 🕮 Fig. 7.4, p. 240.

Predictive testing—✍ refer to Clinical Genetics

When a familial mutation has been defined, predictive testing can be offered to members of the extended family. When a mutation is first identified in an affected individual, the Genetics department may give the person a 'to whom it may concern' letter to distribute to their relatives that outlines the genetic diagnosis and recommends that they seek a referral to Clinical Genetics for further information and an opportunity to discuss their risk and risks to their children and the option of predictive genetic testing.

Since the consequences of a predictive test may be profound, the first appointment for those referred requesting predictive testing is often used to explore the reasons for the request, the potential impact of a positive result on the individual's life/family, their coping strategies and support network. For new patients, taking blood for a predictive test is often deferred until a subsequent appointment.

Management

Breast surveillance

- **MRI (magnetic resonance imaging)**: NICE recommend annual MRIs for *BRCA1/2* mutation carriers aged 30–49 inclusive (🕮 see Fig. 7.2).
- **Mammography**: has a proven survival advantage in women in the age group 50–65yrs.
- **Clinical breast examination**: in situations where mammography is contraindicated and breast MRI is not available, clinical examination by a breast surgeon may be offered (e.g. screening very young women (<30yrs of age) with a very early onset family history.

Ovarian surveillance

- CA125 (cancer antigen 125) screening and ovarian USS. Of unproven efficacy; clinical trials are in progress and in this context it is offered from age 35yrs to mutation carriers who elect against prophylactic oophorectomy (see below).

Prophylactic salpingo-oophorectomy

- Present evidence suggests that all women who are carriers of a *BRCA1* or *BRCA2* mutation should strongly consider this intervention once their families are complete.
- In a prospective study of 170 carriers of *BRCA* mutations with a mean follow-up of 2yrs, there was an important reduction in breast cancer risk, with breast cancer developing in only 4.3% of the women who had undergone oophorectomy compared with 12.9% in the surveillance group.
- Ovarian cancer developed in 3.1% of women who underwent prophylactic oophorectomy compared with 6.9% of women who underwent surveillance.

- Opinion is divided on the use of hormone replacement therapy (HRT) after prophylactic oophorectomy; the decision to use oestrogens should be based on a consideration of symptoms that affect future health and the quality of life. Some centres routinely recommend HRT after prophylactic oophorectomy until the age of 50yrs.

Prophylactic mastectomy

In a small study (*N* = 139) of women with *BRCA1* or *BRCA2* mutations, 76 women chose prophylactic mastectomy, and the remainder surveillance (annual mammography and clinical exam). Over 3yrs no cases of breast cancer occurred in the mastectomy group, whereas 8 breast cancers occurred in the surveillance group. On the basis of an exponential model the yearly incidence of breast cancer in the surveillance group was 2.5%. Prophylactic mastectomy has an efficacy of at least 90% in women classified as high risk on the basis of a family history of breast cancer.

Prophylactic mastectomy is a highly personal decision. Up to 30% of women who undergo the procedure will have surgical complications. The protective effects of reducing cancer risk (and thereby the toxicity of treatment and chance of dying from breast cancer) must be weighed against possible surgical complications and psychological problems.

Chemoprevention

Various agents are under trial.

- **Tamoxifen**: a retrospective case-analysis showed that treatment of *BRCA1* and *BRCA2* mutation carriers with tamoxifen after surgery for breast cancer reduced the incidence of cancer in the contralateral breast by 50%.
- **Oral contraceptive pill (OCP)**: a case-control study showed a 60% reduction in frequency of ovarian cancer after 6yrs use, but there are concerns that OCPs could also increase the risk of breast cancer in women with a family history of the disease. *BRCA1/2* mutation carriers who ever used oral contraceptives have an apparently sustained increased risk of breast cancer (adjusted hazard ratio (HR) = 1.47; 95% CI, 1.16–1.87).

Physical exercise and avoidance of obesity in adolescence.

A large study of Ashkenazi Jewish women with inherited mutations in *BRCA1/2* found that physical exercise and lack of obesity in adolescence were associated with significantly delayed breast cancer onset.

Support groups

Breakthrough Breast Cancer: ℘ www.breastcancergenetics.org.uk
Breast Cancer Genetic algorithm NICE: ℘ www.nice.org.uk
Useful resource for Families and Primary Care Workers:
Familial breast cancer CG 41 2006: ℘ www.nice.org.uk

Breast cancer in men

Breast cancer in men is rare, accounting for 0.8% of diagnoses of all breast cancers, but often men present late because of lack of awareness or embarrassment, or both. Risk factors include:
- Family history: *BRCA2* mutations predispose men to breast cancer.
- Jewish ancestry: the *BRCA2* mutation 6174delT is found in 1–1.5% of Ashkenazi Jews.
- Benign breast conditions.
- Age.
- Klinefelter syndrome (47,XXY) (📖 see Chapter 8, Klinefelter syndrome (47,XXY), p. 298).

Men with *BRCA1*

Male *BRCA1* mutation carriers have a modestly increased risk for prostate and pancreatic cancer, but they do not have a substantially increased risk for breast cancer.

Men with *BRCA2*

- Male *BRCA2* mutation carriers are at increased risk of breast cancer (~6% by 70yrs).
- *BRCA2* mutation carriers are also at increased risk of
  - prostate (RR >5) (📖 see Prostate cancer, p. 282)
  - pancreatic cancer (RR 3–5 times)
  - gallbladder/bile duct cancer
  - melanoma of the skin or eye.

Management in primary care

- Immediate referral to surgeon on suspicion of a cancer.
- Code patient's notes.
- Code, with appropriate consents, notes of other family members. See ch.1 p. 8.
- 🖋 If there is a family history of breast/ovarian/early onset prostate cancer—refer to Clinical Genetics.

Cancer surveillance methods

Strategies for cancer surveillance are continually evolving. This section summarizes some of the approaches in common use for surveillance for some of the more common cancers. This section contains information on:

- Breast surveillance*
- Endometrial surveillance
- GI surveillance (including colorectal*)
- Ovarian surveillance
- Prostate surveillance

* indicates population screening available in the UK for selected age groups.

Breast surveillance (📖 see Fig. 7.2, p. 237)

Mammography

Mammographic screening has been shown to reduce mortality in women aged 50–64yrs from the general population. ***NICE guidelines*** for the care of women at risk of familial breast cancer include the following recommendations:

- Surveillance is not recommended for women at increased risk under age 30.
- Annual MRI for women aged 30–49 who are *BRCA1/2* mutation carriers.
- Mammographic surveillance over the age of 50 can be performed every 3yrs, e.g. as for all women as part of the UK NHS Breast Screening Programme. More frequent surveillance over age 50 should only be carried out as part of a research study.

Breast MRI

Contrast enhanced magnetic resonance imaging (CEMRI) provides information about tissue vascularity that is not available from mammography. In many breast cancers there is neovascularity and the pattern and time course of enhancement after injection of IV contrast material (e.g. gadolinium) can determine the likelihood of malignancy. MRI can detect otherwise occult breast cancer in high-risk patients and is most beneficial in those at highest risk, e.g. carriers of *BRCA* mutations.

Breast self-examination

A large, well-conducted randomized control trial showed conclusively that regular breast self-examination does *not* lead to a reduction in mortality due to breast cancer compared with no screening at all. Moreover, self-examination leads to more breast biopsies and diagnoses of benign breast disease. Nonetheless, 'breast awareness' should be encouraged so that women understand the importance of promptly reporting any unusual changes in their breasts to their doctor.

Endometrial surveillance

There is currently no proven efficacious method of surveillance for endometrial cancer in HNPCC (📖 see Hereditary non-polyposis colorectal cancer (HNPCC), p. 262). Various forms of biopsy-based surveillance are possible, e.g. pipelle aspiration, but the evidence base for their use is lacking. Progestagen-containing intrauterine devices, e.g. Mirena coil, may prove to be efficacious. Prophylactic hysterectomy after the menopause or after a woman has completed her family is a possibility, especially in carriers of an *MSH6* mutation, but this can complicate surveillance for bowel cancer (see below).

GI surveillance

Upper GI endoscopy

The complication rate of upper GI endoscopy performed for surveillance is unknown, largely because the vast majority of such examinations are performed in symptomatic individuals for diagnosis, e.g. oesophageal varices, bleeding peptic ulcers, late-presenting cancers.

Colonoscopy

Patients scheduled for colonoscopy have bowel preparation beforehand, consisting of a low-residue diet for 48h and then a liquid diet for 24h before the procedure, followed by laxatives, e.g. Picolax®. Most are lightly sedated for the procedure, which, although it is usually uncomfortable to some degree, is only rarely painful. If suspicious lesions are seen, they can be biopsied. Small polyps are usually excision biopsied; those with a stalk can be snared; larger polyps can often be removed piecemeal if snaring is not possible.

- Complications are more likely in the elderly and those with co-morbidity or existing disease, e.g. ulcerative colitis.
- Complications include: bleeding in 3/10 000, perforation in 1/1000 and death in 1/10 000. Complications are increased after polypectomy.
- Colonoscopy will miss approximately 6% of polyps, usually those <1cm.
- The background rate of death from colorectal cancer (CRC) at age 50–54yrs is 1.8/10 000).

Flexible sigmoidoscopy

Requires less bowel preparation than a colonoscopy (e.g. sachet of Picolax® on day before study or phosphate mini-enema on morning of study) but reaches, at most, as far as the splenic flexure. The procedure takes 10min and is usually performed without sedation. Polypectomy as for colonoscopy, except that if significant lesion/s are found (CRC, polyps larger than 5mm, three or more adenomas, adenomas 5mm or smaller with a villous component of more than 20%, or severe dysplasia) then a colonoscopy will be required to examine the rest of the colon. Flexible sigmoidoscopy may be of considerable utility for population screening, but is not recommended as a surveillance method in familial CRC instead of colonoscopy. It may be used in screening for polyps in familial adenomatous polyposis (FAP), but this will be as part of a surveillance programme also involving proctoscopy, rigid sigmoidoscopy, and colonoscopy.

Faecal occult blood

The NHS Bowel Cancer Screening Programme is now being rolled out nationally and will achieve nationwide coverage in England by 2009. Screening will be offered every 2yrs to all men and women aged 60–69yrs and on request to those over 70yrs.

The programme hubs operate a national call and recall system to send out faecal occult blood (FOB) test kits, analyse samples and dispatch results. Each hub is responsible for co-ordinating the programme in their area and works with up to 20 local screening centres. The screening centres provide endoscopy services and specialist screening nurse clinics for people receiving an abnormal result. Screening centres are also responsible for referring those requiring treatment to their local hospital multidisciplinary team (MDT).

Ovarian surveillance

Routine ovarian cancer screening for the general population is not currently recommended as there is no research evidence to date to support its use.

Potential screening methods for ovarian cancer are either transvaginal ovarian USS or detection of elevated levels of the tumour marker CA125 in the blood. The small proportion of patients diagnosed with stage I ovarian cancer have a good prognosis, in contrast to the majority who present with advanced disease. The relationship between survival rates and stage thus provides the rationale for such screening. However, the impact of screening on ovarian cancer mortality of any target population has yet to be confirmed.

The UK Familial Ovarian Cancer Screening Study (UKFOCSS) is under way to assess the efficacy of annual surveillance with CA125 and transvaginal USS in the high-risk population. The primary objective is to develop an optimized surveillance strategy for ovarian cancer in terms of the most appropriate screening tests and criteria for interpretation of results, screening interval, morbidity, and cost in the high-risk population.

Prostate surveillance

There is no national screening programme for prostate cancer in the UK, but since prostate specific antigen (PSA) testing became available in the 1990s, *ad hoc* screening of asymptomatic men has taken place. The PSA involves a blood test and is the most acceptable and reliable test available, but:

- **Lack of specificity**. Only about a quarter to a third of asymptomatic men with an abnormally high PSA levels will have prostate cancer.
- **Lack of sensitivity**. Up to 20% of all men with prostate cancers have normal PSA levels.
- The PSA test has not been standardized.

Colorectal cancer (CRC)

See also Familal adenomatous polyposis (FAP) and Hereditary non-polyposis colorectal cancer (HNPCC), p. 256 and 262.

CRC is a common disease.
- In incidence it is the third most common cancer in males (after lung and prostate cancers in males and breast and lung cancer in females).
- Lifetime risks in 1996 in the UK were 1:18 for males and 1:20 for females.
- Genetic susceptibility accounts for 5–10% of CRC, but germline mutations in known single genes account for only 1–2% of cases.
- A family history of the disease confers a significantly increased risk to relatives.

The hallmarks of genetic predisposition to bowel cancer are:
- *Young age at diagnosis.* The mean age of diagnosis in sporadic CRC is 60–70yrs (in HNPCC, the mean age of diagnosis of CRC is 44yrs, and in FAP it is 39yrs).
- *Family history.* Both of CRC and tumours at other sites, especially endometrial, ureter, renal pelvis.
- *Rare tumours*, e.g. small bowel cancers, skin sebaceous tumours, desmoids.
- *Multiple primary tumours* in one individual, e.g. endometrial and CRC.

CRC is a common disease, but the risk of developing it is markedly skewed towards elderly people: <1% of cases develop the disease <45yrs (and <0.1% at <35yrs). In addition, most (~70%) sporadic CRCs occur in the rectum and sigmoid colon, with about 10% in the caecum and the rest elsewhere in the colon.
- *Adenomas and polyps.* Colorectal adenomas are common. Up to one-third of those in their 70s may harbour one or two, but only 1:1000 of the population develop three or more. Large, multiple, dysplastic adenomas and villous (or tubulovillous) histology are all associated with an empiric increased risk to the individual of a CRC. While most (>95%) CRCs develop from adenomas; only a minority of adenomas will develop into CRC.
- *Metaplastic (hyperplastic) polyps* are similarly common. They are often found in association with adenomas, with or without a CRC, and they can undergo adenomatous change. So-called serrated adenomas have features of both adenomas and metaplastic polyps. Patients with a multiplicity of these other sorts of polyp are at increased empiric risk of CRC.
- *Small bowel carcinomas.* Small bowel carcinomas are very rare in the general population (<0.003%), but occur in cancer predisposition syndromes. Duodenal cancers occur in FAP; jejunal and ileal carcinomas occur in HNPCC at ~300× the rate in the general population. So, because of their rarity, small bowel cancers are very significant. Other predisposing causes include coeliac disease and Crohn disease.

- **Ashkenazi Jews.** CRC is significantly more common in this population group due to a variety and combination of genetic factors.
- **Mismatch repair.** Defective mismatch repair occurs in 15% of all colon cancers. In ~5% of all tumours it is caused by mutation in the mismatch repair genes (e.g. *MLH1, MSH2, MSH6* and *PMS2*), 🕮 see Hereditary non-polyposis colorectal cancer (HNPCC), p. 262.

Consultation plan in general practice

History
- Three-generation family tree with particular emphasis on history of tumours, benign and malignant, and documentation of age of diagnosis.
- Have they any symptoms, e.g. a change in bowel habit, that are causing them concern? If yes, explore symptoms further and refer to a gastroenterologist/colorectal surgeon for further evaluation.
- Ask specifically about skin lesions in the individual and family: most patients don't regard them as tumours and won't spontaneously report them.

Examination
- Routine abdominal examination if symptomatic.
- Examine skin and refer to a dermatologist as appropriate—sebaceous adenomas often masquerade as common skin lesions.

Management plan in general practice

- ✍ Referral to appropriate surgical team if cancer suspected.
- ✍ Referral to Genetics of an individual with a strong family history, for full family tree and cancer enquiries.
- Code patient's notes.
- Code, with appropriate consents, notes of other family members.
  🕮 See Chapter 1, Confidentiality and consent, p. 8.

Genetics

✍ Indications for referral to Clinical Genetics
- One first-degree relative diagnosed with CRC at 45yrs or less.
- Two first-degree relatives (including both parents) or 1 first-degree and 1 second-degree relative with CRC on the same side of the family diagnosed at any age.
- Three relatives with CRC all on the same side of the family (at least one should be a first-degree relative).
- Families with cases of colorectal and endometrial cancer on the same side of the family (at least one should be a first-degree relative).
- Family history of FAP or HNPCC.

Management

Surveillance for those at increased risk
🕮 See also Cancer surveillance methods, p. 246.

Following referral to Clinical Genetics, your patient's risk is likely to be stratified to one of the following risk groups. The intensity of surveillance is adjusted according to the level of risk. The following is an example of the approximate levels of surveillance that may be recommended.

- **High-risk**—HNPCC: colonoscopy every 2yrs, starting at 25–30yrs.
- **High–moderate risk:** colonoscopy every 5yrs, starting at 45yrs (or 5yrs before age of earliest-onset CRC in family).
- **Low–moderate risk:** one-off colonoscopy at 55yrs. If an adenomatous polyp should be found, then adenoma surveillance guidance applies. A single, small adenoma found in a member of the general population does not usually warrant follow-up more frequently than another colonoscopy 10yrs later, but if an individual found to have an adenoma has a family history, the risk is sufficient to warrant colonoscopy 3yrs later.
- **Low risk:** those whose empiric risk does not justify screening intervention should be reassured that their level of risk does not merit surveillance over and above that recommended for the general population. If population screening is available, then individuals should be encouraged to participate.

Predictive testing

Not currently feasible, unless a condition with a known genetic basis has been diagnosed, e.g. FAP, HNPCC, in which case, see relevant section.

Population-based screening

- The NHS Bowel Cancer Screening Programme is now being rolled out nationally and will achieve nationwide coverage by 2009. Screening will be offered every 2yrs to all men and women aged 60–69yrs and on request to those over 70yrs.
- The programme hubs operate a national call and recall system to send out faecal occult blood (FOB) test kits, analyse samples, and dispatch results. Each hub is responsible for co-ordinating the programme in their area and works with up to 20 local screening centres. The screening centres provide endoscopy services and specialist screening nurse clinics for people receiving an abnormal result. Screening centres are also responsible for referring those requiring treatment to their local hospital multidisciplinary team (MDT).

Education

Educate your patients about the symptoms of CRC so that they are aware when to seek medical advice and investigation. The most significant symptoms are:

- Rectal bleeding.
- A persistent change in bowel habit, usually to looser or more frequent bowel actions.
- Abdominal pain and/or abdominal mass.
- Unexplained anaemia (present with tiredness).

Diet and other environmental or lifestyle influences

As well as a family history, there are numerous other genetic/environmental influences on CRC risk that patients increasingly enquire about. The magnitude of risk associated with, for example, a diet rich in red meat, or, probably more importantly, poor in fruit and vegetables is about the same as having a single first-degree relative with an adenoma, i.e. 2×, and not quite as great as having a single first-degree relative with CRC (2.8×). How much effect these factors have in those individuals with high penetrance genes, rather than those with 'moderate' risk, remains to be established, but undoubtedly common genetic variation plays an important part in how an individual interacts with environmental factors. There is no evidence that proprietary dietary supplements make any difference.

Update family history

Emphasize the importance of notifying the Genetics department of any new diagnoses in the family, as these may significantly change the risk assessment.

Support group

Cancerline UK: ℘ www.cancerlineuk.net/index.asp

Confirmation of diagnosis of cancer

In cancer genetics, risk assessment usually depends critically on the information reported in the family history. If management decisions, e.g. prophylactic surgery or invasive screening procedures, are going to be based on that information it is important to confirm its accuracy. In a perfect world every cancer diagnosis would be confirmed but, in practice, limited time and resources mean that this is usually impracticable.

Remember when taking a history:
- Reported cases of breast cancer in close relatives are rarely wrong (inaccurate in 5%).
- Reported cases of abdominal, and especially gynaecological, cancers are inaccurate in 20%.
- 'Stomach' cancer can mean almost anything abdominal.
- 'Liver' cancer is usually secondary.
- 'Womb' cancer in lay terms often includes cervical as well as endometrial tumours.

Management of 11% of families referred to a genetic service is likely to be changed as a result of information obtained from cancer confirmation.

In practice it may be considered reasonable, at least in high-risk families, to confirm:
- All cases of colorectal and gastrointestinal tract cancer.
- All cases of ovarian cancer.
- At least one key diagnosis in a family where prophylactic surgery or screening is being considered.
- At least one diagnosis in a family member in whom mutation analysis is initiated on the basis of the family history (rather than immunohistochemical or other histopathological findings in the tumour or clinical features in the proband).

Getting the correct information may be a difficult and lengthy process and this should be explained to patients when they are referred to Clinical Genetics by PCPs. Patients will usually be sent a 'Family History' form to complete so that some of the work to verify diagnoses can be completed ahead of an appointment. Sometimes patients feel upset or overwhelmed by the level of detailed information requested by Clinical Genetics and never return their family history form. Support from a member of the primary care team to complete the form may be helpful in minimizing delays.

Patients should be encouraged to seek help from their primary care team or from the Clinical Genetics department if they have difficulty completing a 'Family History' form that has been sent to them as part of the risk assessment process.

Hierarchy of reliability of confirmation
1. Pathology report. The 'gold standard'.
2. Cancer registry report.
3. Hospital discharge summary.
4. Death certificate. For relatives who died a long time ago, this may be the only accessible document.

Familial adenomatous polyposis (FAP)

Familial polyposis, Gardner syndrome (old term for FAP with extracolonic features), familial (adenomatous) polyposis coli (FPC/FAPC), adenomatous polyposis coli (APC).

- **Classical FAP** is defined when >100 polyps are found in the colorectum at endoscopy (sigmoidoscopy or colonoscopy) or on pathological examination of the colon (after colectomy). Prevalence is 1:8500. Dominantly inherited classical FAP is caused by mutation in the *APC* (5q22.2) gene, and somatic mutations in this gene are also seen in the early stages of sporadic colon cancer.
- **Attenuated FAP (AFAP).** There are a considerable number of individuals and families with generally <100 but >2 adenomas. These are grouped under the term 'attenuated FAP'. Some cases are due to mutations in the *APC* gene (as for classical FAP) but others follow autosomal recessive inheritance and are caused by biallelic mutation in the *MUTYH* gene.
- **Colorectal adenomas.** Up to 30% of the general population will develop an adenoma or two by the age of 70yrs, but only 1:1000 of the population will develop more than two adenomas. Multiplicity of adenomas is empirically associated with a significantly increased risk of colorectal cancer (CRC).

Multisystem disease: extracolonic features

FAP is a multisystem disorder. Individuals develop multiple adenomas of both the colorectum and duodenum, with concomitant risk of cancer. Fundic gland polyps develop in the stomach. Desmoid tumours are liable to develop in connective tissue and mesentery, especially in or around the trunk. Congenital hypertrophy of the retinal pigment epithelium (CHRPE) develops in the eye in some families (while it may be a helpful diagnostic sign, it does not affect vision). Sebaceous cysts occur at greater frequency, as do osteomata, dental (dentiginous) cysts, and supernumerary teeth. An increased risk of cancer at several extracolonic sites is also observed, e.g. adrenals, primary brain, thyroid (papillary cancer), primary liver (hepatoblastoma), and hepatobiliary tree.

Consultation plan in primary care

History
- Three-generation family tree with particular emphasis on history of tumours, benign and malignant, and documentation of histological proof of diagnosis, i.e. >100 adenomas.
- Who has been screened, or operated on? What? When? Where?
- Is the family already known to a familial cancer or polyposis registry?

Examination
- If patient declares, or is found to have, an abdominal mass, refer to a gastroenterologist or colorectal surgeon.
- Gastrointestinal tract. Refer to a gastroenterologist or colorectal surgeon (📖 see 'Surveillance and management', p. 258).
- Check for sebaceous cysts, especially scalp and trunk: most patients disregard them and won't spontaneously report them.
- Examine the mouth and jaws: teeth, cysts, osteomata.

Management in primary care

- Appropriate referral to a GI surgeon for a new case.
- ✍ Referral to Genetics for a patient with a significant history of familial disease or a new diagnosis of FAP.
- Code patient's notes.
- Code, with appropriate consents, notes of other family members.
  📖 See Chapter 1, Confidentiality and consent, p. 8.

Investigations in secondary care

- **Colonoscopy.** There must be over 100 adenomas in the colorectum to diagnose FAP. If there are fewer than 100 adenomas, then AFAP or 'multiple adenomas' can be diagnosed. Microadenomas in the colorectal mucosa, i.e. adenomas confined to a single crypt ('monocryptal' or 'single-crypt' adenomas), are a hallmark of FAP/AFAP (but they are found in both *APC*- and *MUTYH*-associated polyposis).
- **Upper GI endoscopy**. Multiple fundic gland polyps in the stomach are characteristic of FAP, but are benign.
- **Clinical Genetics** may arrange for:
  - *APC* mutation analysis
  - chromosome analysis in cases with learning disability and/or dysmorphic features (looking for deletions of 5q incorporating the *APC* gene).
  - *MUTYH* mutation detection if *APC* negative and consistent with AR inheritance. (Blood from parents and/or other relatives may be useful.)

Genetics

Risk assessment

- FAP follows AD inheritance with a 50% risk to offspring of an affected individual. There is a high new mutation rate.
- There is almost complete penetrance with 50% of FAP patients developing polyps by 15yrs and 95% by 35yrs.
- MUTYH follows AR inheritance with a 25% risk to siblings, but a minimal risk to offspring of an affected individual (unless the partner is a relative or someone with a FH of MUTYH).

Predictive testing—✍ refer to Clinical Genetics

If the familial mutation is known, predictive genetic testing can be offered to children of an affected parent.

Predictive genetic testing is usually offered just before colorectal screening would commence, at 10yrs of age. Testing at this age ensures that screening is targeted to those who need surveillance, while those not at risk can be reassured.

Prenatal diagnosis—✍ refer to Clinical Genetics

Technically possible if the familial *APC* mutation is known.

Surveillance and management

📖 See also Cancer surveillance methods, p. 246.

Without regular surveillance and expert management, FAP has a poor prognosis. PCPs have a crucial role to play in ensuring that all patients with FAP, or at risk for FAP, receive regular specialist surveillance from the age of 10yrs.

Colorectal surveillance

- Most individuals with *APC*-associated FAP will start to develop colorectal adenomas in their teens. Thus, surveillance is geared to the detection of these in those at risk with a view to offering prophylactic surgery in a timely manner. In those with FAP who have not had a prophylactic colectomy, CRC can occur under 20yrs of age.
- Surveillance strategy will depend on local resources and discussion with the surgical team/endoscopist. This will usually involve annual or 6-monthly sigmoidoscopy from early/mid-teens with occasional colonoscopy.
- In AFAP, a regime similar to that for HNPCC is usually more appropriate, i.e. 2-yearly colonoscopy.

Surgical management

Surgical opinion varies, but most plan for prophylactic colectomy in affected individuals between the ages of 16 and 20yrs to minimize risk of malignancy. For the majority of patients, colectomy and ileorectal anastamosis (with rectal surveillance until mid-life when a proctectomy with ileoanal pouch formation is performed) may be preferred.

The best outcomes are obtained in specialist centres and it is important for FAP patients to engage with the care of an appropriate surgical team at an early stage.

Upper gastrointestinal tract

Most patients will have gastric fundic polyps, which are entirely benign, but the significant lesions are duodenal adenomas—seek specialist advice.

Desmoid tumours

FAP patients are at significantly increased risk of desmoid tumours, and about 10% will develop clinically evident disease. Desmoid disease may be triggered by surgery. Desmoids are histologically benign, but may become clinically problematic as they encroach on, and encase, vital organs and structures, particularly in the case of intra-abdominal tumours.

Non-surgical treatment

Although surgical management of FAP is the mainstay, a number of trials have been, or are being, carried out into possible disease modifying and chemotherapeutic options.

Support group

FAP support group: ℘ www.fapsupportgroup.org

Gastric cancer

Gastric cancer is the second largest cancer burden worldwide. In the UK, the lifetime risk in the general population is:

- 2.3% for males, average age at diagnosis: 72yrs.
- 1.2% for females, average age at diagnosis: 75yrs.

Survival rates are low (10% at 5yrs), due to late presentation and diagnosis. In contrast to the West, Japan has introduced systematic mass screening programmes with oesophagogastroduodenoscopy (OGD), leading to the increased detection of gastric cancers confined to the mucosa or submucosa. Survival rates for patients with early gastric cancer are >90% at 5yrs.

Gastric cancer can be classified histopathologically into two distinct types: intestinal and diffuse (linitis plastica type). The major risk factor for intestinal gastric cancer identified so far is *Helicobacter pylori* infection. However, whether *H. pylori* eradication is an effective cancer prevention measure is not yet proven.

Approximately 10% of cases of gastric cancer involve familial clustering. Cancer predisposition syndromes to consider include:

- Hereditary non-polyposis colorectal cancer (HNPCC) gives a 5% lifetime risk (☐ See Hereditary non-polyposis colorectal cancer (HNPCC), p. 262).
- Peutz–Jeghers syndrome.
- Hereditary diffuse gastric cancer (see below).

Most large familial gastric cancer kindreds show no evidence of HNPCC. Mean age at diagnosis is 54yrs, but there is wide variation. No close association with *H. pylori* has been demonstrated to date.

Hereditary diffuse gastric cancer (HDGC)

HDGC accounts for just 1–3% of gastric adenocarcinomas. Histology is diffuse or 'linitis plastica' type. Hereditary diffuse gastric cancer has a high penetrance (70–80% for gastric cancer and 39% for breast cancer in females) and a high mortality rate. It is AD and caused in ~35% of families by inactivating mutations in the *CDH1* (E-cadherin) gene. It has a strikingly young age of onset at 38yrs compared with 60–70yrs for sporadic gastric cancer.

Consultation plan in primary care

History
Three-generation family tree with specific enquiry for all forms of cancer, with age at diagnosis.

Examination
Not usually helpful in an asymptomatic family member.

Management in primary care

- Referral to surgical team if cancer suspected.
- Referral to Genetics if an asymptomatic individual presents with a strongly positive family history.
- Code patient's notes.
- Code, with appropriate consents, notes of other family members.

Genetics

Risk assessment—✍ refer to Clinical Genetics if multiple affected family members

Relatives of gastric cancer patients have a two- to threefold increased risk of developing gastric cancer. The risk is elevated for both genders.

- The lifetime risk in the general population is 2.3% for males and 1.2% for females.
- The risk with 2 affected relatives is 1 in 8 to 1 in 10.
- The risk with 3 affected relatives is 1 in 3.

Surveillance

- 📖 See also Cancer surveillance methods, p. 246.
- Consider *H. pylori* screening and eradication. Consider regular endoscopy (ineffective for diagnosis of diffuse gastric cancer). Consider prophylactic total gastrectomy in HDGC.

Hereditary non-polyposis colorectal cancer (HNPCC)

Lynch syndrome type 1: site-specific colorectal cancer; Lynch syndrome type 2: family cancer syndrome

HNPCC is a familial cancer syndrome which predisposes to **colorectal** cancer, **endometrial** cancer and a variety of other tumour types, e.g. **ovarian**, **gastric**, upper **urothelial** (ureter and renal pelvis), **biliary** cancers, brain tumours (**gliomas**) and **small-bowel** tumours, together with **sebaceous** tumours of the skin.

HNPCC accounts for about 1% of colorectal cancers, and its prevalence is of the order of 1:3000. HNPCC follows AD inheritance and, once a diagnosis is made in a family, it is common for multiple affected family members to be identified either retrospectively, when it is recognized that they were affected by tumours in the HNPCC spectrum, or prospectively through predictive testing.

HNPCC is caused by a mutation in one of the components of the DNA mismatch repair (MMRep) system that results in the accumulation of un-repaired DNA mismatches predisposing to tumour formation. Germline mutations in *MSH2* and *MLH1* account roughly equally for >90% HNPCC. A small number of families (<5%) have mutations in *MSH6*, while <1% have mutations in *PMS2*.

- *Muir–Torre syndrome:* a subset of HNPCC where sebaceous skin tumours (rare tumours of the skin) occur together with a tumour in the HNPCC spectrum, e.g. colorectal cancer (CRC).
- *MUTYH polyposis:* mutations in *MUTYH*, a DNA repair gene, also predispose to colorectal adenomatous polyposis (📖 see Familial adenomatous polyposis (FAP), p. 256).

Pathology

- *Immunohistochemistry:* it is possible to test tumours for loss or abnormality of mismatch repair protein expression by means of immunohistochemistry (IHC).
- Multiple adenomas are uncommon in HNPCC, but they do occur. However, if more than, say, half a dozen are found and there are no other HNPCC-associated tumour types in the family, the possibility of attenuated FAP (📖 see Familial adenomatous polyposis (FAP), p. 256) should be considered.
- Hyperplastic polyps and serrated adenomas are more typical of HNPCC than FAP.
- Unusual and rare tumours may occur in HNPCC.

Tumour spectrum

The major predisposition conferred by HNPCC is to adenocarcinoma of the colon and rectum which occur in both sexes, typically at a younger age than sporadic CRCs. In the general population, most bowel cancers occur in the rectum and sigmoid colon. However in HNPCC they occur equally throughout the large bowel, thus appearing to have a propensity for 'right-sided' lesions.

As well as colorectal, HNPCC also predisposes to endometrial cancer (particularly in *MSH6* families) and a wide variety of tumours at other sites.

Consultation plan in primary care

History
- Three-generation family tree with the history of tumours, benign and malignant.
- Is the family already known to a familial cancer or polyposis registry?

Examination
Look for skin lesions (e.g. sebaceous carcinoma or adenoma; keratoacanthoma). When present they are often on the face.

Management in primary care
- If patient declares or is found to have a mass, refer to a surgeon as appropriate.
- Refer to a dermatologist as appropriate.
- Refer 'at-risk' family members to Clinical Genetics.
- Code patient's notes.
- Code, with appropriate consents, notes of other family members (📖 See Confidentiality and consent, p. 8).

Investigations in secondary care
- Histopathology.
- Tumour testing.
- Mutation analysis of mismatch repair genes (*MLH1*, *MSH2*, *MSH6* and *PMS2*) in an affected member of a family that meets criteria for genetic testing.

Genetics
HNPCC is an AD disorder (📖 see Chapter 2, Autosomal dominant (AD) inheritance, p. 36).

Surveillance
- 📖 See also Cancer surveillance methods, p. 246.
- HNPCC gene carriers are at increased risk of many tumour types.
- Counsel patients that they should have a low threshold for presentation.
- PCPs have a pivotal role in co-ordinating screening.

PCPs should have a very low threshold for onward referral of any symptomatic family member. Members of HNPCC families commonly recall stories of delays in diagnosis, especially in individuals who developed cancer at a young age.

Colorectum

Generally accepted practice is to carry out colonoscopy every 2yrs from the age of 25 to 30yrs in those at 50% prior risk of HNPCC.

Endometrium

- Lifetime risk for endometrial cancer (50%) exceeds that for colorectal cancer (40%) in women with HNPCC, especially those with mutations in *MSH6*.
- There is no proven method of surveillance for endometrial cancer, so women should be warned of its risk and advised to seek help in case of irregular/postmenopausal bleeding, etc. In some centres screening may be offered by means of, for example, pipelle biopsy, but this is not proven to be of benefit.
- Women with *MSH6* mutations, who have completed childbearing, may wish to consider a hysterectomy, though it should be borne in mind that pelvic surgery can make colonoscopy more difficult if adhesions form.

Ovaries

Surveillance by means of annual ultrasound scan (USS) and serum CA125 level is possible but, like endometrial screening, it is not of proven benefit.

Urothelial tumours

Surveillance, e.g. by annual urine cytology, may be offered to families in which such tumours have already occurred, but there is no definite geno-type–phenotype or family concordance data to support this approach and the limited data available suggest that it is of fairly low efficacy.

Stomach

Screening is not usually offered currently in the UK for the modest increased risk for gastric cancer seen in HNPCC.

Skin

Refer to a dermatologist for management of skin lesions if these are present.

Education

Educate your patient about the symptoms of colorectal cancer so that he/she is aware when to seek medical advice and investigation. The most significant symptoms are:

- Rectal bleeding.
- A persistent change in bowel habit, usually to looser or more frequent bowel actions.
- Abdominal mass.
- Fatigue (unexplained anaemia).

Future developments

- It is important to let those at risk of HNPCC know that current recommendations and surveillance regimes are liable to change or revision as knowledge of the disorder advances. Indeed, they may welcome invitations to take part in clinical trials.
- It is possible that advanced imaging techniques, e.g. colonography by MRI, may eventually replace colonoscopy for screening.

Support group

Hereditary Non-Polyposis Colon Cancer: ✆ www.whatnow.org.uk/cancer-forums/hnpcc-or-lynch-syndrome

Lifestyle factors in cancer: smoking, alcohol, obesity, diet, and exercise

Smoking

Smoking is bad for your health, but some of our patients still smoke, although most say they would welcome our support to break the habit. Carcinogenic effects of tobacco cause cancer of the lung, pancreas, bladder and kidney, and (synergistically with alcohol) the larynx, mouth, pharynx (except nasopharynx), and oesophagus. Recent evidence suggests that the prevalence of several other types of cancer (stomach, liver, and cervix) is also increased by smoking.

About 60% of cancers amongst smokers are due to smoking. The rapid increase in the lung cancer incidence rate among continuing smokers ceases when they stop smoking—the rate remaining roughly constant for many years in ex-smokers.

> Tobacco causes one-third of all cancer deaths in developed countries. PCPs can make a significant difference by helping patients to stop smoking.

Alcohol

- Alcohol increases the risk of cancers of the oral cavity, pharynx, larynx, oesophagus, liver, and breast.
- GPs should enquire about alcohol intake and give advice on 'safe' levels of drinking (<2 units/day).

Obesity

There is now a consensus that cancer is more common in those who are overweight. A meta-analysis conducted in 2008 found that a $5kg/m^2$ increase in BMI was strongly associated with oesophageal adenocarcinoma (RR 1.5) and renal cancer (RR ~1.3) in both men and women. In men a $5kg/m^2$ increase in BMI was strongly associated with thyroid (RR = 1.33) and colon (RR = 1.24), cancers. Whereas in women a $5kg/m^2$ increase in BMI was strongly associated with endometrial (RR = 1.59) and gallbladder (RR = 1.59) cancer and is also associated with breast cancer.

Overall, 10% of all cancer deaths among American non-smokers (7% in men and 12% in women) are caused by excess weight; 5% (3% in men and 6% in women) of all incident cancers in the European Union might be prevented if no one had a BMI > 25.

Diet

Diet-related factors are thought to account for 30% of cancers in developed countries. Adequate intakes of fruit and vegetables (5 portions a day) probably lower the risk for several types of cancer, especially cancers of the gastrointestinal tract. The significance of other factors, e.g. red meat, fibre, and vitamins, is currently unclear.

Exercise

Regular exercise reduces the risk of colon cancer and probably also of breast cancer, although the quantitative effect is uncertain.

General lifestyle advice

Advice to members of the general population is therefore

- Not to smoke.
- To maintain a healthy weight.
- To restrict alcohol consumption.
- To eat a conventionally balanced diet, ensuring an adequate intake of fruit, vegetables, and cereals.

The extent to which such advice can modify the risk of cancer in individuals who carry, or are at risk of carrying, a mutation in a cancer-predisposing gene is uncertain. However, any reduction in risk, even if very small, may be of benefit, and it will be this group of patients who are highly motivated to follow advice.

Multiple endocrine neoplasia (MEN)

Multiple endocrine neoplasia type 1 (MEN1)

MEN1 accounts for 10% of patients with primary hyperparathyroidism who require surgery.

MEN is an AD cancer syndrome affecting primarily parathyroid, entero-pancreatic, endocrine, and pituitary tissues. MEN1 is caused by inactivating germline mutations in *MEN1*, a tumour suppressor gene encoding menin, a novel nuclear protein.

In most patients hyperparathyroidism is the first manifestation of MEN1, but this is not the case in up to 10% of mutation carriers. Unlike sporadic cases of primary hyperparathyroidism, tumours are typically present in one or more parathyroid glands and at a young age (25–35yrs). Disease-specific mortality in MEN1 is largely from the effects of pancreatic islet cell tumours (e.g. gastrinomas and insulinomas) and malignant thymic carcinoid.

Anterior pituitary tumours occur in 30% of MEN1 patients. Associated tumours that occur in MEN1 include adrenal cortical tumours (5%), carcinoid tumours (4–10%), lipomas (1%), facial angiofibromas (88%), and collagenomas (72%).

Multiple endocrine neoplasia type 2 (MEN2)

MEN2 is an AD cancer predisposition syndrome characterized by the association of medullary thyroid cancer (MTC) and phaeochromocytoma.

It is caused by activating germline mutations in the *RET* proto-oncogene. MEN2 has a prevalence of 1/30 000. MTC can occur in those as young as 4yrs, so screening is usually commenced at 6 months of age.

The ability of an MTC to oversecrete calcitonin, occasionally together with other hormonally active peptides, e.g. adrenocorticotrophic hormone (ACTH) or calcitonin-gene related peptide (CGRP), leads to unexplained diarrhoea, symptoms of Cushing's syndrome, or facial flushing in many patients with advanced disease. Metastatic spread occurs both locally to regional lymph nodes and to distant sites, e.g. the liver in advanced disease. Phaeochromocytomas may present with hypertension and episodes of palpitation, sweating, headache, anxiety, and nausea.

Other conditions to consider

- *Familial medullary thyroid carcinoma (FMTC)*. A subtype of MEN2. An AD condition characterized by MTC, usually diagnosed in middle-age, without other features of MEN2. Caused by mutations in the *RET* proto-oncogene.
- *Hyperparathyroidism, jaw tumour syndrome (HPJT)*. A rare AD disorder characterized by the combination of parathyroid tumours, causing hyperparathyroidism and fibro-osseous tumours of the jaw bones. It is caused by mutations in the parafibromin gene (*HRPT2*).

Consultation plan in primary care

History

Three-generation family tree with specific enquiry for presence of endocrine tumours, age of death, and cause of death.

Examination

May occasionally have unusual physical features, i.e. mucosal neuromas on lips and tongue, full lips, Marfanoid habitus (MEN2B).

Management in primary care

- Code patient's notes.
- Code, with appropriate consents, notes of other family members.
  - 📖 See Chapter 1, Confidentiality and consent, p. 8.

Genetics

✐ Referral to Clinical Genetics (for assessment and genetic testing) should be made for:

- Any patient with MTC or two or more MEN1/2-associated endocrine tumours.
- Any patient <30yrs of age with one MEN1/2-associated tumour.
- Any **first-degree relative** of someone with MEN1/2.
- Any patient with mucosal neuromas (MEN2).

Risk assessment

- **MEN1/2:** AD with 50% risk to offspring of an affected individual or mutation carrier.
- In MEN1 most are penetrant by 20yrs and >90% are penetrant by 30yrs; but some after age 40yrs.
- In MEN2 penetrance is 70% by 70yrs.

Predictive testing—✐ refer to Clinical Genetics

- **MEN1**. Genetic testing for MEN1 in the index cases gives useful information and confirms the clinical diagnosis, but rarely alters management. However, predictive genetic testing for at-risk family members is of great value in determining which family members are at risk and should be offered annual biochemical surveillance.
- **MEN2 and familial MTC**. Test to determine which family members are at risk and who should be offered prophylactic thyroidectomy.

Prenatal diagnosis—✐ refer to Clinical Genetics

Technically feasible by chorionic villus sampling (CVS) if the familial mutation is known.

Management

All patients with MEN1/2, or at risk for MEN1/2, need to be under regular specialist review to ensure periodic biochemical and endocrine monitoring and proactive surgical intervention to minimize morbidity.

MEN1
- Surgery for hyperparathyroidism includes subtotal or total parathyroidectomy.
- Proton pump inhibitors or somatostatin analogues are the main management for oversecretion of most enteropancreatic tumours except insulinomas.
- Surgery on gastrinomas is generally not indicated, and surgery for other enteropancreatic tumours is controversial.

MEN2 and FMTC
- Where the familial mutation is known, predictive genetic testing should be offered at a young age.
- Prophylactic thyroidectomy is the cornerstone of management for individuals with a mutation, but the timing of surgery is controversial and should be guided by the tertiary-care team. Patients with MEN2 require lifelong surveillance for phaeochromocytoma.

Support group
Association for Multiple Endocrine Neoplasia Disorders (AMEND): ℜ www.amend.org.uk

Neurofibromatosis type 2 (NF2)

Central neurofibromatosis, bilateral acoustic neurofibromatosis

NF2 is an AD disorder caused by inactivating mutations in the tumour suppressor gene 'merlin' (schwannomin) on 22q. Merlin's function as a tumour suppressor has not been elucidated. Schwannomas are benign solitary tumours of the peripheral nerve sheaths. The occurrence of multiple schwannomas usually implies hereditary disease.

> Vestibular schwannomas (acoustic neuromas), intracranial meningiomas, spinal tumours, peripheral nerve tumours, and presenile lens opacities are common in NF2.

NF2 is much less common than NF1, but is often a more serious condition with a significant disease burden. The morbidity and mortality of NF2 are largely due to bilateral vestibular schwannomas which present with hearing loss and tinnitus or vertigo and to other CNS tumours.

The mean age of first symptoms is 22yrs and the mean age of diagnosis is 27yrs; 31.5% of patients are diagnosed at <20yrs. Life expectancy may be shortened. The risk of mortality is inversely related to the age at diagnosis, with patients diagnosed at a young age generally having a worse prognosis.

Clinical features

- **CNS tumours:** vestibular schwannomas, meningiomas, spinal tumours (meningiomas, schwannomas), astrocytomas (usually in brainstem ± upper cervical cord), ependymomas (usually in brainstem ± upper cervical cord).
- **Peripheral nervous system:** peripheral schwannomas, peripheral neuropathy (glove and stocking or mononeuritis).
- **Skin:** NF2 plaques (slightly raised, roughened skin lesions that may be slightly pigmented; overlying skin is often hairy), nodular schwannomas, NF-like cutaneous neurofibromas, *café au lait* spots (CALs)—usually only a few, e.g. 1–3.
- **Eyes:** posterior subcasular cataracts, cortical cataracts, retinal hamartomas.

Differential diagnosis

Multiple schwannomatosis is a rare AD disorder caused by mutations in the *INI1* gene and characterized by multiple schwannomas without the involvement of the vestibular nerve characteristic of NF2. It is a milder condition with a better prognosis than NF2.

Genetics

- **Familial.** AD with 50% risk to offspring. There is strong intrafamilial correlation in the course of the disease, but marked interfamilial variability.
- **De novo.** About half of all patients are founders with clinically unaffected parents. A significant proportion of such patients are mosaic for their NF2 mutation, i.e. it is present in some cells/tissues

and not others. Almost all individuals with mosaicism have relatively mild disease.

Risk assessment

AD with 50% risk to offspring of an affected individual. Penetrance is age-dependent and is almost complete by 60yrs.

Predictive testing—✍ refer to Clinical Genetics

Possible if the familial mutation is known. If there is no mutation, but there are several affected family members and the diagnosis is typical with bilateral vestibular schwannomas, it may be possible to do predictive testing by linkage. Predictive testing in childhood is warranted since surveillance of 'at-risk' individuals begins in early childhood.

Surveillance of family members—✍ refer to Clinical Genetics

Parents <60yrs of age should be referred for assessment by a specialist, comprising:

- Careful examination of skin.
- Ophthalmological assessment for posterior subcapsular and cortical cataracts and CHRPE or astrocytic hamartomas.
- Cranial and spinal MRI with gadolinium enhancement and imaging of IAMs (internal auditory meatus).

Consultation plan in primary care

History

Three-generation family history with specific enquiry for diagnosis of neurofibromatosis, deafness, neurosurgery.

Examination

Examination of the skin for NF2 plaques, *café au lait* spots (CALs), cutaneous neurofibromas, schwannomas.

Management in primary care

- ✍ Refer to Clinical Genetics if the diagnosis is suspected or if there is a close family history.
- ✍ Refer to Neurosurgery if a patient is symptomatic.
- Code patient's notes.
- Code, with appropriate consents, notes of other family members.
  📖 See Chapter 1, Confidentiality and consent, p. 8.

Investigations in secondary care

- DNA for mutation analysis of *NF2*.
- Cranial and spinal magnetic resonance imaging (MRI) with gadolinium enhancement and imaging of IAMs.
- ✍ Refer to Ophthalmology (for assessment for ocular features of NF2, see above).

Management

Patients with NF2 will receive care from a team with expertise in skull-base surgery, usually comprising a neurosurgeon, ear, nose, and throat (ENT) surgeon, audiologist, clinical geneticist, etc.

NF2 patients who are treated in specialist centres have a significantly lower morbidity and mortality than those treated in non-specialist centres.

Early microsurgery for small tumours results in optimal preservation of hearing and facial nerve function. Complete removal of a large vestibular schwannoma usually renders the patient completely deaf on the side of surgery with a considerable risk for facial palsy. Brainstem implants may offer hope for some patients. Surgery for lesions other than vestibular schwannomas is usually undertaken only when indicated by symptoms.

Surveillance

For mutation carriers and 'at-risk' individuals, i.e. offspring of an affected parent in whom predictive genetic testing is declined or not possible, regular surveillance is important. This is usually organized through a multi-disciplinary clinic in a tertiary centre and will include:

- Ophthalmological assessment in early childhood.
- Annual review for symptomatic lesions until early teens.
- Screening for vestibular schwannomas from early teens.
- Full cranial and spinal MRI at 15yrs and again at 30yrs.

Support group

The Neurofibromatosis Association: ℑ www.nfa.zetnet.co.uk

Ovarian cancer

Most GPs will have experienced the late presentation of a woman with ovarian cancer, and the poor prognosis that ensues. The wish for 'genetic testing' by her first-degree relatives is often raised.

The lifetime risk of ovarian cancer in the general population is 1 in 70 or 1.4%. The majority of women with a family history of ovarian cancer have a single first-degree relative affected with ovarian cancer. If there is no significant cancer history in other members of the family (e.g. breast or bowel), the estimated relative risk of developing ovarian cancer is fairly small at 3. In northern Europe and North America this equates to a cumulative risk of 4% by age 70yrs. The relative risk of ovarian cancer in a monozygotic (MZ) twin of an affected woman is 6, i.e. twice the sibling risk, indicating that much of the excess familial risk is due to genetic factors rather than shared environmental factors.

Inherited mutations of *BRCA1* in particular, also *BRCA2* (☐ see *BRCA1* and *BRCA2*, p. 238), and to a lesser extent the mismatch-repair (MMRep) genes (HNPCC), are known to confer predisposition to ovarian cancer. Together they account for close to half of the excess familial risk of ovarian cancer. No gene that confers increased susceptibility to ovarian cancer alone has yet been identified.

Mutations in *BRCA1* are thought to be responsible for the majority of families with breast/ovarian and site-specific ovarian cancer. Approximately 6–8% of all cases of ovarian cancer are attributable to *BRCA* mutations. Very early age at diagnosis is not a feature of familial ovarian cancer.

Carriers with a mutation in *BRCA1* (☐ see *BRCA1* and *BRCA2*, p. 238 and Fig. 7.3, p. 239) have an increased risk of ovarian cancer. The risk for any individual is affected by both genetic modifiers and environmental exposures, but approximate averages are as follows:
- 39% risk to age 70yrs of ovarian cancer.
- Ovarian cancer risks in *BRCA1* carriers are low below age 40yrs (in absolute terms); thereafter the incidences are 1% between 40 and 59yrs and 2% after age 60yrs.

Women with a mutation in *BRCA2* (☐ see *BRCA1* and *BRCA2*, p. 238 and Fig. 7.4) have an increased risk of ovarian cancer. The risk for any individual is affected by both genetic modifiers and environmental exposures, but approximate averages are as follows:
- 11% risk to age 70yrs of ovarian cancer.
- Ovarian cancer risk in *BRCA2* carriers are very low below age 50yrs but then increase sharply in the 50–59yr age group, perhaps declining somewhat thereafter.

Women at high risk of developing ovarian cancer

Such women:
- Have a first-degree relative with ovarian cancer at any age who herself has a first-degree relative with breast cancer diagnosed at <50yrs or vice versa.
- Have a first-degree relative with ovarian cancer who herself has a first- or second-degree relative with ovarian cancer.

- May also be at high risk if they are in a family in which the affected individuals are connected by a second-degree relationship through an unaffected male, e.g. paternal aunt and paternal grandmother.

Is the diagnosis correct?
- 📖 See Confirmation of diagnosis of cancer, p. 254.
- Ovarian cancer is easily misreported by families (the actual diagnosis may prove to be a benign lesion, teratoma, adenocarcinoma of the bowel, uterine cancer, secondaries).

Consultation plan in primary care

History
Three-generation family tree with particular emphasis on history of cancer (especially ovarian, breast, and bowel) and documentation of age at diagnosis.

Examination
Not usually appropriate to do pelvic exam, but check normal screening (smears, mammogram, BP, etc. up-to-date).

Management in primary care
- If family history meets high risk criteria outlined in the tinted box above, ✍ refer to Clinical Genetics.
- Code patient's notes.
- Code, with appropriate consents, notes of other family members. 📖 See Chapter 1, Confidentiality and consent, p. 8.

Investigations in secondary care
- DNA for *BRCA1/2* mutation analysis from an affected member of a family meeting the high-risk criteria (see above).
- DNA for MMRep genes if the family has pedigree suggestive of HNPCC (📖 see Hereditary non-polyposis colorectal cancer (HNPCC), p. 262), especially if the ovarian cancer is mucinous or endometrioid.

Genetics
Risk assessment
Will be discussed in the clinic, but the patient and her family may want to discuss this with the primary care team, too.
- **Single relative affected <30yrs with no other significant family history** (e.g. breast cancer or other cancers suggestive of a familial cancer syndrome). A study found no *BRCA1/2* mutations amongst women with ovarian cancer diagnosed at <30yrs and no tendency to greater familiality. Overall risks are likely to be similar to those of the sister of an older proband, i.e. two- to threefold increased lifetime risk for ovarian cancer.
- **Single relative affected >30yrs with no other significant family history** (e.g. breast cancer or other cancers suggestive of a familial cancer syndrome). Sister of a woman with 'sporadic' ovarian cancer has a threefold increased lifetime risk for ovarian cancer.

- **High-risk women.** High chance of a dominant genetic susceptibility to ovarian and breast cancer.
- The risks of both breast and ovarian cancer are higher in *BRCA1* carriers than *BRCA2* carriers, but the difference is much more marked for ovarian cancer and for breast cancer diagnosed at young ages, i.e. before 50yrs.

Predictive testing—✍ refer to Clinical Genetics
Possible for those families in whom the causative mutation has been defined.

Management

- **Women with a single affected relative.** While the risk of developing ovarian cancer is higher than those of a similar age who are at population risk (relative risk (RR) 3 for first-degree relatives), this increased risk amounts to a cumulative risk of 4% by age 70yrs. In the absence of formal evidence of its efficacy, screening is not currently recommended at this level of risk.
- **High risk women and BRCA1/2 carriers.** The risk of ovarian cancer among *BRCA1* or *BRCA2* mutation carriers decreases with parity (reduction in the odds of ovarian cancer is 12% per birth).

Prophylactic laparoscopic salpingo-oophorectomy
Although the risk of ovarian cancer in carriers of *BRCA* mutations is considerably lower than the risk of breast cancer in these carriers, the absence of reliable methods of early detection and the poor prognosis of advanced ovarian cancer make prophylactic bilateral salpingo-oophorectomy (BSO) an option that all female carriers should consider after their families are complete. There is also an important reduction in breast cancer risk, with a breast cancer hazard ratio of 0.32 after prophylactic BSO compared with the surveillance-only group.

Salpingo-oophorectomy should be considered rather than oophorectomy, given reports of tumours arising in the Fallopian tubes in carriers of *BRCA* mutations. There is a residual risk for primary peritoneal ovarian cancer after oophorectomy.

The risk of developing ovarian cancer at <40yrs is low, even in women at high genetic risk. Oophorectomy in premenopausal women precipitates an abrupt menopause. Important side-effects include hot flushes, disturbed sleep, vaginal dryness, and increased risk of osteoporosis and heart disease. Hormone replacement therapy (HRT) may be needed in the short term to counteract these side-effects. Oestrogen-only HRT is used where possible; in women who retain their uterus it may be combined with topical progesterone (via an intrauterine Mirena® coil).

The NIH Consensus Statement on Ovarian Cancer recommended that women at risk of inherited ovarian cancer undergo prophylactic oophorectomy after completion of childbearing or at age 35yrs.

Chemoprevention
Although the combined oral contraceptive pill (OCP) reduces the risk of ovarian cancer in the general population, in women with a family history of ovarian cancer and, possibly, in *BRCA1/2* carriers, concerns about

enhanced breast cancer risk mean that the OCP should not currently be recommended as an option for reducing the risk of ovarian cancer.

Surveillance

- 📖 See also Cancer surveillance methods, p. 246.
- ***Breast surveillance.*** Site-specific ovarian cancer and breast/ovarian cancer are currently regarded as a continuum. Due to the high incidence of *BRCA1/2* mutations in high-risk ovarian cancer families, even those in whom an affected family member screens negative for *BRCA1/2* mutations should be managed as if they were at high risk of breast cancer.
- ***Serum CA-125 estimation and ovarian ultrasound scan (USS).*** Early-stage cancers can be identified by a programme of annual serum CA-125 estimation and ovarian ultrasonography (transvaginal USS), but there is a high false-positive rate (with consequent anxiety and surgical intervention). This approach may also fail to detect ovarian cancers at a curable stage (significant false-negative rate). The outcomes of current trials are urgently needed to inform practice in this area.

Phaeochromocytoma

The adrenal medulla and ganglia of the sympathetic nervous system are neural crest derivatives. They synthesize and secrete catecholamines (adrenaline, noradrenaline, etc.). Phaeochromocytomas usually arise in the adrenal medulla, but can arise outside the adrenals, in the sympathetic chain, where they may be called paragangliomas. Paragangliomas that originate in the sympathetic nervous system are commonly found in the retroperitoneum, but can also occur in the thorax. Paragangliomas that originate in the parasympathetic nervous system can occur adjacent to the aortic arch, neck, and skull base as local 'non-functioning' masses. They are also known as 'glomus tumours' or chemodectomas when they arise in the neck.

Classical clinical features of phaeochromocytoma are paroxysmal headache, sweating, and palpitations accompanied by hypertension due to the pressor effects of catecholamine release.

Germline mutations in the succinate dehydrogenase subunit genes (*SDHB*, *SDHC*, and *SDHD*) can cause susceptibility to both phaeochromocytomas (adrenal and extra-adrenal) and parasympathetic-derived head and neck paragangliomas. 84% of multifocal tumours and 59% of phaeochromocytomas presenting at <19yrs of age are due to germline mutations in a variety of genes, including *VHL, RET, SDHB, SDHC, SDHD, NF1*.

Consultation plan in primary care

History
Three-generation family tree.

Examination
- Blood pressure.
- Marfanoid body habitus and mucosal neuromas (multiple endocrine neoplasia type 2B).
- Thyroid mass (MEN2).
- Carotid-body tumour (familial paraganglioma).
- *Café au lait* spots, axillary freckling, and dermal neurofibromas (neurofibramotosis type 1).
- Observe gait, and observe eyes for nystagmus and past-pointing/dysdiadochokinesia (cerebellar signs in von Hippel–Lindau (VHL) secondary to cerebellar haemangioblastoma).

Management in primary care

- Referral to physician.
- Code patient's notes.
- Code, with appropriate consents, notes of other family members.
  See Chapter 1, Confidentiality and consent, p. 8.

Investigations in secondary care
- 24h urine collection for vanillylmandelic acid (VMA).
- Onward referral to Clinical Genetics for assessment of diagnosis, discussion of genetic testing, and assessment of risks to other family members.

- Ophthalmology referral for retinal angiomas (VHL) if no specific syndrome identified.
- Most patients with phaeochromocytoma will have had recent intra-abdominal imaging (usually magnetic resonance imaging (MRI)) as part of their diagnosis which should identify pancreatic cysts, renal-cell cancers (VHL).

Genetics

Risk assessment

If specific syndrome, or germline mutation is identified, the genetics clinic will offer screening to all first-degree family members.

Predictive testing —✍ refer to Clinical Genetics

- If a specific germline mutation is identified, first-degree relatives will be offered testing by Genetics in order to target subsequent surveillance.
- Genetic conditions predisposing to phaeochromocytoma include:
  - multiple endocrine neoplasia (📖 see Multiple endocrine neoplasia (MEN), p. 268)
  - von Hippel–Lindau (VHL) (📖 see von Hippel–Lindau (VHL) disease, p. 288)
  - familial paraganglioma (*SDHB/SDHC/SDHD*)
  - neurofibromatosis (NF1) (📖 see Chapter 5, Neurofibromatosis type 1 (NF1), p. 156).

Surveillance

In genetic conditions predisposing to phaeochromocytoma, screening is usually done by analysing 24h urine samples for VMA, although plasma catecholamine analysis may be available in some centres. Advice on frequency of testing will be given to PCPs by the tertiary-care team.

Prostate cancer

Prostate cancer is the most common cancer in men in the UK and is second to lung cancer as a cause of cancer death in males. Like all common cancers, it increases with age and about 60% men are aged >70yrs at diagnosis. The lifetime risk is 1 in 14. Many men are diagnosed when the disease is widespread, but the 5yr survival after diagnosis is 70%.

There are some ethnic differences, with African and Caribbean men at greater risk than Europeans, who have a greater risk than men from Asia. Some families show clustering of prostate cancer, and in some there is a history of breast cancer in female relatives. The breast cancer gene *BRCA2* (📖 see *BRCA1* and *BRCA2*, p. 238) is an important single-gene cause of increased risk, though *BRCA2* mutations are only found in about 2% of men who present at age <55yrs. However, men with inherited mutations of *BRCA2* are not only at 5 times more risk of prostate cancer (the relative risk is even higher at younger ages) but it is also often of a more aggressive type.

The cumulative risk for prostate cancer in men with *BRCA2* is:
- 0.1% by age 50yrs
- 1.6% by age 60yrs
- 7.5% by age 70yrs
- 19.8% by age 80yrs

Mutations in the *BRCA1* gene have a smaller effect, increasing a man's risk of prostate cancer by less than twofold.

The current IMPACT (**I**dentification of **M**en with a genetic predisposition to **P**rost**A**te **C**ancer: **T**argeted) study is evaluating the benefits of prostate screening in male *BRCA1* and *BRCA2* mutation carriers and controls.

Consultation plan in primary care

History
- Three-generation family tree with specific enquiry for breast, ovarian, prostate, and other associated cancers.
- Specific questioning for prostatic symptoms and bone pain.

Examination
- Prostate exam if indicated.
- Consider skeletal X-rays.

Management in primary care

- ✍ Referral to Urology for management of prostatic cancer.
- ✍ Referral to Genetics if strong family history of prostate cancer or strong family history of tumours in the *BRCA1/2* spectrum e.g. breast/ovary, etc. (📖 see *BRCA1* and *BRCA2*, p. 238).
- Code patient's note if *BRCA1/2* mutation found.
- Code, with appropriate consents, other family members' notes. 📖 See Chapter 1, Confidentiality and consent, p. 8.

Surveillance

- Three screening tests for prostate cancer are available (digital rectal examination (DRE), transrectal ultrasound (TRUS), and the measurement of prostate specific antigen (PSA) levels), but all have problems.
- There is no UK screening programme for prostate cancer but in the USA screening by PSA is encouraged in men over 50yrs, particularly in African Americans.
- In the UK, informal screening of asymptomatic men takes place (e.g. in 'Well Men' clinics) but there is at present no national population screening for prostate cancer in the UK as the available screening methods do not currently meet criteria for establishing such a programme.
- Of the three, the PSA test, a blood test, is the most acceptable and reliable, but it fails to be a useful population screening test mainly because of:
  - Lack of specificity. Only about a quarter to a third of asymptomatic men with abnormally high PSA levels will have prostate cancer. Up to two-thirds of men with elevated PSA levels will not have prostate cancer but will suffer the anxiety, discomfort, and risk of follow-up investigations.
  - Lack of sensitivity. Up to 20% of all men with prostate cancers have normal PSA levels.

Retinoblastoma

Retinoblastoma (RB) is an embryonic neoplasm of retinal origin caused by mutations in a tumour suppressor gene. RB affects approximately 1/20 000 live births and arises predominantly in children <7yrs of age (90% of diagnoses are made at <5yrs).

An RB develops according to Knudson's two-hit hypothesis when both *RB1* alleles are deleted or mutated (🕮 see Fig. 7.5). Patients with inherited forms of RB inherit the first hit, a hit on the other allele of the *RB* gene then triggers a tumour to develop (🕮 see Fig. 7.5). Inherited RB tends to be bilateral or multifocal whereas sporadic RB is unilateral and unifocal. However, there are exceptions to this situation, where patients carrying a germline *RB* mutation present with a solitary tumour, or do not develop retinoblastoma at all.

Genetic predisposition to RB is inherited as an AD trait. The penetrance (i.e. the chance that a mutation carrier will develop a retinoblastoma) can vary. Most mutations are associated with a high (>90%) penetrance, but some mutations have a much lower penetrance.

Genetics

- ***Genetic or hereditary RB*** is defined as a germline mutation affecting all cells in the body and a single somatic hit to the *RB1* gene then initiates tumorigenesis. This will include all trilateral, bilateral, and multifocal RB. It will also include 10% of unilateral/unifocal RB. It follows autosomal dominant inheritance (50% risk to offspring), but with incomplete penetrance. For inactivating mutations, penetrance is estimated at 90%. Mosaic individuals have reduced penetrance (60%) and expressivity.
- ***Non-genetic/non-hereditary RB*** occurs when the two hits to the *RB1* gene have occurred only in the tumour and are not present in other cells. This will include the majority of unilateral/unifocal RB.

> ✑ Genetic counselling in retinoblastoma is complex; refer patients with a history of RB, or a family history of RB to Clinical Genetics if they have not received recent genetic advice.

Predictive testing—✑ refer to Clinical Genetics

- Where a mutation is identified, cascade testing of the family is indicated, starting with parents and siblings and including the extended family as indicated.
- Predictive testing of 'at-risk' neonates is appropriate because of the burden of frequent screening by examination under anaesthesia (EUA) in the early years of life.
- Linkage analysis can be helpful in families where there is clearly familial RB but no mutation has been identified.

Prenatal diagnosis—✑ refer to Clinical Genetics

Prenatal diagnosis by chorionic villus sampling (CVS) is available in those families in which the *RB1* mutation is known or when a family is informative for linkage. Pre-implantation genetic diagnosis (PGD) may also be an option for some families.

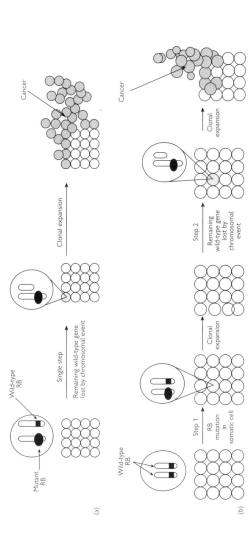

Fig. 7.5 Knudson's hypothesis. (a) In individuals with an inherited predisposition to retinoblastoma every somatic cell contains one intact *RB* allele and one mutant *RB* allele. A single somatic mutation is therefore sufficient for loss of RB activity, with a subsequent clonal expansion of the double mutant cell and tumour formation. (b) In normal individuals both copies of *RB* must be targeted by somatic mutation for RB function to be disrupted. Since the somatic mutation rate is low, the risk of two *RB* mutations occurring in the same cell is low. This explains the later onset and unifocal nature of retinoblastoma cases that occur in the absence of a family history. (Taken from Warrell (2003) *Oxford Textbook of Medicine, 4th edn*, p. 230, by permission of Oxford University Press.)

Consultation plan in primary care

History

Three-generation (or more extensive) family tree, documenting RB and all other types of tumour.

Examination

- Check for red reflex at 8-week neonatal check, or if parents report a problem. An abnormality requires immediate referral to Ophthalmology
- Brief examination of skin of older patients with hereditary RB if appropriate.
- Parents of a child with RB should always be examined by an experienced ophthalmologist to look for spontaneously regressed tumour.

Management plan in primary care

- The treatment of an infant/child for RB (including radiotherapy, chemotherapy, possible enucleation of the affected eye) puts huge strains on the child, their parents, and their siblings. PCPs are in a position to offer ongoing support, as well as pointing to other sources of help and advice:
  - health visitors (HV)
  - SENCO
  - visual aid services.
- ✍ Refer to Clinical Genetics.
- Code patient's notes.
- Code, with appropriate consents, notes of other family members.
  ☐ See Chapter 1, Confidentiality and consent, p. 8.

Investigations in tertiary care

- DNA sample for *RB1* mutation analysis. Mutation identifiable in ~90% of families with bilateral or familial RB. For children with unilateral RB, mutation analysis will have a pick-up rate of only ~8%.
- Karyotype with fluorescent *in situ* hybridization (FISH) (☐ see Chapter 3, Genetic investigations, p. 74) for *RB1*. Approximately 3% have an interstitial deletion of 13q14 (many of the children with deletions have associated dysmorphic features and/or developmental delay, but a significant proportion do not).
- Possible linkage exclusion testing alongside mutation analysis, e.g. if several siblings are being screened as a result of a new diagnosis in a child, or if particular family circumstances make sibling screening difficult.
- Tumour mutation analysis. This will be considered when mutation testing on blood is negative.

Management

At present chemotherapy is the first-line treatment, followed by local treatments such as plaques or cryotherapy for accessible tumours, or lens-sparing radiotherapy. Treatment is aimed a preserving sight as far as possible, but enucleation may be offered as treatment for a large unilateral tumour or if disease is hard to control by other treatments.

Surveillance

Screening of children at risk of RB

- Any child with an increased risk of RB (including siblings of a child with isolated unilateral RB in whom the risk is only 1%) should be offered EUAs from the age of 2–3 weeks until the age of 5yrs under the care of a specialist opthalmologist. The examinations are offered at decreasing frequency and most 'at-risk' children undergo 14 EUAs.
- Genetic testing can be very helpful in targetting surveillance to those at high risk and enabling surveillance to be avoided or discontinued if found not to carry the familial mutation.

Second tumours

Survivors of RB who carry a germline mutation in *RB1* are at greatly increased risk for a variety of other tumours, which include sarcomas, melanoma, and brain tumours:

- Radiotherapy as part of RB treatment further increases the mortality from second tumours.
- The tumours most commonly develop in the second to fourth decades.

Surveillance for second non-RB primaries

Increased level of awareness by patient and GP (with accelerated referral if any concern).

Support group

Retinoblastoma Society: ☎ 020 7600 3309; ⌕ www.rbsociety.org.uk

von Hippel–Lindau (VHL) disease

VHL disease is an AD disorder characterized by a predisposition to a wide variety of tumours:

- Haemangioblastomas of the cerebellum and spinal cord (probability 84% by age 60: average age at presentation 33yrs).
- Retinal angiomas (probability 70% by age 60)—mostly present in children and young adults.
- Renal cell carcinoma (probability 69% by age 60).
- Phaeochromocytoma.
- Renal, pancreatic, and epididymal cysts.

The gene for VHL on 3p25 encodes a tumour-suppressor protein involved in the oxygen sensing pathway in cells. Approximately 20% of patients with VHL have no family history and are due to new dominant mutations.

> VHL is a genetic disorder which places a considerable burden on the individual and their family. Complications of the disorder accrue over time and patients will benefit from long-term support from their primary care team as they encounter new problems.

Genetics

Risk assessment

AD, with 50% risk that offspring will inherit the disease-causing mutation. There is considerable variation within families carrying the same mutation. Penetrance is age-dependent and the mean age at first diagnosis (in those not undergoing surveillance) is 25yrs.

Predictive testing—⇗ refer to Clinical Genetics

Possible if the familial mutation is known. Usually this is considered just prior to the commencement of regular surveillance at 5yrs of age.

Prenatal diagnosis—⇗ refer to Clinical Genetics

Technically feasible by chorionic villus sampling (CVS) at 11 weeks' gestation if the familial mutation is known, but not commonly requested.

Investigations and surveillance

- Annual blood pressure from age 5yrs.
- Annual direct and indirect ophthalmoscopy for detection of retinal angiomas from age 5yrs. More frequent screening may be indicated if angiomas are present.
- Annual renal imaging (MRI or ultrasound scan (USS)) from age 16yrs. More frequent renal USS or follow-up MRI imaging may be indicated if there are abnormalities on the renal scan.
- Annual 24h urine collection for VMA from 11yrs.
- MRI brain scans every 3yrs from age 15yrs. Patients should be aware that in general, CNS lesions are only removed if symptomatic.

Consultation plan in primary care

History
- Detailed three-generation family tree with specific enquiry about renal tumours, brain tumours, and visual loss. Extend the family tree of affected individuals as far as possible.
- Detailed past medical history.
- Enquiry re. current symptoms.

Examination
- Blood pressure (BP).
- If diagnosis is suspected, careful neurological examination, and refer immediately if cerebellar signs.
- Fundoscopy.

Investigations in primary care

Consider sending 24h urine collection for vanillylmandelic acid (VMA).

Management plan in primary care

- Refer immediately to Neurology if cerebellar signs.
- Refer for ophthalmic assessment if fundoscopy suspicious.
- Refer to Genetics if a patient presents with a family history.
- Code patient's notes.
- Code, with appropriate consents, notes of other family members. ☐ See Chapter 1, Confidentiality and consent, p. 8.
- GPs need to be aware of the surveillance, and from whom the co-ordinated screening and action on results is to be expected (☐ see 'Investigations and surveillance', p. 288).

Long-term complications
- *Cerebellar haemangioblastoma*. Approximately 30% of all cerebellar haemangioblastomas occur as part of VHL The younger the patient at diagnosis, the more likely that the patient has VHL. Most haemangioblastomas of the craniospinal axis can be safely and completely excised by surgery, but resection is usually deferred until the onset of symptoms.
- *Retinal angiomas*. Solitary retinal angiomas can occur sporadically or be associated with VHL disease. Virtually all patients with multiple retinal angiomas have VHL.
- *Renal cysts and renal cell carcinoma*. Renal cysts may be detected from the second decade. Renal cell carcinoma is often, but not invariably, associated with cysts. Renal cell carcinoma may be multifocal and bilateral in VHL. Tumours are usually treated with partial nephrectomy.

Ongoing surveillance is crucial in VHL from age 16yrs because of the high risk of renal cell carcinoma.

Support group
VHL Family Alliance: ☞ www.vhl.org

Chromosomes

Introduction

Chromosomal disorders cover a huge spectrum from those that are benign and have no implications for health except with regard to reproduction (e.g. many balanced translocations) to those that cause profound developmental delay. Some have only mild or minimal effects on health, and frequently remain undiagnosed (e.g. XYY), whereas others cause multiple congenital anomalies and severe limitation of lifespan (e.g. trisomy 18). In order to communicate sensitively and effectively with patients and their families it is important to know where in this spectrum the chromosome disorder that affects your patient/family lies. The sections in this chapter are designed to provide the necessary information. The following may be helpful sources of additional information:

- 📖 Chapter 4, Regional genetics services in the UK, p. 82.
- The Rare Chromosome Disorder support group 'Unique' ⌀ www. rarechromo.org is an excellent source of information about a whole range of chromosomal disorders. They provide informative booklets, a helpline, and a strong network of support for families.

Chromosome anomalies

These are classified as:

- **Numerical:** the presence of an additional chromosome as in Down syndrome (3 copies of chromosome 21) or the absence of a chromosome as in Turner syndrome (45X).
- **Structural:** a change of some kind to the structural integrity of a chromosome by:
  - the *deletion* of part of a chromosome, e.g. del 22q11 in DiGeorge syndrome/velocardiofacial syndrome (📖 see Figs. 8.1 and 8.2)
  - the *duplication* of part of chromosome
  - the *inversion* of part of a chromosome—two breaks form on a single chromosome and the middle section is flipped round
  - the *translocation* of part of a chromosome to another chromosome. This can result in a *balanced* translocation if chromosomal content is maintained, or *unbalanced* if there is a net loss or gain of chromosomal material (📖 see Translocations, p. 306).

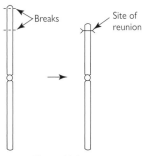

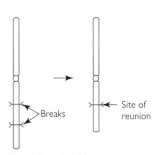

Fig. 8.1 Terminal deletion. (Reproduced with permission of Oxford University Press, Young, *Medical Genetics*, 2005.)

Fig. 8.2 Interstitial deletion. (Reproduced with permission of Oxford University Press, Young, *Medical Genetics*, 2005.)

Down syndrome (trisomy 21)

The incidence of trisomy 21 conceptions increases strikingly with maternal age (☐ see Chapter 9, Maternal age, p. 380). There is a high incidence of spontaneous loss of trisomy 21 pregnancies. Between ~11 weeks and term, 43% of affected pregnancies are spontaneously lost, and between ~16 weeks and term, ~23%. The natural prevalence of ~1/600 affected live births has decreased to a current incidence in the UK of ~1/1100 live births, due to an increase in antenatal screening, prenatal diagnosis, and termination of some affected pregnancies.

Genetics

The chromosomal basis for Down syndrome can be summarized as follows:

- **Trisomy 21:** 95% of cases arise from meiotic non-disjunction, giving rise to trisomy 21 (☐ see Fig. 8.3).
- **Translocation Down syndrome:** 2% of cases result from Robertsonian translocation (☐ see Fig. 8.6) especially rob(14;21) of which 50% are familial (inherited). These are clinically indistinguishable from Down syndrome due to trisomy 21, and the only significant difference is in the recurrence risk for future pregnancies (☐ see Robertsonian translocation, p. 308).
- **Mosaic Down syndrome:** 2% of cases result from mosaicism. In these individuals there is a mixture of normal cells and Down syndrome cells. In a boy with mosaic Down syndrome this would usually mean a combination of 46,XY with 47,XY + 21 cells. A girl with mosaic Down syndrome would usually have a mixture of 46,XX and 47,XX + 21. Because these individuals have a proportion of normal cells, they generally have a milder clinical picture than individuals with trisomy 21 in all of their cells. However, the ratio of normal to Down syndrome cells in blood is not a reliable indicator of the ratio in other tissues, e.g. brain or heart, and cannot be used to predict severity in anything but the most general terms (☐ see Chapter 2, Mosaicism, p. 46).

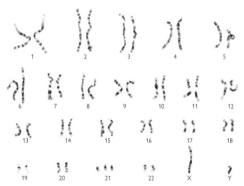

Fig. 8.3 Trisomy 21 G-banded karotype. (Reproduced from Firth, Hurst and Hall (2005). *Oxford Desk Reference—Clinical Genetics*, with permission from Oxford University Press.)

Risk assessment

The person providing genetic advice regarding future pregnancies should have seen the cytogenetic report in order to confirm: (i) the diagnosis of Down syndrome and (ii) the chromosomal basis for this.

- The risk of recurrence of trisomy 21 is affected by maternal age and parental germline mosaicism. Overall, advising a 'slightly less than 1% recurrence risk' (0.8%) for women <39yrs, with an age-related risk thereafter, seems reasonable (📖 see Chapter 9, Maternal age, p. 380).
- If an individual has Down syndrome due to trisomy 21, there is no increased risk to his/her second- and third-degree relatives, e.g. children of siblings, aunts, uncles, etc.
- If a woman with +21 becomes pregnant, the risk of +21 in the offspring is ~50% (fertility in men with +21 is exceptionally rare).

Parents are not usually offered karyotype analysis if the karyotype shows trisomy 21 (47,XX+21 or 47,XY+21), or if the karyotype shows mosaic +21 Down syndrome. However, parental karyotyping is essential if the karyotype shows translocation Down syndrome.

Family history of Down syndrome
- ***Single affected relative.*** If a sibling, aunt, or uncle has Down syndrome, try to obtain the karyotype of the affected individual or refer to Clinical Genetics. If it shows trisomy 21, there is no added risk to your patient arising from this. If the karyotype is not obtainable and the mother was <40 at the time of the affected child's birth, offer your patient a karyotype to exclude the very small possibility of a Robertsonian translocation involving chromosome 21.
- ***More than one affected relative on same side of family*** raises the possibility of a Robertsonian translocation involving chromosome 21 (e.g. rob(14;21)), *karyotype of your patient is essential* unless the family has already been carefully investigated.

Antenatal screening
📖 See Chapter 9, Antenatal screening for genetic disorders, p. 324.

Risk of Down syndrome is increased by:
- Increased nuchal fold thickness at 10–12 weeks' gestation on USS.
- Abnormal levels on maternal serum screening, e.g. triple test (alpha-fetoprotein (AFP), beta human chorionic gonadotrophin (β-hCG), unconjugated oestriol (uE_3)), at 14–16 weeks' gestation.
- Current research suggests that it is likely that over the next few years screening for Down syndrome by analysis of cell-free fetal nucleic acids (e.g. cffDNA or cffRNA) in maternal blood may become possible.

Prenatal diagnosis
Definitive testing is possible by CVS at 11–12 weeks or amniocentesis at 15–16 weeks. Both are invasive tests and carry a small risk of miscarriage (~1%).

Consultation plan in primary care

History

- Draw a family tree—if the karyotype is already known to be trisomy 21, only a brief family tree is required.
- Ask about any other affected family members.
- Age of the mother at the time of the birth of her Down syndrome child.
- Have any other family members already been seen by genetic services?

Examination (of the neonate)

- Facial features with upslanting palpebral fissures, flat facial profile, epicanthic folds, short nose with depressed nasal bridge.
- Brachycephaly and patent posterior fontanelle.
- Dermatoglyphics: single palmar creases and sandal gap between hallux and 2nd toe.
- Hypotonia: e.g. marked head lag as a newborn, hypotonia contributes to delayed motor milestones in infancy.
- Heart: careful clinical assessment, including an echocardiogram, must be done by a paediatric cardiologist during infancy, due to the high incidence of congenital heart disease (40–50%).
- Growth parameters: height, weight, OFC—plot on Down syndrome specific charts; see ◎ www.growthcharts.com

Initial management in primary care

Suspicion that a neonate that you are seeing for the first time may have Down syndrome would require a timely consultation with a paediatrician. To substantiate the diagnosis, rapid FISH analysis for +21 followed by karyotyping will be performed to confirm/refute the diagnosis.

Ongoing management in primary care

- The patient's GP computer notes should be coded for
  - Down syndrome
  - learning disability
  - Carers' register.
- The parents' notes should also be appropriately coded, including the Carers' register.
- If the patient is newly registering post-diagnosis (e.g. just moved into your Practice Area) as well as the above coding, enquire about the involvement of other relevant professionals (social services, Learning Disability Community Team, SENCO, etc.) and refer to a community paediatrician/adult learning disability team.

Key areas to consider

- Ophthalmological assessment (refractive errors and cataracts are common).
- Hearing assessment.

- Obesity.
- Periodontal disease.
- Coeliac disease.
- Thyroid function.
- Early signs of dementia.

These could all be included in relevant yearly checks.

Also be aware of arthritis, atlantoaxial subluxation, diabetes mellitus (1%), leukaemia (0.6%), obstructive sleep apnoea, seizures (8%).

Impact on patient and/or family

- If the diagnosis is made antenatally, PCPs, as well as specialists, may support the parents facing a decision about the continuation of the pregnancy. The support group ARC (℘ www.arc-uk.org) may be a useful contact for the couple, as well as fetal medicine personnel and midwifery staff. An appointment with a community paediatrician specializing in developmental paediatrics may be helpful if the couple require further information to inform their decision.
- Parents will be deeply affected by this diagnosis and will need ongoing support, and ongoing explanations, long term.
- The risk to future pregnancies, and to the extended family, depends on the genetic basis of the Down syndrome which will be investigated by the Paediatric and/or Genetics teams (📖 see 'Risk assessment', p. 295).

Support groups

Down Syndrome Association: ℘ www.downs-syndrome.org.uk
MDS UK—Mosaic Down syndrome support group: ℘ www.mosaicdownsyndrome.org
US National Down Syndrome Society: ℘ www.ndss.org

Klinefelter syndrome (47,XXY)

Klinefelter syndrome has a prevalence of 1/600–1/800 male births. There is a significant maternal age effect, with 47,XXY being more common with advanced maternal age, increasing from 1/2500 live births at maternal age 33yrs to 1/300 at 43yrs.

47,XXY is usually either diagnosed prenatally as an unexpected finding at amniocentesis/chorionic villus sampling (CVS) or in adult life during investigation of male infertility. The majority probably remain undiagnosed. Males with Klinefelter syndrome have a normal lifespan.

Genetics

Recurrence risk

- **Parents** of boys with XXY are not routinely karyotyped. The recurrence risk is low, <1%.
- **Offspring**: 47,XXY men are generally infertile. For the few that are fertile or use intracytoplasmic sperm injection (ICSI) to achieve a pregnancy, there may be an increased risk of aneuploidy (both for sex chromosomes and for +21) and pre-implantation genetic diagnosis (PGD) or prenatal diagnosis should be offered.

Prenatal diagnosis

- Prenatal diagnosis should be offered to parents, but there is a fine balance between the very small risk of recurrence and the risk of procedure-associated pregnancy loss.
- Prenatal diagnosis is indicated if a patient with Klinefelter fathers a pregnancy because of the increased risk for aneuploidy.

Consultation plan in primary care (postnatal presentation)

History

- **Developmental milestones,** including speech and language: may be mildly delayed but in the majority of boys development is within the normal range. A tendency towards passive and unassertive behaviour has been noted frequently.
- **Schooling:** there is a modest decrement in intelligence quotient (IQ) of 10–15 points when compared with siblings, but IQ varies widely: 67–133. The majority of 47,XXY (two-thirds) will have more problems with reading and spelling than their 46,XY peers.
  In one study, 70% received additional educational support (usually part-time support in mainstream school). Most XXY boys have less-skilled jobs than their fathers, but there is no increase in unemployment. Variation is wide and some 47,XXY men will follow professional careers.
- **Fertility:** 47,XXY men are generally infertile. Occasionally, men with 47,XXY have a few sperm in their testes, even when none are present in the ejaculate.

Examination

- **Height:** men with 47,XXY tend to be rather tall, with final adult height 186cm (compared with 177cm for 46,XY).

- *Age-related pubertal development:* boys enter puberty normally. By midpuberty the testes begin to involute, and boys develop hypergonadotrophic hypogonadism with decreased testosterone production. Testes are small in adult life and men with Klinefelter syndrome are, with occasional exceptions, infertile. 47,XXY males are no more likely to be homosexual than 46,XY males. Men with 47,XXY have, with the exception of small testes, normal genitalia and normal sexual relations.

Investigation

Semen analysis: most will be azoospermic but, rarely, mosaicism may allow production of sperm and subsequent fertility.

Impact on patient and/or family

Adult presentation usually confines the impact of the diagnosis to issues of fertility.

Management in primary care

- Advise parents that, if their son shows developmental, behavioural, or educational difficulties, they should have a low threshold for asking for professional help, as early intervention can improve outcome.
- In general, disclosure of the karyotype on a 'need to know' basis is advised so that the child is not treated differently or regarded differently by others. Telling a child about his 47,XXY karyotype should be a gradual process extending over many years, with parents being supported in this by health professionals.
- Refer to a paediatric endocrinologist at around 10yrs of age for monitoring of growth and measurement of testosterone, follicle-stimulating hormone (FSH), and luteinizing hormone (LH). If studies suggest hypergonadotrophic hypogonadism, testosterone supplementation should be offered. Testosterone supplementation (usually given as intramuscular (IM) injections every few weeks or transdermal patches applied daily) improves self-esteem, facial hair growth, and libido. It also has a protective effect in reducing the risk of osteoporosis.
- For management of infertility, refer to a reproductive medicine specialist for consideration of artificial insemination by donor (AID) or assisted conception with *in vitro* fertilization (IVF) and ICSI. Sperm for ICSI may be obtained from ejaculate or testicular biopsy.
- *Some* of the literature mentions an increased risk of cancer in 47,XXY males. One study of men with Klinefelter found that the overall cancer incidence is not increased and concluded that no routine cancer screening seems justified. Breast cancer is more common in XXY men than in XY men (relative risk 20); however, mean age at diagnosis was 72yrs and the actual risk (approximately 3%) remains much lower than in females. There is a very small (<1%) risk of primary mediastinal germ cell tumours that may present with precocious puberty, or respiratory symptoms at age 10–30yrs.

Investigation in secondary care
- Karyotype.
- Measurement of testosterone, follicle-stimulating hormone (FSH), and luteinizing hormone (LH) from early adolescence.

Support groups
Klinefelter's Syndrome Association UK: ℜ www.ksa-uk.co.uk
Klinefelter's Syndrome and Associates: ℜ www.genet.org/ks

Rare chromosomal disorders

Introduction

Given the complexity of DNA, the inherent risks in its replication and the hazards of meiosis, it is not surprising that there are a large number of rare chromosomal disorders. They are briefly mentioned here, without full discussion.

Refer to 📖 Chapter 3, Chromosome basics, p. 60 for notes on chromosome nomenclature. Chromosome deletions and duplications (📖 see Figs. 8.1 and 8.2, p. 293).

22q11 deletion syndrome (includes DiGeorge syndrome, velocardiofacial syndrome)

22q11 deletion syndrome affects ~1/6000 live births. The condition may present to a variety of different health professionals, e.g. PCPs, speech and language therapist, paediatricians, and there is often considerable delay in establishing the diagnosis. Clinical features include:

- Communication and language difficulties.
- Behavioural, psychological, and psychiatric problems.
- Developmental delay.
- Cardiovascular abnormalities (75% significant congenital heart disease).
- Palatal abnormalities, e.g. cleft palate, submucous cleft palate, or velopharyngeal insufficiency, may cause nasal regurgitation during feeding in infancy and hypernasal speech.
- Recurrent infections due to impaired T-cell-mediated immunity.
- Hypocalcaemia due to hypoparathyroidism—may present in infancy or later, e.g. adolescence or adult life.

Genetics

- Approximately 90% occur *de novo* and 10% are inherited.
- If either parent is found to carry the 22q deletion, the recurrence risk is 50% for future pregnancies. The affected child will have a 50% risk of transmitting the deletion to his/her offspring in any pregnancy.
- If neither parent carries the 22q deletion, the recurrence risk is very small (~1%).
- Prenatal diagnosis possible by chorionic villus sampling (CVS) at 11–12 weeks or amniocentesis at 15–16 weeks.

Other well-defined chromosome deletion syndromes

Angelman syndrome del(15q11–13): maternal homologue deleted ♒ www.angelmanuk.org/
Prader–Willi syndrome del(15q11–13): paternal homologue deleted ♒ www.pwsa.co.uk/
Smith–Magenis syndrome del(17p11.2): ♒ www.smith-magenis.co.uk
Williams syndrome del(7q11.23): ♒ www.williams-syndrome.org.uk/

In general, a duplication of chromosomal material is better tolerated than a deletion.

If de novo apparently isolated deletion or duplication

Recurrence risk is very low.

Prenatal diagnosis—🖎 refer to Clinical Genetics
Prenatal diagnosis may be offered/requested for reassurance and is possible by CVS at 11–12 weeks/amniocentesis at 15–16 weeks. Both invasive procedures carry a small (~1%) risk of miscarriage.

If apparently identical deletion/duplication in parent
Recurrence risk
If an individual carrying the deletion/duplication reproduces, the risk in each pregnancy for a child carrying the deletion/duplication is 50%.

Prenatal diagnosis—🖎 refer to Clinical Genetics
Possible by CVS/amniocentesis and may be considered by those families in which the deletion/duplication is the cause of abnormality.

Trisomies

Edwards' syndrome (trisomy 18)
Trisomy 18 is associated with a high rate of spontaneous loss in pregnancy and very poor outcomes in surviving infants. Trisomy 18 has an incidence of 1/7900 live births with a strong female excess. 85% are maternal in origin and there is a strong maternal age effect (as for trisomy 21).

Clinical features
The most striking features in the newborn are small for dates, short sternum, and congenital heart disease (CHD).
- **Growth retardation.** Mean birth weight 2240g (weight, length, and occipital-frontal circumference (OFC) <3rd centile), with postnatal failure to thrive.
- **Dysmorphic features.** Prominent occiput, simple ears, irregular ribs on CXR, rocker-bottom feet.
- **Congenital anomalies.** At least 90% have CHD, usually ventricular septal defect (VSD) ± valve dysplasia.
- **Developmental disability.** Developmental quotient (developmental age/chronological age) averages 0.18, i.e. severe to profound developmental delay, but falls further in older children.
- **Short life expectancy.** Median life expectancy is 4 days and survival beyond the first year of life is exceptional.

Genetics
Sibling recurrence risk is very low at 0.55%. For mothers aged >37yrs, the risk for a +21 pregnancy exceeds that for a recurrence of +18.

Prenatal diagnosis
Prenatal diagnosis by CVS/amniocentesis should be offered but, in view of the low recurrence risk, some couples may prefer the option of surveillance of the pregnancy by a combination of:
- First trimester screening: USS at 10–14 weeks' gestation.
- Second trimester screening: maternal serum screen (AFP), unconjugated oestriol (typically low in +18 pregnancies), and human chorionic gonadotrophin.
- Detailed fetal anomaly: USS at 19–20 weeks' gestation.

Combining the above it should be possible to detect in excess of 80% of affected pregnancies, reducing the already low recurrence risk of 1/200 to closer to 1/1000.

Patau syndrome (trisomy 13)

Patau syndrome is associated with a high rate of spontaneous loss in pregnancy and a very poor outcome in surviving infants due to a combination of multiple congenital anomalies (e.g. cleft lip, congenital heart disease, holoprosencephaly) and severe/profound mental retardation.

Genetics

Sibling recurrence risk is low at ~0.5%. For mothers aged >37yrs, the risk for a +21 pregnancy exceeds that for a recurrence of +13.

Prenatal diagnosis

Prenatal diagnosis by CVS/amniocentesis should be offered but, in view of the low recurrence risk, some couples may prefer the option of surveillance of the pregnancy by a combination of:

- Nuchal scan at 12 weeks.
- Detailed fetal anomaly: USS at 16 weeks' and 19–20 weeks' gestation.

Because of the high incidence of structural malformation in Patau syndrome, there is a high detection rate (~90%) on fetal anomaly USS.

Support groups

Unique—The Rare Chromosome Disorder Support Group: ☎ 01883 330766; 🖰 www.rarechromo.org
SOFT UK (Support organization for Trisomy 18, 13 and related disorders): 🖰 www.soft.org.uk
ARC (Antenatal Results and Choices): ☎ 020 7631 0285; 🖰 www.arc-uk.org

Translocations

Approximately 1/700 individuals carries a chromosome translocation. In the example below, there is no net loss or gain of genetic material, and this is referred to as a **reciprocal balanced** translocation (☐ see Fig. 8.4).

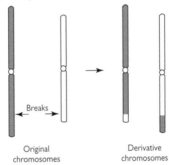

Breaks

Original
chromosomes

Derivative
chromosomes

Fig. 8.4 Reciprocal translocation. (Reproduced from Young, *Medical Genetics* (2005), Figure 2.15a, p. 40, with permission from Oxford University Press.)

Such rearrangements are commonly unique to a family and may come to light during the investigation of babies and children with congenital malformations, developmental delay, and/or learning disability, or in the work-up of patients with recurrent miscarriage or subfertility. They may occasionally be identified on karyotyping performed for maternal age indications, increased nuchal translucency, or abnormal ultrasound scan (USS) findings. Determining whether the finding is incidental or causative, in the case of investigation of abnormal USS findings, is crucial.

The terminology is as follows.
- **De novo.** If the abnormality is not found in either parent, it is described as de novo (also, silently, consider the possibility of non-paternity).
- **Familial.** Inherited from a parent.

The investigation and risk assessment of translocations, however discovered, demands expert genetic advice.

Balanced autosomal reciprocal translocations are common, carried by >0.1% of the population, and usually harmless. However, in simplistic terms, following meiosis there are four possible outcomes to any pregnancy of a carrier of a balanced autosomal reciprocal translocation. These are a pregnancy with:
- A *normal* karyotype.
- A *balanced* autosomal reciprocal translocation (as in the parent).
- An *unbalanced* product of the translocation, resulting in spontaneous pregnancy loss, e.g. miscarriage or intrauterine (fetal) death (IUD).
- An *unbalanced* product of the translocation that is viable, resulting in a child with a high likelihood of learning disability with/without congenital anomalies.

Where there *is* net loss or gain of genetic material, this is referred to as an **unbalanced** translocation. Unbalanced translocations tend to be severe in their effect, often causing serious abnormalities (☐ see Fig. 8.5).

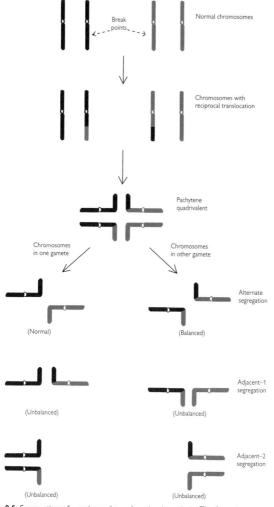

Fig. 8.5 Segregation of a reciprocal translocation in meiosis. The four chromosomes form a quadrivalent in pachytene in meiosis I. Alternate segregation results in all gametes having either a normal or a balanced chromosome complement. Both adjacent-1 (non-homologous centromeres segregate together) and adjacent-2 (homologous centromeres segregate together) segregation result in all gametes having an unbalanced chromosome complement. (Reproduced from Young (2005). *Medical Genetics*, Fig. 2.17, p. 45, with permission from Oxford University Press.)

Robertsonian translocations

A **Robertsonian translocation** is named after W.R.B. Robertson who first described fusion of acrocentric chromosomes in insects (📖 see Fig. 8.6).

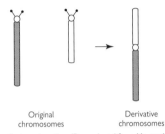

Original
chromosomes

Derivative
chromosomes

Fig. 8.6 Robertsonian translocation. (Reproduced from Young (2005). *Medical Genetics*, Fig. 2.7, p. 45, with permission from Oxford University Press.)

The human acrocentric chromosomes that may be involved in a Robertsonian translocation are numbers 13, 14, 15, 21, and 22. The fused chromosome contains the long arms of the two component chromosomes but lacks some or all of the short arms. The short arms contain the nucleolar organizing regions (NOR) but, as there are other copies of these genes, their loss does not have a phenotypic effect. Thus, though a carrier of such a translocation has only 45 chromosomes, they will be balanced as they effectively have a full complement of functional chromosomes. One example is the Robertsonian translocation rob(14;21), the cause of 2% of Down syndrome, but other Robertsonian translocations, e.g. rob(13;14), will give similar outcomes, in this case with Patau syndrome (due to three copies of chromosome 13) replacing Down syndrome. There are four possible outcomes to pregnancy. These are a pregnancy with:

• A *normal* karyotype; e.g. 46,XX or 46,XY.
• A *balanced* Robertsonian translocation (as in the parent), e.g. 45,XX rob(14;21); or 45,XY rob(14;21).
• An *unbalanced* product of the translocation resulting in spontaneous pregnancy loss (e.g. miscarriage), e.g. 46,XX rob(14;21) + 14 or 46,XY rob(14;21) + 14 will both effectively result in an additional chromosome 14 which is not viable.
• An *unbalanced* product of the translocation that is viable, resulting in a child with a high likelihood of learning disability with/without congenital anomalies, e.g. 46,XX rob(14;21) + 21 or 46,XY rob(14;21) + 21, which both result in Down syndrome due to the additional chromosome 21.

Consultation plan in primary care

PCPs should consider including in their referral to Genetics:
• Three-generation family tree.
• History of recurrent miscarriage/ IUD/subfertility.
• History of learning disability, developmental delay, congenital anomaly.
• Has any family member been seen by Genetics? Where and when?

Management in general practice

This will clearly be on an individual basis but, for any child with a chromosome rearrangement ensure that:
• The child's notes are marked with this information.
• The child's parents know that they should request an appointment in the Genetics clinic when the child is in his/her mid-teens.

Genetics

Investigations
• Karyotyping, including parents of an affected child.
• Possible analysis of genes at the breakpoint, e.g. FISH, array-CGH.

Recurrence risk—✎ refer to Clinical Genetics
• For an individual known to carry a translocation, seek expert advice to assess the risk of a viable imbalance.
• In a child affected with a *de novo* change, the risk to future siblings is very small, but prenatal diagnosis will usually be offered.

Prenatal diagnosis—✎ refer to Clinical Genetics
Possible by CVS at 11–12 weeks or by amniocentesis at 15–16 weeks. Both techniques are invasive and incur a small risk of miscarriage (~1%).

Support groups

Unique—The Rare Chromosome Disorder Support Group: ☎ 01883 330766; 🖱 www.rarechromo.org
ARC (Antenatal Results and Choices): ☎ 020 7631 0285; 🖱 www.arc-uk.org

Triple X syndrome (47,XXX)

47,XXX may be diagnosed incidentally at amniocentesis/CVS. It occasionally comes to light later in life, but usually as an incidental finding. The incidence is 1/1000 to 1/1200 female births, with significant maternal age effect. It is substantially underdiagnosed and the majority of 47,XXX women are unaware of their karyotype.

Clinical features

- A normal female appearance is usual from birth through to old age.
- Tall stature is a consistent finding.
- Full-scale intelligence quotient (IQ) averages 10–15 points less than that of siblings. Mental retardation is not associated with 47,XXX.
- Sexual development and puberty are normal.
- Most 47,XXX women are fertile and have chromosomally normal babies. There may be a slightly increased risk for premature ovarian failure (POF).

Genetics

- Parents of girls with 47,XXX are not routinely karyotyped. The recurrence risk is low, <1%.
- Offspring risk: the risk for chromosome anomaly in women with 47,XXX is very low, <1%.
- Prenatal diagnosis should be offered to parents and to women with 47,XXX but there is a fine balance between the very small risk of recurrence and the risk of procedure-associated pregnancy loss.

Support group

Unique—The Rare Chromosome Disorder Support Group: ☎ 01883 330766; ✆ www.rarechromo.org

Turner syndrome (45,X and variants)

Introduction

Turner described the features of this syndrome in 1938, and in 1959 it was found that girls with Turner syndrome (TS) had an absent X chromosome (45,X karyotype). It affects 1 in 2500 live female births. The majority (up to 99%) of TS conceptions are lost as spontaneous abortions. The rate of intrauterine lethality between 12 and 40 weeks' gestation is ~65%. Diagnosis may be missed in childhood, but in general terms:

- One-third of TS is diagnosed in the neonatal period.
- One-third in childhood.
- One-third in adolescence.

In some females with TS there may be a normal X chromosome and a structurally rearranged X chromosome. In addition, mosaicism is frequently present, particularly when multiple tissues are tested (📖 see Chapter 2, Mosaicism, p. 46).

Physical features

There is considerable phenotypic variation in TS. In some girls there may be few features other than short stature to suggest the diagnosis. The phenotype can be sufficiently subtle that a karyotype is routinely included in the evaluation of girls with short stature because otherwise this diagnosis may be missed.

- **Short stature** and **gonadal dysgenesis** are the two features found in the majority of females with TS. The untreated mean adult height is 147cm, but this is increased following growth hormone (GH) therapy in childhood. Physical features such as the short, broad, webbed neck, ptosis, and low hairline are secondary to fetal oedema/hydrops and may be absent. Motor milestones may be slightly delayed.
- **Cardiovascular malformations** are found in 15–50%, particularly coarctation of the aorta and ventricular septal defect (VSD).
- **Oedema of the hands and feet** is a common finding in the newborn with TS.
- **Renal anomalies** including horseshoe kidney, other structural abnormalities, and agenesis are found in about one-third.
- **Puberty and sexual development.** Poor growth, with no pubertal growth spurt, and absent or minimal breast development is usual. Some women have a few periods and this is more likely in the presence of a 46,XX cell line.
- **Education.** Intelligence is usually normal but mean intelligence quotient (IQ) is generally 10–15 points lower than that of siblings. Mild speech and language delay is common. Individuals with TS have relative difficulty on measures of spatial/perceptual skills, visual–motor integration, visual memory, and attention. Most girls with TS attend mainstream schools.
- **Behaviour.** Social adjustment problems are common. Girls with TS may also have subtle perceptual difficulties, e.g. difficulties with facial affect recognition.
- **Employment.** Most women with TS lead independent adult lives.
- **Fertility and pregnancy.** The majority of women with TS are infertile. *In vitro* fertilization (IVF) with donor oocytes has resulted in successful pregnancy for some women with TS. In women with Turner syndrome,

the risk for aortic dissection or rupture during pregnancy may be 2% or higher, and the risk of death during pregnancy is increased as much as 100-fold. It is imperative that patients are assessed by a cardiologist (including echocardiogram) and advised of the potential cardiovascular risks before attempting to become pregnant (see below).

- **Deafness.** High-frequency sensorineural hearing loss is very common and may be a premature variant of presbycusis.
- **Cancer.** Breast cancer is very uncommon in women with TS.

Genetics

Recurrence risk

After the birth of a child (or the loss of a pregnancy) with 45,X the risk of recurrence is very low.

Offspring risk

- Natural fertility is rare. Prenatal diagnosis should be offered because of the increased risk for trisomy 21 and 45,X.
- Women carrying structural rearrangements are at risk for a similarly affected female or a more severe problem in a male fetus, which may not be viable. Prenatal diagnosis is possible by either CVS or amniocentesis.

Prenatal diagnosis

Recurrence risk is very low (<1%). Prenatal diagnosis based on this indication should be offered by CVS at 11–12 weeks or amniocentesis at 15–16 weeks, but the risk of recurrence is less than the procedure associated miscarriage risk of ~1%. USS for nuchal translucency (NT) at 10–14 weeks, to examine for evidence of hydrops, is a non-invasive screening test which, if normal, may reduce the already small recurrence risk.

Consultation plan in primary care

History

- Developmental milestones.
- Deafness.
- Obstetric and gynaecological history.

Examination

- Height/length.
- Neck short, broad, webbed; low posterior hairline.
- Hands and feet: puffiness/oedema. Short metacarpals/metatarsals, especially 4th. Small nails.
- Chest. Widely spaced nipples; chest described as shield-shaped. Breast development.
- Cardiovascular system. Delayed femoral pulses, heart murmurs, raised blood pressure.
- Skin. Pigmented naevi.
- Secondary sexual development and external genitalia (if appropriate).

Management in primary care

Recognition, or suspicion, of Turner syndrome will require a subsequent referral to a paediatrician. Ongoing management of the affected girl and her family will be largely supportive. To offer effective support, a working knowledge of probable secondary-care management at different life stages is described.

Investigation in secondary care

- A karyotype that includes counting 30 cells to establish if there is mosaicism. Parental karyotypes are not requested in the presence of non-mosaic 45,X. Maternal karyotypes are indicated when a girl has 46,XX and a structurally abnormal second X. Mosaicism involving 46,XY in the presence of a female phenotype requires consideration of the risk of gonadoblastoma in the residual gonadal tissue.
- Possible fluorescent *in situ* hybridization (FISH) studies in girls with a ring X chromosome.
- Echocardiogram.
- Renal ultrasound scan (USS).
- Audiogram.

Management in secondary care

Antenatal/neonatal TS

When TS has been detected due to the presence of fetal oedema/hydrops, there is a high chance that the pregnancy will be lost naturally. Women in whom the pregnancy is ongoing, will be scanned for cardiac and renal anomalies. When detected incidentally, with no associated hydrops, the survival may be longer and the phenotype milder. In the newly diagnosed neonate the same scans are indicated. Parents will be given information about future surveillance (📖 see p. 315).

Childhood

All girls known to have TS should be under the care of a paediatric endocrinologist. Short stature, due to a combination of the loss of growth genes on the X and an absent pubertal growth spurt, can be partially corrected by growth hormone (GH) in childhood, but the overall gain in height is comparatively small (<5cm). Recurrent otitis media is common, affecting ~two-thirds of girls, and a sensorineural dip in hearing that progresses over time has been observed as early as 6yrs of age. Careful surveillance for deafness is important to facilitate language acquisition and schooling.

Adolescence

Oestrogen replacement therapy may be initiated at the usual age of puberty, with blood pressure monitoring. Deafness and autoimmune disease may present in this age group. Schooling and emotional difficulties may require management.

Adults with TS

In addition to primary ovarian failure, adults with TS are also susceptible to a range of disorders, including osteoporosis, hypothyroidism, and renal and gastrointestinal disease. The problems of adult life are the following.

- ***Primary ovarian failure*** (📖 see Chapter 9, Amenorrhoea, infertility, and premature ovarian failure (POF), p. 320). Sex hormone replacement can be continued. Ovum donation provides an option for some women with TS to become pregnant.
  The prevalence of osteoporosis and bone fractures is not increased significantly in women with TS who are treated with standard oestrogen

therapy. However women <150cm in height are likely to be misdiagnosed with osteoporosis when bone density is measured, unless adjustments for body size are made.

- *Autoimmune diseases.* Hypothyroidism is a common problem; also diabetes mellitus (15%) and inflammatory bowel disease.
- *Obesity.* Ensure that hypothyroidism has been excluded.
- *Deafness.* High-frequency sensorineural hearing loss is very common and may be a premature variant of presbycusis.
- *Reduced life expectancy.* The life expectancy in TS is reduced due to obesity and cardiovascular disease, mainly ischaemic heart disease but also aortic dissection, which is more common in individuals with pre-existing coarctation.
- *Bowel.* Bleeding and protein loss due to telangiectasiae.

Surveillance

With the aim of improving life expectancy and reducing morbidity, it is recommended that women stay under the care of an endocrinologist, or specialist with experience of TS or, preferably, a multidisciplinary Turner clinic to co-ordinate surveillance. PCPs are likely to be able to contribute to the suggested screening tests that include:

- Annual assessment of weight and blood pressure. Consider tests of glucose and bone metabolism, liver function tests, renal function if symptomatic.
- Thyroid function tests—baseline and then as required.
- Cardiovascular risk profile—increased risk for ischaemic heart disease.
- Cardiac review—increased risk for aortic dissection (baseline echocardiogram as a young adult, then as required).
- Bone density scan—baseline as a young adult, then as required.
- Hearing test (audiometry).

Support group

Turner Syndrome Support Society: ✆ www.tss.org.uk

47,XYY

An extra Y chromosome is found in approximately 1 in 1000 male births. There is no advanced paternal age effect. From cytogenetic study of series of consecutive live births, it appears that the great majority of cases of 47,XYY (at least 85%) probably remain undiagnosed throughout life.

Clinical features

- **Puberty.** The growth spurt is prolonged, with a final mean height of 188cm (91st–98th centile). Secondary sexual development is normal, but the onset may be delayed by about 6 months compared to that of controls.
- **Educational.** There is a small but significant lowering of the intelligence quotient (IQ) scores, with the mean 10–15 points lower than that of siblings, but remaining within the normal range. Most boys with 47,XYY will attend mainstream school.
- **Behaviour.** Behavioural problems are more common in males with XYY, especially in those with learning difficulties. Much attention has been paid to the association of criminal behaviour and XYY. The mean IQ scores are lower in those with criminal convictions (mainly property offences rather than crimes against persons), and lowered intelligence appears to be the major risk factor for antisocial and criminal behaviour. There is no association between 47,XYY *per se* and criminality.
- **Fertility.** Most men with XYY are fertile and the majority of sperm in 47,XYY men are chromosomally normal.

Genetics

- **Recurrence risk.** Fathers of boys with XYY are not routinely karyotyped. The recurrence risk is low, <1%.
- **Offspring risk.** The majority of sperm in 47,XYY men are chromosomally normal and XYY men are not reported to have an increased risk of sons with XYY or XXY.
- Prenatal diagnosis should be offered, but there is a fine balance between the very small risk of recurrence and the risk of procedure-associated pregnancy loss.

Support group

Unique—The Rare Chromosome Disorder Support Group: ☎ 01883 330766; ✍ www.rarechromo.org

Fertility, pregnancy, and newborn

Introduction

It was the best of times, it was the worst of times.

The opening line of Charles Dickens's novel *A Tale of Two Cities* sums up obstetrics in general practice. To look after a woman from pre-conception counselling to a good delivery with a healthy baby is one of the most satisfying aspects of general practice. When things go wrong; the misery of infertility, the desolation of recurrent miscarriage, the despair from the decision to abort an abnormal fetus and the tragedy of an unex-plained intra-uterine death, affect not just the woman and her partner but often the community you serve. Being there to support that patient, her partner, and the wider family and friends is essential general practice. The emotional toll on you, as the care giver, should not be underestimated.

This chapter deals with specific issues relating to genetics, fertility, and congenital malformations.

Further information

Arulkumaran S, Symonds I, and Fowlie A (ed.) (2009) *Oxford Handbook of Obstetrics and Gynaecology*. Oxford University Press.
Arulkumaran S (ed.) (2009) *Emergencies in Obstetrics and Gynaecology*. Oxford University Press.

Amenorrhoea, infertility, and premature ovarian failure (POF)

Primary amenorrhoea

The four most common causes of primary amenorrhea are:
- Gonadal dysgenesis, including Turner syndrome (TS) (48.5%).
- Congenital absence of the uterus and vagina (CAUV) (16.2%).
- Gonadotrophin-releasing hormone (GnRH) deficiency (8.3%).
- Constitutional delay of puberty (6.0%).

These require specialist assessment by a paediatric endocrinologist/reproductive medicine specialist with expertise in adolescent medicine.

> The girl and her family will benefit from support from their PCP during the process of investigation and after a diagnosis is reached, particularly if this has long-term implications for her fertility.

Infertility

Infertility is defined by the failure to conceive after 12 months of unprotected intercourse, and affects an estimated 14% of the population of reproductive age in the UK. Despite advances in the diagnosis of causes of subfertility, inability to conceive remains unexplained in 25–30% of fully investigated couples.

Premature ovarian failure (POF)

The median age at menopause in Western populations is approximately 51yrs. This has not changed since Hippocrates' time. A menopause that occurs at ages 40–45yrs is considered 'early' and occurs in ~5% of women.

> POF is defined as cessation of menses with hypergonadotrophic amenorrhoea below the age of 40yrs.

POF occurs in ~1% of women in the general population. Amongst women with idiopathic sporadic POF, ~2% carry a fragile X pre-mutation (📖 see Chapter 5, Fragile X syndrome, p. 122). Amongst women with familial POF, ~14% carry a FMR1 pre-mutation.

Differential diagnosis of genetic causes

X-chromosome abnormalities: Turner syndrome (TS), mosaic Turner syndrome, X-chromosome rearrangements

45,X karyotype giving rise to female phenotype with short stature and streak gonads. Typically, in TS menopause precedes menarche, and there is no evidence of ovarian function, but occasional individuals with TS may menstruate briefly. This, and POF, may be more likely in women with mosaic TS and rearrangements of the X chromosome. 📖 See Chapter 8, Turner syndrome (45,X and variants), p. 312.

Other causes of gonadal agenesis/dysgenesis (including 46,XY)

- Approximately 80% of XY females with gonadal dysgenesis are of unknown aetiology. They often have a uterus and streak gonads.
- Complete androgen insensitivity syndrome (CAIS) Women have a female phenotype with a 46,XY karyotype. There is primary amenorrhoea due to absent uterus and, on examination, there is absent/sparse pubic and axillary hair. CAIS is caused by mutations in the androgen receptor gene (AR) on the X chromosome. Women and families with CAIS need sensitive discussion with a paediatric endocrinologist/adolescent gynaecologist as the diagnosis can be deeply unsettling to a teenage girl. Referral to a clinical geneticist is also indicated as her female siblings and other maternal female relatives may also be affected or carriers of the familial mutation in the AR gene.

Congenital absence of uterus and vagina (CAUV)

Also known as Mayer–Rokitansky–Kuster–Hauser syndrome or Müllerian aplasia. Prevalence is 1/4000–1/5000 females. Patients with CAUV are genetically and phenotypically female, with 46,XX karyotype, normal ovaries, breast development, and female patterns of body hair. In most CAUV patients, the uterus, cervix, and upper two-thirds of the vagina are absent. Most cases are isolated with only occasional reports of familial occurrence.

Fragile X pre-mutation carrier

Approximately 24% of female fragile X pre-mutation carriers will undergo premature menopause (cessation of menses at <40yrs). This information may be helpful to carrier women for reproductive planning. 📖 See Chapter 5, Fragile X syndrome, p. 122.

Congenital adrenal hyperplasia (CAH)

Non-classical CAH may present with polycystic ovarian syndrome and subfertility in adult life.

Survivor of radiation- and chemotherapy-treated childhood cancer

Approximately one in every six female survivors develops POF.

Consultation plan in primary care

History

- Family history (including age of menarche/menopause of mother, older sisters, etc.).
- Enquire about breast development, menarche, and menstruation (if any).
- Enquire about possible eating disorders, e.g. anorexia nervosa?

Examination

- General physical exam (height, weight, and BMI).
- Assessment of secondary sex characteristics.
- Examine briefly for physical features of Turner syndrome (TS), e.g. short, broad, webbed neck and low posterior hairline, wide carrying angle, shield-shaped chest, heart murmur, and pulses (aortic coarctation).

(Continued)

Investigations
- Blood tests: follicle-stimulating hormone (FSH), luteinizing hormone (LH), prolactin, thyroid function tests (TFTs), and serum progesterone.
- Pelvic ultrasound scan (USS) might be done in secondary care as appropriate.
- Karyotype and/or FMRI might be done in secondary care as appropriate.

Investigation and management in secondary care
- The **geneticist's role** is to explain the genetic basis of the disorder causing infertility/amenorrhoea. Depending on the specific diagnosis, if ART using the patient's own ova could be used to achieve a pregnancy, then advice about reproductive implications is also appropriate.
- Management of the amenorrhoea and infertility is the remit of a specialist in reproductive medicine.
- ART enables pregnancy in some patients. Women with ovarian failure may use donated ova to achieve a pregnancy. Women with CAUV may undergo oocyte retrieval and *in vitro* fertilization (IVF) and have their fetus carried by a surrogate mother.
- Women with POF should be given hormone replacement therapy (HRT) until at least the age of 50yrs.
- The **PCP's role** is to support the affected female through the difficult process of coming to terms with the diagnosis. Family therapy may be required.

Support groups
Müllerian aplasia: rosagroup@yahoo.co.uk
CHILD: The National Infertility Support Network: ☎ 01424 732361; ℅ www.child.org.uk

Antenatal screening for genetic disorders

Antenatal screening in the UK is offered through a variety of approaches (📖 see Fig. 9.1):
- Family history.
- Screening for Down syndrome.
- Fetal anomaly screening programme.
- Sickle cell and thalassaemia screening programme.

Screening tests in pregnancy should follow the general rules:
- They are offered to a population only after it has been proved that they are effective.
- Resources are available to deliver a high-quality service to the population as a whole.
- They are performed at a stage in pregnancy when effective management or treatment is possible.
- The potential benefits of the screening test outweigh any possible risks from the test. For example, a positive result from a non-invasive screening test may lead to the offer of an invasive test to determine whether the fetus is affected. (Since invasive testing carries a small risk of miscarriage, the threshold for invasive testing determines both the percentage of affected pregnancies identified and the percentage of normal pregnancies miscarried following an invasive test, e.g. CVS/amniocentesis.)

Family history

This is the simplest and sometimes the most important screening test! Its efficacy depends upon the diligence of the midwife/PCP/obstetrician taking the family history and recognizing when a genetic referral is indicated (📖 see Chapter 2, Taking a family history, p. 52).

A three-generation family tree should include enquiry about consanguinity, neonatal death, malformations, handicaps, and ethnicity. Refer to Clinical Genetics if indicated.

Screening for Down syndrome

In the UK the National Screening Committee (2008) has recommended that screening in pregnancy for Down syndrome should achieve a detection rate (DR) for Down syndrome of >75% of affected pregnancies with a screen positive rate (SPR) of <3%, improving to a DR of >90% with a SPR of <2% by 2010. Screening for Down syndrome is now offered to women of all ages and there is no additional routine maternal age screening for trisomies. There are a various approaches:
- *First trimester combined test.* This is the preferred method for women who book before 14 weeks. This test is only valid up to 13 weeks + 6 days of pregnancy with the optimal time for testing between 11 + 0 to 13 + 0 weeks. The test uses the combination of nuchal translucency measurement with serum biochemistry to measure

beta-hCG and pregnancy-associated plasma protein A (PAPP-A). Maternal age, gestation and other factors such as weight are also factored in, to compute a risk estimate for Down syndrome. Women with a risk of 1 in 150 or above are offered a CVS to obtain the fetal karyotype. Rapid testing by FISH or QFPCR may be available to women at particularly increased risk.

- **Late bookers quadruple test.** Not all women book for pregnancy care in the first trimester. This is the recommended screening test for late bookers. It is a serum biochemical test measuring hCG (all types), unconjugated oestriol (uE$_3$), AFP, and inhibin A, and can be undertaken between 15 + 0 and 20 + 0 weeks. Women with a 1 in 200 risk or higher are offered amniocentesis.
- **Cell-free free fetal DNA.** Current research suggests that it is likely that over the next few years screening for Down syndrome by analysis of cell-free fetal nucleic acids (e.g. cffDNA or cffRNA) in maternal blood may become possible.

Serum screening abnormalities can suggest an increased risk for other abnormalities, e.g. low maternal oestriol (see Low maternal serum oestriol, p. 375) and Edwards syndrome—trisomy 18 (see Chapter 8, Rare chromosomal disorders, p. 302), but only the trisomy 21 risk will be reported from the first trimester combined test.

Fetal anomaly screening programme

This is an ultrasound-based screening programme performed between 18+0 and 20+6 weeks to examine fetal growth and development. There is guidance to sonographers about the detail required. The recommendations are under revision but include a systematic check of some of the external features of the baby and some of the internal organs, e.g. heart. See Imaging in prenatal diagnosis, p. 366.

Neural tube defects (NTD)

Serum AFP is not routinely offered if anomaly scanning is used to screen for NTD.

Infectious diseases

- Hepatitis B (Hep B), HIV, rubella and syphilis testing is performed in the UK.
- Routine cytomegalovirus (CMV) and toxoplasmosis, hepatitis C and Group B streptococcus screening are not routine or recommended in UK.

Haemoglobinopathies

- In areas of high prevalence of sickle cell disease (>1.5 per 10 000 pregnancies), there is universal screening by high-performance liquid chromotography (HPLC) to identify carriers of sickle and thalassaemia. Use of the family origin questionnaire (FOQ) at www.sickleandthal. org.uk can help to identify the likelihood of alpha-thalassaemia.
- In areas of low prevalence of sickle cell disease, all pregnant women should be screened for thalassaemia using the MCH. Women with levels of <27 picograms, and at high risk using the family origin questionnaire, should be screened for thalassaemia. If at high risk of sickle cell disease from the FOQ, request HPLC.

Further information

🔗 www.screening.nhs.uk

NHS Fetal Anomaly Screening Programme-Screening for Down's syndrome: UK NSC Policy recommendations 2007-2010: Model of Best Practice (2008). Available at 🔗 www.fetalanomaly.screening.nhs/publications

🔗 www.nscfa.web.its.manchester.ac.uk

Antenatal care. Routine care for the healthy pregnant woman. NICE clinical guideline 62 (March 2008). Available at 🔗 www.nice.org.uk

Family origin questionnaire: 🔗 www.sickleandthal.org.uk

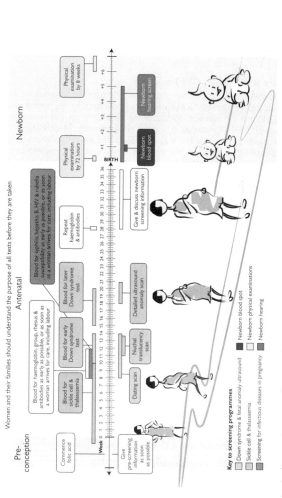

Fig. 9.1 Screening timeline—optimum times for testing. Screening timeline version 2, March 2008. (Reproduced with permission of the UK National Screening Committee www.screening.nhs.uk/an ©2008.) (Also see p. 412.)

Assisted reproductive technology

Assisted reproductive technology (ART) has revolutionized the treatment of infertility. Treatment with ART now accounts for 1–3% of all births in many Western countries. In conjunction with single-cell genetic analysis based on polymerase chain reaction (PCR) or fluorescent *in situ* hybridization (FISH) it has also made pre-implantation genetic diagnosis (PGD) possible for some genetic disorders.

In vitro fertilization (IVF)

Controlled stimulation of the ovaries with exogenous gonadotrophins leads to the recruitment of many follicles (monitored by ultrasound scan (USS)). When the number and size of the developing follicles is deemed appropriate, oocyte maturation is triggered hormonally. 34–38h later, the oocytes are collected by transvaginal USS-guided aspiration of the follicular fluid. The oocytes are then fertilized *in vitro* with the partner's sperm and any resulting morphologically sound embryos are transferred into the woman's uterus 2 days later.

In a study, 9.0% of infants conceived with IVF had a major birth defect diagnosed by 1yr of age, compared with 4.2% of the normal population. Excess defects were observed in multiple, singleton, and term singleton births. Risk of low birth weight (not due to prematurity) was 2.6 times that of the general population for singletons.

> Use of ART roughly doubles the risk of having a term singleton with low birth weight or a child with a major birth defect and greatly increases the risk of multiple pregnancy with increased risk of prematurity and consequent low birth weight. There is an increased risk for imprinting disorders such as Beckwith–Weidemann syndrome after IVF and ICSI but, despite the increased relative risk, the absolute risk appears to be low.

Intracytoplasmic sperm injection (ICSI)

ICSI involves the injection of a single sperm directly into a mature oocyte. ICSI is favoured for fertility patients where there is male factor infertility, including azoospermia, oligozoospermia, and poor morphology or motility. Additionally, ICSI is used for PCR-based PGD techniques, to avoid the risk of extracting extra sperm, buried in the zona pellucida, at embryo biopsy, which would contaminate the assay.

8.6% of infants conceived with ICSI have a major birth defect diagnosed by 1yr of age, compared with 4.2% of the normal population.

Pre-implantation genetic diagnosis (PGD)

Most couples requesting PGD do so because they wish to avoid the possibility of terminating a pregnancy following prenatal diagnosis. Others may require ART anyway to circumvent a fertility problem that may be caused by a genetic disorder, e.g. congenital bilateral absence of the vas deferens (CBAVD), as well as the presence of a genetic risk to the offspring.

PGD was first introduced for sexing embryos in the case of X-linked genetic disorders in 1990. In 1992 the first case of a live-born girl after successful PGD for the single-gene disorder, cystic fibrosis, was reported. In 1995 the successful outcome of a pregnancy following PGD for Duchenne muscular dystrophy was achieved.

While PGD is an attractive option to couples facing a high risk for a genetic disorder, in practical terms it can be a challenging option to pursue. Problems include: the need for IVF (🕮 see p. 328), the high cost of IVF & PGD, limited availability of these highly specialist and expensive services, difficulty in access due to provision in only a few specialist centres, limited data on long-term outcomes, etc.

Outcome of liveborn babies

Evidence suggests that human embryo development *in vitro* is not affected by biopsy at the 8-cell stage, but on-going pregnancies should be closely monitored by USS. In the very small number of pregnancies that have been followed through and published, the perinatal mortality rate was 1%. Prematurity was the most commonly reported neonatal complication (37%), which in turn was related to the number of multiple pregnancies. Overall, the congenital malformation rate was 6.6% (3.9% major; 2.7% minor).

Many centres are not able to offer PGD to couples with rare mutations that may be family specific, although the development of SNP genotyping may permit PGD once the causal gene has been identified.

Regulation of PGD

The regulation of PGD worldwide varies from country to country. In many countries where regulations do apply, the bodies responsible for ART will also regulate PGD. The UK Human Fertilisation and Embryology Act (HFE Act 1990) came into being and, in accordance with the Act, the Human Fertilization and Embryology Authority (HFEA) regulates all ART, including PGD, in the UK.

Success rate

The pregnancy and live-birth success rates of PGD are comparable to those for infertile couples undergoing ART (22% per embryo transferred). Given that the majority of couples referred for PGD are fertile, the chance of success must be discussed with couples in detail prior to the start of treatment.

Side-effects of treatment

The occurrence of ovarian hyperstimulation syndrome (OHSS) is relatively common, but can vary in its clinical severity from mild to severe and life-threatening. In its mildest form it is likely to occur in 8–23% of cases and, in its severe form, in 0.1–2% of cases.

Misdiagnosis

There have been reports of misdiagnoses in PGD cycles. The technology of single-cell analysis is complex and demanding and all couples are made aware of the chance of this happening. There are several possible reasons for misdiagnosis, including:

- Mosaicism: this may occur if the cell analysed is not representative of the embryo biopsied.
- Allele drop-out (ADO): this results in effective amplification of only one of the two parental alleles being studied.
- The need to apply large numbers of PCR (DNA amplification) cycles to obtain sufficient DNA for diagnosis creates scope for contamination.

Cost

In the UK, funding for PGD is not centrally organized within the NHS. Most local health authorities will apply their policy for funding IVF treatment to PGD and this may vary from area to area. Couples who are unsuccessful in their application for health authority funding will face a costly bill of several thousand pounds per cycle, making treatment inaccessible for many.

Special issues

- ***HLA tissue typing for bone marrow transplantation (BMT).*** One of the most controversial uses of PGD, for which the HFEA (UK) has just granted one ART centre a licence to practise, is that of HLA typing to provide a compatible bone-marrow-matched child for a sibling with a genetic disorder.

Congenital infections

The fetus with a maternally acquired infection may present during pregnancy with ultrasound scan abnormalities such as:
- Hydrops/fetal ascites (particularly parvovirus).
- Poor fetal growth.
- CNS features of reduced brain growth, intracranial calcification, brain cysts, ventriculomegaly.
- Hyperechogenic bowel (📖 see Fetal abnormalities: hyperechogenic bowel (hyperechoic bowel), p. 352).
- Oligohydramnios.

Neonates and babies may present to midwives, PCPs, or paediatricians with a low birth weight, small occipital-frontal circumference (OFC), lethargy, failure to thrive, petichiae/rash, or prolonged jaundice, along with neurological and developmental problems.

This section reviews the following congenital infections:
- Cytomegalovirus (CMV)
- Parvovirus
- Rubella
- Toxoplasmosis
- Varicella.

Cytomegalovirus (CMV)

CMV is by far the most common serious intrauterine infection, with an incidence of symptomatic disease at birth of 0.1%. CMV is a member of the herpes virus family; primary disease is more likely to lead to congenital infection than recurrent infection. The virus is transmitted by close personal contact (saliva, genital tract, breast milk).

The severity of infection is related to gestation at the time of infection: those fetuses acquiring infection in the first trimester have relatively severe consequences, whereas those infected during the third trimester may be asymptomatic. Of the 10% with signs, there is a significant mortality and about 20% with typical features die in the perinatal period.

Parvovirus B19 (fifth disease, slapped cheek syndrome)

This virus was identified in 1975 and is the cause of the common childhood infectious disease, fifth disease, also known as 'slapped cheek syndrome'. The name 'fifth disease' arose because it was the fifth cause of a superficial red rash of childhood to be identified. If a woman is infected in early pregnancy she has an additional 10% risk of miscarriage. The main risk in mid-trimester is the development of fetal hydrops secondary to anaemia. Intrauterine transfusion may be used to manage affected fetuses with progressive hydrops.

Rubella

Maternal rubella infection at 8–10 weeks' gestation results in fetal damage in up to 90% of infants and multiple defects are common; by 16 weeks gestation the risk of damage declines to ~10–20%, and fetal damage is rare after this stage in pregnancy.

Some affected infants appear normal at birth, but sensorineural deafness is detected later, and before immunization programmes were introduced, congenital rubella syndrome (CRS) was an important cause of congenital deafness.

Rubella re-infection can occur in individuals with either natural or vaccine-induced antibody. Occasional cases of CRS after re-infection in pregnancy have been reported. Although the risk to the fetus cannot be quantified precisely, it is considered to be low.

Rubella vaccine

The vaccine virus is *not* transmitted from vaccinees to susceptible contacts. Thus there is no risk to pregnant women from contact with recently immunized subjects. Active surveillance in the USA, UK, and Germany has found no case of CRS following inadvertent immunization shortly before or during pregnancy.

- Termination of pregnancy (TOP) following inadvertent immunization should *not* be recommended (UK Department of Health 1996).
- Nevertheless, rubella vaccine should not be given to a woman known to be pregnant, and pregnancy should be avoided for 1 month after immunization (UK Department of Health 1996).

Women found to be rubella virus antibody negative on antenatal screening should be immunized after delivery and before discharge from the maternity unit in order to provide protection in a subsequent pregnancy (Department of Health 1996).

Toxoplasmosis

Congenital toxoplasmosis is caused by a parasite, *Toxoplasma gondii*. The maternal signs and symptoms of toxoplasmosis include fever, tiredness, and lymphadenopathy, although the infection is often asymptomatic. In the pregnant mother, the infection is caught by eating anything infected or contaminated with the parasite such as:

- Raw or undercooked meat.
- Food contaminated with cat faeces or with contaminated soil.
- Unpasteurized goats milk.

The fetus is infected across the placenta from an infected mother. The brain and retina are particularly affected.

The rate of transmission depends on the point in gestation at which the mother acquires the infection. In a recent European review, none of the mothers infected in the first trimester had affected babies ($n = 45$), there was transmission in 17% of mothers with seroconversion or probable infection in the second trimester, and a transmission rate of 35% with infection in the third trimester. Overall there is a ~40% chance of fetal infection from affected mothers. 80–90% of infants with congenital toxoplasmosis are asymptomatic at birth and thus careful clinical assessment, particularly of the eye and central nervous system (CNS), is required. Antibiotic treatment during pregnancy can reduce the rate of complications.

Making a firm antenatal diagnosis can be difficult due to problems timing the onset of the infection, because IgM titres stay positive for years in some cases. Diagnosis of toxoplasmosis should be made in conjunction with colleagues in microbiology and a national reference laboratory.

Varicella

Varicella (chickenpox) is an acute highly infectious disease that is transmitted by personal contact or droplet spread. The incubation period is 2–3 weeks. Chickenpox is usually a mild illness in childhood, but can be more serious in adults, especially pregnant women who are at risk of fulminating varicella pneumonia.

Women who develop chickenpox during the first 20 weeks of pregnancy have a 1–2% risk of having a baby with congenital varicella infection. The syndrome comprises congenital limb hypoplasia, skin scarring usually involving one or a few dermatomes, and damage to the eyes and central nervous system (CNS).

Most cases of congenital varicella syndrome follow maternal varicella at 8–20 weeks' gestation. The risk of congenital varicella syndrome after maternal herpes zoster is very low.

Management of the mother

Maternal varicella can be a serious and even fatal condition (risk of pneumonitis and encephalitis).

- PCPs must seek advice from an infectious diseases expert or virologist and give consideration to the use of aciclovir.
- If a pregnant woman has no history of chickenpox or zoster and has recently been in contact with a case of chickenpox or zoster, take a 10mL clotted blood sample for varicella zoster virus (VZV) IgG assay. Pregnant woman with no immunity to VZV should be offered zoster immune globulin (ZIG) in these circumstances.

Consultation plan in primary care

History
- Detailed information regarding dating of the pregnancy.
- Date as accurately as possible the day(s) of contact.
- Verify the diagnosis in the infected individual (where possible).
- Enquire for symptoms of infection in the mother.

Examination
As indicated by mother's health and gestation of the pregnancy.

Investigations
Serology (10mL clotted sample for specific IgM/IgG assay) for congenital infection under consideration.

Management in primary care

Seek advice from an infectious disease expert and/or fetal medicine specialist.

Investigation and management of congenital infections in secondary care

Prenatal

- **Ultrasound scan** for abnormalities described:
  - hydrops
  - brain: reduced BPD and head circumference for gestational age, venticulomegaly, intracranial calcification
  - hyperechogenic bowel.
- **Polymerase chain reaction (PCR)** for virus/parasite DNA in amniotic fluid and/or blood.
- **Maternal serology** (IgM indicating recent infection, IgG immunity and comparison with booking bloods).
- Post-mortem.

Postnatal

- Appropriate microbiology investigations to confirm congenital infection.
- Blood count, platelets, liver function, etc. for baby.
- Brain imaging of all symptomatic babies.
- Audiological assessment and follow-up of baby.
- Ophthalmology referral (cataract, chorioretinitis, pigmentary retinopathy (rubella)) for baby.
- Cardiac echo for baby with congenital rubella.

PCPs should ensure that the woman has adequate contraceptive protection until it is safe for her to proceed with another pregnancy.

Drugs in pregnancy

The *British National Formulary* has an excellent section on prescribing in pregnancy. In general, any woman on regular prescribed medication should discuss the pros and cons of that medication **before** becoming pregnant. If in doubt, seek advice from the UK National Teratology Information Service (NTIS), which provides information and advice about all aspects of toxicity of drugs and chemicals in pregnancy throughout the UK, or its equivalents in Europe, the USA, and Canada (📖 see p. 339 for websites).

Angiotensin-converting enzyme inhibitors (ACE inhibitors)

All ACE inhibitors are contraindicated in pregnancy. Early exposure may not be associated with abnormalities, but ACE inhibitors may decrease fetal renal function, leading to oligohydramnios. Prolonged renal failure and hypotension in the newborn, decreased skull ossification, hypocalvaria, and renal tubular dysgenesis have been reported.

Anticonvulsants

📖 See Fetal anticonvulsant syndrome, p. 360.

Seizure disorders are one of the most common neurological problems affecting women of childbearing age. Approximately 0.4% of pregnant women take anticonvulsant medication during pregnancy. Sodium valproate (Epilim®), phenytoin (Epanutin®), carbamazepine (Tegretol®), and phenobarbitone all have teratogenic potential. A range of newer anticonvulsant agents such as lamotrigine, vigabatrin, topiramate, etc. have been introduced over the past 10–15yrs, but experience in pregnancy is slight and their teratogenic potential is unclear.

> For any woman with epilepsy who is contemplating pregnancy, the risks of anticonvulsant therapy must be weighed against the risks of seizure-induced morbidity and mortality, both to the mother and the unborn fetus.

Emphasize to the mother that she should not stop or change her medication without prior discussion with her neurologist. Maternal morbidity includes the physical risks of accidents and the social consequences of active epilepsy (e.g. loss of driving licence) and the risk of sudden unexplained death in epilepsy (SUDEP), a documented cause of death in maternal mortality statistics in recent years. Fetal morbidity in epilepsy is largely related to the risks of the mother falling, the risks of status epilepticus during pregnancy and seizures during delivery (1–2% of women with epilepsy will have a convulsion during delivery), and the risks due to teratogenic effects of anti-epileptic drugs. Overall, there is a fairly solid consensus that treatment with anticonvulsants in pregnancy (epilepsy or mood disorder), is associated with an overall two- to threefold increased risk of congenital malformation. The risks are greater for combination therapy and for higher doses.

Management

Discuss with her neurologist prior to conception. If her seizures are well controlled consider:

- A reduction in dose/simplification of therapy (monotherapy rather than polytherapy).
- A change of dosing regime: total dose of valproate (and possibly other drugs) should be divided and given 3 to 4 times a day to minimize high peak concentrations of the parent drug or its metabolites. Slow-release preparations are available.
- Possible withdrawal of anticonvulsants (if the mother has not had a seizure for several years).

Addition of 5mg folic acid/day prior to conception and up to the 12th week of gestation.

Support group

National Fetal Anti-convulsant Syndrome Association: ℘ www.facsline.org

Carbimazole

Choanal atresia, hypoplastic nipples, and developmental delay may occur after first-trimester exposure to carbimazole (or its active metabolite methimazole), used in the treatment of maternal hyperthyroidism (e.g. Graves disease). This is likely to be a rare but significant effect.

Cocaine

An increased incidence of spontaneous abortion, placental abruption, prematurity, intrauterine growth retardation (IUGR), and neurological deficits has been documented. Congenital limb deficiency and intestinal atresia may be a consequence of drug-induced fetal vascular disruption. Exposure to cocaine and its derivatives, e.g. 'crack', is connected with clear drug-induced effects: an increased incidence of abruptio placentae, maternal and neonatal intracranial haemorrhage, and possibly urogenital defects.

Fluconazole

Risk of Antley–Bixler craniosynostosis after high dose in first trimester.

Lithium

A recent review of pooled data suggests an increased risk of Ebstein anomaly of the tricuspid valve (10–20 times that in the general population where it occurs in 1/20 000 cases). There is an increased relative risk of 1.2 for all congenital anomalies and of 3.5 for cardiac anomalies in the babies exposed to lithium. Lithium has also been reported to affect neonatal thyroid function. A 5-yr follow-up of 60 children exposed to lithium in the second and third trimesters found no significant differences in developmental anomalies compared with non-exposed siblings. The danger of coming off lithium to a woman with severe bipolar affective disorder must not be underestimated and all aspects of a contemplated pregnancy should be discussed in full with the consultant psychiatrist before conception.

Oral contraceptive pill (OCP)

No association between first-trimester exposure to oral contraceptives and malformation in general or external genital malformations was noted in two meta-analyses.

Retinoids

Women are advised not to get pregnant on retinoid treatment because of its severe teratogenic effect. There is no similar advice for men and no male data are available.

Retinoid embryopathy results in some, or all, of the following abnormalities: CNS defects (hydrocephalus, optic-nerve blindness, retinal defects, microphthalmia, posterior fossa defects, and cortical and cerebellar defects); craniofacial defects (microtia or anotia, low-set ears, hypertelorism, depressed nasal bridge, microcephaly, micrognathia, and agenesis or stenosis of external ear canals); cardiovascular defects (transposition of the great arteries (TGA), tetralogy of Fallot, ventricular septal defect (VSD), atrial septal defect (ASD)); thymic defects (ectopia and hypoplasia or aplasia; and miscellaneous defects (limb reduction, decreased muscle tone, spontaneous abortion, and behavioural anomalies).

Warfarin

- Warfarin and other coumarin derivatives cross the placenta and can cause:
  - bleeding in the fetus
  - an embryopathy (chondrodysplasia punctata with nasal hypoplasia and/or stippled epiphyses) after exposure between 6 and 12 weeks' gestation
  - CNS malformations can occur after exposure during any trimester.
- The risk of a poor outcome is 80% when the mean daily dose of warfarin is >5mg, but <10% when the mean daily dose is <5mg.
- Warfarin does not induce an anticoagulant effect in an infant who is breastfed and therefore can be used safely postpartum. Nevertheless, to be on the safe side, the infant should receive 1mg vitamin K orally 2–3 times a week in the first 4 weeks of life. To avoid any possible complication, the coagulation status should be checked at about 10–14 days, at least in premature infants.
- Unfractionated and low molecular weight heparins do not cross the placenta and are not secreted into breast milk.

Patients with prosthetic heart valves

Pre-pregnancy counselling from a cardiologist and obstetrician with expertise in fetomaternal medicine is advised. The precise safety of warfarin during pregnancy continues to be debated, but it is probably appropriate to withhold warfarin between 6 and 12 weeks' gestation because of the risk of embryopathy, and from 34 weeks' gestation because of the risk of postpartum haemorrhage (PPH). Recommended options include:

- Once-daily low molecular weight heparin to maintain the activated partial thromboplastin time (APTT) within therapeutic range throughout the pregnancy.

- Warfarin throughout the pregnancy except for the first trimester (either for the entire trimester or between 6 and 12 weeks' gestation) and from 34 weeks' gestation, when warfarin should be replaced by unfractionated or low molecular weight heparin.

When coumarins have been used after 6 weeks post-conception or throughout pregnancy, fetal risks should be assessed by detailed ultrasound scan (USS), but termination of pregnancy is not necessarily to be recommended.

Further information

UK: National Teratology Information Service (NTIS): ☎ 0191 232 1525; ⌨ www.ncl.ac.uk/pharmsc/entis.htm

Europe: European Teratology Information Services (ENTIS): ⌨ www.entisorg.com

Canada: Motherisk Program: ☎ (416) 813 6780; ⌨ www.motherisk.org

USA: OTIS Organisation of Teratology Information Services: ☎ (866) 626 6847; ⌨ www.otispregnancy.org

Fetal alcohol syndrome (FAS)

- The incidence of FAS varies depending on geographical location, but may be 1% of all live births. Quantitative structural MRIs in children with FAS have shown structural abnormalities in several regions of the brain, including the cerebellum, corpus callosum, and the basal ganglia. The changes are more frequent and severe in children with dysmorphic facial features.

Both high regular intake of alcohol and binge drinking can cause FAS and alcohol related neurodevelopmental disorder (ARND).

- The critical time period extends throughout pregnancy.
- FAS is associated with high-dose exposure (estimated blood alcohol concentrations to ≥100mg/dL) delivered at least weekly for at least several weeks in the first trimester. (1 unit (8g alcohol) = 1 small glass of table wine = 0.5 pints of beer, lager, or cider = 1 measure of sherry or vermouth. Standard bottle of spirits = 32 units; standard bottle of wine = 9–10 units; can of extra-strong lager = 4 units.)
- There is a continuum of risk, with population-based studies showing that chronic low-dose exposures to 1.5 units/day can be associated with reduction in intelligence quotient (IQ) and increased rates of attention deficit disorders and learning problems. These changes are too subtle to detect in an individual, but at higher levels of exposure probably merge with ARND.

Clinical features of FAS

- *Facial features*: short palpebral fissures, flat midface, long and featureless philtrum (area between upper lip and nose), thin vermilion of upper lip.
- *Growth retardation*: low birth weight for gestational age (less than 2.5 centile), decelerating weight over time not due to nutrition, disproportionately low weight for height.
- *CNS neurodevelopmental anomalies*: microcephaly or decreased cranial size at birth, structural brain anomalies, e.g. partial or complete agenesis of corpus callosum, cerebellar hypoplasia.
- *Impaired fine motor skills*: sensorineural deafness, poor hand–eye co-ordination, poor tandem gait.
- *Behavioural/cognitive/learning deficits*: learning difficulties, deficits in school performance, poor impulse control, problems in memory, attention, and judgement.
- *Alcohol-related birth defects*: congenital heart disease, developmental anomalies of the renal tract.

Consultation plan in primary care

History

- Draw a brief family tree and document parental heights (useful for calculating target parental centile range in assessment of short stature).
- Obtain a detailed account of maternal alcohol intake throughout pregnancy. If you strongly suspect FAS clinically, you may need to seek information on maternal alcohol intake from several sources.
- Take a careful history of exposures in pregnancy, including medical and recreational drugs.
- Document the birth weight. Are other birth measurements recorded, e.g. occipital-frontal circumference (OFC)?
- Developmental history.

Examination

- Growth parameters. Height, weight, OFC (measure head size and height of parents for comparison).
- Facial features.
- Neurological examination, including developmental assessment.

Management in primary care

Unless the maternal alcohol problem is successfully treated the recurrence risk in a subsequent pregnancy is high.

Investigations in secondary care

As it is often difficult to exclude other causes, refer to a specialist for:
- Karyotype.
- FRAX (fragile X syndrome) unless microcephalic.
- Consider cranial magnetic resonance imaging (MRI) scan.

Support group

National Organization for Fetal Alcohol Syndrome: ✆ http://www.nofas-uk.org/

Fetal anomalies

Introduction

This section reviews some of the more common fetal anomalies. These may present unexpectedly, often during routine fetal anomaly scanning. Often there is no family history, or it only becomes evident with hindsight.

A precise diagnosis is vitally important in order to advise about appropriate management and also recurrence risks.

The diagnosis and investigation of a fetal anomaly is often an intensely stressful time for the pregnant woman and her partner. The PCP has an important role in reinforcing information and advice from the fetal medicine service and spending time with the pregnant woman to support her emotionally during this time. The support group Antenatal Results and Choices (ARC) ℰ www.arc-uk.org may be a very helpful resource in such circumstances.

Consultation plan in primary care

History
- Enquire specifically about consanguinity—when present this increases the chance that an autosomal recessive (AR) genetic syndrome underlies the fetal anomaly.
- Enquire about infections, medication, maternal illness, trauma, bleeding disorders in mother.
- Detailed three-generation family tree. Extend further on maternal side if possible. Enquire specifically for other relatives with congenital malformations, miscarriage, unexplained stillbirths, or mental handicap.

Examination and investigations
These will usually be undertaken in secondary/tertiary care.

In the event of severe anomalies incompatible with life or with a very poor prognosis, the woman may need to make a decision about whether to continue with the pregnancy. In the event of a termination of pregnancy or fetal death, discussions with the fetal medicine team may include the request for a post-mortem to try to make a diagnosis in order to provide accurate genetic counselling for a future pregnancy.

After delivery or termination, ensure adequate contraception until the risks for the next pregnancy are clear.

This section will provide some basic background information on some of the common structural fetal anomalies:

- Anterior abdominal wall defects
- Cleft lip and/or palate
- Club foot (talipes)
- Congenital cystic lung lesions
- Congenital heart disease (CHD)
- Dandy–Walker malformation
- Diaphragmatic hernia
- Nuchal translucency, cystic hygroma, and hydrops
- Hyperechogenic bowel (hyperechoic bowel)
- Renal tract anomalies
- Short and/or bowed limbs
- Ventriculomegaly

Fetal anomalies: anterior abdominal wall defects

The overall prevalence is 4.3/10 000 births. The frequent use of antenatal ultrasound scan (USS) and maternal serum alpha-fetoprotein (AFP) has led to increased detection. The sensitivity of USS detection is ~95% for both gastroschisis and exomphalos.

Gastroschisis

Gastroschisis involves herniation of gut through an abdominal wall defect to one side (usually the right) of the umbilicus. It is strongly associated with young maternal age, mothers under 20yrs being 12 times more likely to have infants with gastroschisis. The total prevalence of gastroschisis has changed from 0.29/10 000 births in 1974 to 1.66/10 000 in 1998. The speed at which the increase has occurred suggests environmental rather than genetic risk factors.

Exomphalos (omphalocele)

This is a midline defect with herniation of abdominal contents into the base of the umbilical cord, confined by an amnioperitoneal membrane. In a large exomphalos, liver as well as intestine may be present in the sac. In two-thirds of cases there are other structural anomalies, especially congenital heart disease (CHD). Exomphalos is a feature of Beckwith–Wiedemann syndrome (BWS; large placenta/polyhdramnios, fetal macrosomia, macroglossia, nephromegaly, neonatal hypoglycaemia).

The pregnancy will be monitored closely and delivery planned for ~37 weeks' gestation. Perinatal management involves delivery in a high-risk unit.

Consultation plan in primary care

(📖 see Fetal anomalies, p. 342)

Support group

GEEPS (Gastrochisis, Exomphalos, Extrophies Parents' Support Group): 🖱 www.geeps.co.uk

Fetal anomalies: cleft lip and palate

In the majority of children a cleft is an isolated malformation, although newborn surveys found an associated malformation in about 20–30%. The risk of associated problems is lowest for cleft lip, at about 8%. There are many syndromes that may have a cleft as a feature, and the aim of the fetal anomaly scan is to exclude these as far as possible.

Cleft lip

Cleft lip, with or without cleft palate, is found in 1/700–1/1000 births. It is unilateral in 80%, with the left side more commonly affected, and bilateral in 20%. Males are more likely to have severe disease with alveolar (gum) and palatal involvement. There is a spectrum of abnormality ranging from a small notch in the upper lip lateral to the midline, to a bilateral cleft extending up to the nostrils and into the gums and palate. Cleft lip is sometimes seen at the 20-week fetal anomaly scan.

Cleft palate

Cleft palate occurs in 4 per 10 000 births. The spectrum ranges from a bifid uvula, to submucous cleft palate (palatal mucosa intact but underlying muscle deficiency) with velopharyngeal insufficiency (regurgitation of milk through the nose in babies and nasal speech in older children), to cleft soft palate, narrow V-shaped cleft and finally wide U-shaped central cleft involving the hard palate. Isolated cleft palate is extremely difficult to detect antenatally, even with expert ultrasound scanning, so most cases are diagnosed postnatally.

Pierre–Robin or Robin sequence

The Robin sequence is defined as a U-shaped palatal cleft in association with micrognathia and glossoptosis (retrodisplacement of the tongue in the pharynx) causing upper airway obstruction. It occurs with a frequency of 1/8500 births. Babies usually need extra assistance with feeding. There is a substantial chance of an underlying syndrome, e.g. Stickler syndrome (see Chapter 5, Stickler syndrome, p. 170), 22q11 deletion (diGeorge syndrome) (see Chapter 8, Rare chromosomal disorders, p. 302).

Consultation plan in primary care

(see Fetal anomalies, p. 342)

Investigation and management in secondary care

- If, after careful USS assessment, the fetus appears to have an isolated CL/P, further investigations are not routinely performed but mothers are referred to the Cleft Lip and Palate team to discuss postnatal management.
- If other anomalies are present, then a karyotype, including del 22q11 is performed.

Support group

Cleft Lip and Palate Association: www.clapa.com

Fetal anomalies: club-foot (talipes)

Club-foot usually occurs as an isolated anomaly (77%) but, particularly when bilateral, it may reflect an underlying neurological or neuromuscular disorder. It may also be a feature of a chromosomal disorder (e.g. trisomy 18), syndrome, skeletal dysplasia, or neural tube defect (NTD). Club-foot may be a consequence of oligohydramnios: early amniocentesis <14 weeks, liquor leak, or renal abnormality.

- Talipes is bilateral in ~60% and in nearly 50% of bilateral cases, talipes occurs in association with other defects (higher figure in postnatally ascertained babies). Adverse outcomes are more frequently associated with bilateral talipes than with unilateral talipes.
- Talipes equinovarus (TEV) is the most common type. The spectrum of disorder ranges from mild positional deformity that corrects easily in the first week or two of life to completely rigid deformity. 50% respond to conservative treatment (stretching exercises and strapping/splinting), 50% require surgery. It is about twice as common in males.

Consider investigating mother for myotonic dystrophy if any suggestive features on history/examination (📖 see Chapter 5, Myotonic dystrophy, p. 152).

Consultation plan in primary care

(📖 see Fetal anomalies, p. 342)

Support group

STEPS: ☎ 0871 717 0044; 🖱 www.steps-charity.org.uk

Fetal anomalies: congenital cystic lung lesions

These are rare and present on ultrasound scan (USS) as a cystic or solid mass in the chest, which needs to be differentiated from a congenital diaphragmatic hernia. Causes of congenital cystic lung lesions include:
- Congenital cystic adenomatoid malformation (CCAM).
- Pulmonary sequestration.
- Congenital lobar emphysema (CLE).
- Bronchogenic cysts.

Most cases fare well and many cases of CCAM improve spontaneously or resolve apparently completely *in utero*.

Fetuses with a significant lesion, particularly if associated with mediastinal shift in the third trimester, should be delivered in a unit with facilities for neonatal intensive care and respiratory support, as early surgical treatment may be required.

Consultation plan in primary care

(see Fetal anomalies, p. 342)

Fetal anomalies: congenital heart disease (CHD)

Structural heart malformations occur in 7/1000 live births (0.7%). The earliest presenting feature in pregnancy can be an increased nuchal translucency noted on USS from ~11–12 weeks. Most commonly, CHD occurs as an isolated finding in an otherwise normal individual. However, CHD can occur as part of an enormous number of chromosomal disorders or specific syndromes, or as a consequence of teratogenic exposure. Where a second anomaly is identified, this increases the risk of an associated syndrome.

Women with a congenital heart lesion require specialist care in pregnancy and genetic advice about offspring risks and prenatal diagnosis (e.g. fetal echocardiography).

Trisomies

40–50% of individuals with Down syndrome have a congenital heart defect. At least 90% of individuals with trisomy 18 have CHD and 80% of individuals with trisomy 13 have a cardiac malformation. (📖 See Chapter 8, Down syndrome, p. 294 and 📖 Chapter 8, Rare chromosomal disorders, p. 302.)

22q11 deletion (di George syndrome)

CHD with short stature, cleft palate or velopharyngeal insufficiency (nasal speech), speech delay, may have low calcium, mild learning disability, and immunodeficiency (typically reduced T-cell subsets). The single most common cardiac anomaly amongst children with 22q is VSD. Aortic arch anomalies, such as interrupted aortic arch or truncus arteriosus, are characteristic. A significant proportion of children with Fallot's tetralogy have 22q11 deletions. (📖 See Chapter 8, Rare chromosomal disorders, p. 302.)

Consultation plan in primary care

(📖 see Fetal anomalies, p. 342)

Investigation and management in secondary care

Fetal cardiac scanning (fetal echocardiography)

This is performed in the regional prenatal or fetal medicine department by specialist fetal and paediatric cardiologists to define the anomaly and to give prognostic advice to parents. In most centres fetal echocardiography is offered at 16–20 weeks' gestation to:

- Women who have CHD themselves.
- Women with a family history of CHD, or whose partner has CHD.
- Women whose fetus has an abnormally high nuchal translucency (e.g. 3mm or greater).

In addition, a complete fetal anomaly scan will be done, the maternal serum markers will be reviewed for indications of a trisomy. A CVS or amniocentesis for fetal karyotype, including 22q11 deletion, will usually be offered if congenital heart disease is detected in a fetus.

Support group

Little Hearts Matter, 11 Greenfield Crescent, Edgbaston, Birmingham, B15 3AU; ☎ 0121 455 8982; 🖰 www.lhm.org.uk

Fetal anomalies: Dandy–Walker malformation

A Dandy–Walker malformation (DWM) is a developmental anomaly of the posterior fossa. The cerebellar vermis does not finish its development until 17–18 weeks' gestation and at 15–16 weeks it is not uncommon to find the cerebellar vermis incompletely formed.

Nearly half of fetuses with DWM have a chromosome anomaly, and Dandy–Walker variant is listed as a feature of many syndromes, including autosomal recessive conditions.

Consultation plan in primary care

(📖 see Fetal anomalies, p. 342)

Fetal anomalies: diaphragmatic hernia

- Congenital diaphragmatic hernia occurs in ~1/3700 live births. The diaphragm develops in early embryonic life and is usually fully formed by 9 weeks' gestation. The most common site for diaphragmatic hernia is the left side, through which stomach, bowel, spleen, and liver can pass. Poor prognostic features include early diagnosis, and liver in chest. The main cause of death is pulmonary hypoplasia, due to constrained development of the fetal lungs *in utero*.
- The overall prenatal detection rate by ultrasound scan (USS) is ~60%; most commonly at the 20 weeks' gestation fetal anomaly scan.
- Isolated congenital diaphragmatic hernia has a survival rate in excess of 50% when delivered in a tertiary unit with access to expert neonatal intensive care and paediatric surgical facilities. Long-term complications including feeding difficulties, respiratory problems, and intellectual delay may occur.

Genetic advice and management

Amniocentesis or placental biopsy for karyotype; 14% of pregnancies with diaphragmatic hernia have chromosomal abnormalities.

Consultation plan in primary care

(📖 see Fetal anomalies, p. 342)

Support group

Contact a Family: 🖱 www.cafamily.org.uk/Direct/d28.html

Fetal anomalies: nuchal translucency, cystic hygroma, and hydrops

The reason that chromosomally abnormal fetuses have increased nuchal oedema, cystic hygromas, or hydrops is not well understood. *Cystic hygroma per se* seems to arise as a result of lymphatic dysplasia and is particularly associated with 45,X (Turner syndrome). Increased nuchal fold thickness/ nuchal translucency may resolve spontaneously (even in a karyotypically abnormal pregnancy). Even when fetal lymphoedema resolves, dysmorphism may result from the tissue distension/displacement that occurred during fetal life, e.g. neck webbing, nuchal skin folds, hypertelorism and epicanthic folds, low set ears, wide-spaced nipples.

Nuchal translucency

Subcutaneous accumulation of fluid at the back of the fetal neck is visualized by ultrasound scan (USS) examination at 10–14 weeks' gestation as increased nuchal translucency (NT) thickness. It is associated with chromosomal abnormalities, a wide range of cardiac defects and genetic syndromes, and the measurement is used as part of first-trimester screening for Down syndrome (📖 see Chapter 8, Down syndrome, p. 294).

Hydrops

The presence of skin oedema (over the skull), associated with other serous effusions (ascites, pericardial effusion, hydrothorax) and/or polyhydramnios and/or increased placental thickness.

Fetal hydrops is classified as:
- Immune (fetomaternal alloimmunization) (📖 see Fetomaternal alloimmunization, p. 362).
- Non-immune: where there is a high pregnancy loss rate due to a wide variety of cardiac, infective, genetic, chromosomal, and metabolic conditions.

Genetic advice and management

Every effort will be made to achieve a diagnosis and counsel as for the specific diagnosis.

Consultation plan in primary care

(📖 see Fetal anomalies, p. 342)

Fetal anomalies: hyperechogenic bowel (hyperechoic bowel)

Hyperechogenic bowel, sometimes referred to as 'echogenic bowel', is usually identified as an incidental finding at a routine antenatal ultrasound (USS) examination. The assessment of the echogenicity of the fetal bowel is subjective: to be classed as hyperechogenic the bowel should be of equivalent brightness to the bone of the fetal iliac crests.

Hyperechogenic fetal bowel is detected in 0.1–1.8% of pregnancies during the second or third trimester. Pregnant women may present to their PCP upset as 'something abnormal' has been found on their anomaly scan.

In many fetuses this is a normal variant.

There is a recognized association with intrauterine growth retardation (IUGR) and fetal abnormality. In a large series of fetuses with hyperechogenic bowel, in whom screening for viral infection, karyotyping, and screening for cystic fibrosis (CF) mutations were performed, and there was postnatal follow-up,

- 65.5% had a normal outcome.
- 6.9% had multiple malformations.
- 3.5% had a significant chromosome anomaly.
- 3% had CF.
- 2.8% had a congenital viral infection.

Genetic advice and management

Parents are offered CF carrier testing (because of the 2–3% risk for CF). The CF29 screening kit identifies ~85% of CF mutations, i.e. ~15% are not detectable by routine methods. 📖 See Table 5.1.

- The pregnant woman may be offered an amniocentesis to determine the fetal karyotype (in which case efforts should be made to store amniotic fluid and cultures pending these results, in case both parents are found to be CF carriers and then wish to determine whether the fetus is affected by CF).
- If an abnormal karyotype is discovered, the mother may be referred to Clinical Genetics for explanation and advice.
- She may also be offered maternal serology to investigate for a possible congenital infection.
- If a CF mutation is detected in both parents, the risk for CF in the fetus with hyperechogenic bowel is very high.
- If only one parent is found to be a CF carrier, invasive testing for CF alone will not be performed as there will be no definitive result—if a CF mutation is not identifiable in a parent, it will not be identifiable in the fetus.

- Occasionally testing for fetal CF mutations has already been performed. If this shows a single CF mutation in the fetus with echogenic bowel, there will be ~15% chance that the fetus will have CF. Conversely, if one parent is a known CF carrier (but not affected by CF) and the fetus with echogenic bowel has not inherited the parental mutation, then despite the echogenic bowel, the fetus will be very unlikely to have CF.

Consultation plan in primary care

(□ see Fetal anomalies, p. 342)

Fetal anomalies: renal tract anomalies

Renal tract anomalies are common, comprising ~15% of all prenatally detected congenital anomalies. More than 70% are associated with other anomalies. Renal tract anomalies are found in many syndromes and ~35% of all chromosome anomalies.

The main presentations of renal tract anomalies on fetal ultrasound scan (USS) are:

Renal tract dilatation

- *Mild pyelectasis*. A fetal renal pelvic diameter of >7mm at 18 weeks' gestation is likely to denote a clinically significant degree of dilatation, and follow-up and postnatal investigation are recommended.
- *Congenital urethral obstruction*. In males this is usually due to maldevelopment of the urethra, ranging from complete urethral atresia to posterior urethral valves (PUVs) that form around the membranous/prostatic urethra.
- *Prune-belly syndrome*. In this condition there is abdominal muscle deficiency, megaureter, megacystis, and undescended testis. It is rare, almost all cases are male and the cause is outflow obstruction.
- *Vesico-ureteral reflux (VUR)*. VUR is common (~1% of all live births) and is usually an asymptomatic and self-limiting disease, but babies in whom this is suspected may be started on antibiotic propylaxis until VUR has been formally excluded with appropriate imaging studies.

Cystic or 'bright' kidneys

- *Multicystic dysplastic kidney (MCDK)*. MCDK most commonly presents as an incidental finding on prenatal USS, where it is large and irregularly bright, with cystic areas all but replacing the renal substance. There is a strong association between dysplasia and obstruction and the lower urinary tract should always be assessed carefully. 10% have contralateral renal agenesis. Most MCDKs involute, both pre- and postnatally.
- *Large 'bright' or hyperechogenic kidneys.* The term 'hyperechogenic' or 'bright' kidneys is used to describe renal tissue that is brighter than liver or spleen. This feature is associated with some well-delineated genetic syndromes, the two genetic conditions most frequently diagnosed are:
  - *Autosomal recessive polycystic kidney disease (ARPKD)*. Prognosis is usually poor but mothers will be seen by a paediatrician to discuss postnatal management. In some, the disease phenotype is milder, and dialysis and transplantation are possible.
  - *Autosomal dominant polycystic kidney disease (ADPKD)*. Rarely, ADPKD may present in fetal or neonatal life with large hyperechogenic kidneys; individual cysts may also be detectable (📖 see Chapter 5, Autosomal dominant polycystic kidney disease, p. 100.)

Oligohydramnios

Fetal urine production accounts for the majority of amniotic fluid production from 14 weeks' gestation and any impairment in fetal urine output will manifest as oligohydramnios.

Renal agenesis

- **Unilateral renal agenesis** occurs in 0.15/1000 newborns and bilateral renal agenesis affects 0.12/1000 newborns. Renal agenesis is more common in males (2.45M:1F).
- **Bilateral renal agenesis** presents with severe oligohydramnios beyond 14 weeks' gestation and progresses to the neonatal lethal condition, **Potter sequence** (pulmonary hypoplasia, micrognathia, talipes). There is a high incidence of associated anomalies.

In unilateral renal agenesis there may be hypertrophy of the contralateral kidney. The ipsilateral ureter and Fallopian tube may be absent. Renal agenesis may be an isolated anomaly, may be inherited as a variable dominant condition, or may be a feature of a variety of genetic disorders.

Genetic advice and management

The clinical geneticist will attempt to exclude monogenic, syndromic, and chromosomal causes insofar as this is possible by family history, clinical examination of the fetus/child/parents, genetic and chromosome testing, and parental USS.

Numerous families have been described with autosomal dominant (AD) inheritance of aplasia, dysplasia, and other urinary tract abnormalities, including vesico-ureteral reflux (VUR), duplications, and horseshoe kidneys. Consider referral of parents for renal ultrasound scan (not indicated for unilateral MCKD or mild pyelectasis).

Consultation plan in primary care

(📖 see Fetal anomalies, p. 342)

Fetal anomalies: short and/or bowed limbs

The femur length is measured routinely during the anomaly ultrasound scan (USS) at 18–20 weeks' gestation in order to compare it with other fetal measurements, such as head circumference (HC) and abdominal circumference (AC), to assess proportionate growth.

Bowing of all the long bones, or an isolated long bone, may also be seen at the 20-week fetal anomaly scan. Alternative terms for bowing include 'bent' or 'angulated'. Bowing is often seen in association with limb shortening.

It is common for referrals to be made later than 20 weeks, after it becomes apparent that the femur length growth is falling away from the centile chart.

Differential diagnosis

The major causes of a short femur are:
- Incorrect dates.
- A small, perfectly normal baby.
- Intrauterine growth retardation (IUGR), which would have to be very severe to be detected at 20 weeks.
- A chromosomal disorder.
- A malformation syndrome with IUGR or limb reduction as one of the major features.
- Skeletal dysplasias—some of the dysplasias can be confidently diagnosed prenatally, either by the USS appearance alone, or USS plus genetic testing (e.g. achondroplasia, thanatophoric dysplasia). Some are always lethal conditions, but in others the survival cannot always be predicted; however, poor survival is often seen in conditions characterized by short ribs and a small thorax. Specialist genetic counselling is needed.

Genetic advice and management

If the pregnancy is terminated, a post-mortem with specialist radiology and pathology input is required to make the diagnosis prior to genetic counselling.

Fetal anomalies: ventriculomegaly

Ventriculomegaly in a fetus is an increase in the size of the cerebral ventricles, as measured by ultrasound scan (USS). This finding is associated with an increased risk of fetal chromosomal abnormalities, congenital anomalies and infections, syndromes, perinatal death, and childhood developmental delay. A wide range in the incidence of mild ventriculomegaly is reported in the literature (1.5–20/1000 fetuses). Atrial diameters exceeding 10mm (above 4 SDs) suggest ventriculomegaly, with a low false-positive rate.

- **Mild ventriculomegaly.** The lateral ventricle diameter is 10–12mm.
- **Moderate/ventriculomegaly.** The lateral ventricle diameter is 12.1–15mm.
- Severe ventriculomegaly. The lateral ventricle diameter is >15mm.

True hydrocephalus

- This has a birth incidence of 4–8/10 000 live births and stillbirths. Congenital malformations of the central nervous system (CNS; e.g. spina bifida), infections (congenital infection or meningitis), and haemorrhage can all give rise to hydrocephalus.
- The prognosis for ventriculomegaly depends on the underlying diagnosis. It is important to determine if the ventriculomegaly is isolated or associated with other malformations, as isolated mild ventriculomegaly is associated with a significantly better prognosis than non-isolated mild ventriculomegaly. Additional abnormalities can be detected with a combination of detailed scans and chromosomal analysis; in addition, fetal MRI scanning may be arranged for some pregnancies.
- Isolated mild ventriculomegaly resolves in ~two-thirds before birth, with no apparent neurodevelopmental sequelae.

Differential diagnoses

- **'True' isolated hydrocephalus:** this is secondary to a relative or complete block to cerebrospinal fluid (CSF) flow. This is divided into communicating and non-communicating hydrocephalus. X-linked hydrocephalus with aqueduct stenosis may present in this way.
- **Hydrocephalus with an NTD:** (📖 see Neural tube defects, p. 392) structural brain anomalies that may be associated with, or confused with, ventriculomegaly.
- **X-linked hydrocephalus**: X-linked disorder due to mutation in the gene *L1CAM*. Enquire carefully for a family history. Mutation analysis and carrier testing for a familial mutation are available.

Congenital infection (📖 see Congenital infections, p. 332)

- **Pseudo-TORCH:** an AR condition with intracranial calcification, therefore mimicking congenital infection.

Chromosomal disorders: a large variety of chromosome disorders may present with ventriculomegaly.

Management in secondary care

- Over 80% of fetuses with dilated cerebral ventricles have another abnormality on scan.

- Detailed fetal anomaly USS looking for other intracranial and extracranial anomalies, especially the spine (NTDs).
- Karyotype and specific genetic testing will be considered.
- Congenital infection screen and screening for neonatal alloimmune thrombocytopenia (NAIT).
- Possible fetal magnetic resonance imaging (MRI), particularly used to investigate CNS anomalies.
- Storage of DNA from fetus if pregnancy terminated, in case features of a genetic disorder are found at post-mortem. Detailed post-mortem to include neuropathology. As neuropathology takes extra time (brain requires fixing), ensure that the parents give the correct consent for this procedure. Despite clear appearances of ventriculomegaly on prenatal USS, these appearances may not be confirmed at post-mortem.

Consultation plan in primary care

(📖 see Fetal anomalies, p. 342).

Support group

Association for Spina Bifida and Hydrocephalus (ASBAH): ☎ 01733 555988; 🖰 www.asbah.org

Fetal anticonvulsant syndrome

Seizure disorders are one of the most common neurological problems affecting women of childbearing age. Approximately 0.4% of pregnant women take anticonvulsant medication during pregnancy. Sodium valproate (Epilim®), phenytoin (Epanutin®), carbamazepine (Tegretol®), and phenobarbitone all have teratogenic potential. A range of newer anticonvulsant agents such as lamotrigine, vigabatrin, topiramate, etc. have been introduced over the past 10–15yrs, but experience in pregnancy is slight and their teratogenic potential is unclear.

> For any woman with epilepsy who is contemplating pregnancy, the risks of anticonvulsant therapy must be weighed against the risks of seizure-induced morbidity and mortality, both to the mother and the unborn fetus.

Emphasize to the mother that she should not stop or change her medication without prior discussion with her neurologist. Maternal morbidity includes the physical risks of accidents and the social consequences of active epilepsy (e.g. loss of driving licence) and the risk of sudden unexplained death in epilepsy (SUDEP), a documented cause of death in maternal mortality statistics in recent years. Fetal morbidity in epilepsy is largely related to the risks of the mother falling, the risks of status epilepticus during pregnancy, and seizures during delivery (1–2% of women with epilepsy will have a convulsion during delivery), and the risks due to teratogenic effects of anti-epileptic drugs. Overall, there is a fairly solid consensus that treatment with anticonvulsants in pregnancy (epilepsy or mood disorder), is associated with an overall two- to threefold increased risk of congenital malformation. The risks are greater for combination therapy and for higher doses.

Main features of anticonvulsant embryopathy
- **Major malformations:**
  - heart defects
  - hypospadias
  - club-foot
  - cleft lip or palate (the risk for cleft lip is increased threefold after exposure to phenobarbitone as monotherapy, but is increased only slightly after exposure to phenytoin); 5mg folic acid/day prior to conception
  - neural tube defects—the risk appears to be ~5% with valproate exposure, ~1% with carbamazepine exposure, and not increased for other drugs.
- **Microcephaly** (?noted only after polytherapy).
- **Growth retardation**.
- **Midface hypoplasia**, e.g. depressed bridge of the nose, short nose with anteverted nostrils, and long upper lip; less commonly, a broad bridge of the nose, thin vermilion, small mouth, and a wide philtrum.
- **Hypoplasia** of the fingers, e.g. arch patterns on >5 fingers and/or stiff interphalangeal joints; nail hypoplasia.

- *Cognitive development and behaviour.* Concern is emerging about important adverse effects on cognitive development and behaviour.

Genetic advice

Sibling recurrence risk is high if the woman remains on anticonvulsants and is estimated at 39–55%.

Management

Discuss with her neurologist prior to conception. If her seizures are well controlled consider:

- A reduction in dose/simplification of therapy (monotherapy rather than polytherapy).
- A change of dosing regime: total dose of valproate (and possibly other drugs) should be divided and given 3 to 4 times a day to minimize high peak concentrations of the parent drug or its metabolites. Slow-release preparations are available.
- Possible withdrawal of anticonvulsants (if the mother has not had a seizure for several years).

Addition of 5mg folic acid/day prior to conception and up to the 12th week of gestation.

Support group

National Fetal Anti-convulsant Syndrome Association: ℘ www.facsline.org

Fetomaternal alloimmunization (Rhesus D and thrombocytopenia)

Alloimmunization against blood cell alloantigens

Blood cell alloantigen incompatibility between fetus and mother may occur where the fetus possesses a blood cell alloantigen derived from the father that is not present on the maternal blood cells. Blood cell alloantibodies of the IgG class will cross the placenta and bind their cognate alloantigen.

Red cell blood groups

Rhesus D (RhD)

- About 15% of Caucasian women are RhD negative. Immunization against RhD is rare because of the introduction of RhD prophylaxis. Severe RhD haemolytic disease of the newborn (HDN) occurs in less than 100 cases per annum in the UK (620 000 live births).
- Alloimmunization against red cell alloantigens occurs as a consequence of fetomaternal haemorrhage, which is generally below 4ml of fetal erythrocytes. Abdominal trauma, complications of pregnancy such as vaginal bleeding and abruption, and any invasive procedures carry an increased risk of significant fetomaternal haemorrhage. Such events in RhD-negative women need to be covered with RhD prophylaxis.
- Prevention of RhD immunization is by injection of anti-D immunoglobulin G (RhD prophylaxis) to all RhD negative pregnant women at specified times during pregnancy, and after delivery in case of a RhD positive baby. Once sensitization occurs, RhD prophylaxis is no longer effective.

Red cell alloantigens other than RhD

HDN because of immunization against red cell blood groups other than RhD is rare but may be severe, i.e. in the case of K(ell) immunization. ABO incompatibility cannot cause severe anaemia in the fetus, but frank haemolysis may occur in the group A or B neonate born to a group O mother.

Screening

- A routine screening programme to identify women with immunization against red cell alloantigens other than A and B and to identify all RhD-negative women is in place.
- The aim of this screening programme is to prevent morbidity and mortality due to severe HDN and to provide compatible transfusion support for alloimmunized women.
- Good antenatal care should prevent the occurrence of hydrops fetalis and cases of severe HDN should be managed in partnership with a fetal medicine team with an interest in HDN and the National Blood Service.
- Monitoring of the severity of RhD immunization is by measuring the concentration of anti-D in the maternal serum.
- RhD-negative women require antenatal RhD prophylaxis with a follow-up dose after delivery of a RhD-positive infant.

- The RhD positive father may be homozygous for D (DD), in which case all future children are at risk of RhD immunization, or heterozygous (Dd) with a 50% risk.
- In case of a RhD heterozygous partner, RhD genotyping can be performed on maternal plasma from late in the first trimester.

Clinical features in the fetus

- The fetus becomes anaemic due to haemolysis caused by the maternal IgG anti-D.
- The severity of the anaemia can be determined by periumbilical blood sampling (PUBS).
- Before correction of fetal anaemia became feasible by the transfusion of RhD-negative donor blood, cardiac failure developed as the fetus became more anaemic and, in severe cases, progressed to hydrops fetalis.

The management of the at-risk fetus

Since the technical advance of PUBS, survival rates of severe cases have been excellent. This will all be done in secondary care by a specialist team, but your patient might ask your help about what to expect. The following investigations are routine.

- Prior history of HDN.
- Maternal anti-D quantitation in IU/ml.
- RhD phenotyping of the partner.
- In case of a heterozygous partner, RhD genotyping of the fetus using non-invasive prenatal diagnosis (NIPD) by analysis of free fetal DNA in maternal blood.
- Ultrasound (USS) fetal assessment.
- Fetal haemoglobin (Hb) estimation by PUBS and, if required, correction of anaemia by intrauterine, intravascular transfusion.

The management of the neonate

This will be done by the neonatologists:

- RhD antigen and direct antiglobulin test.
- Full blood count and bilirubin levels.
- In severe HDN the baby rapidly becomes jaundiced, as the immature liver is unable to adequately conjugate the bilirubin and levels of unconjugated bilirubin rise. This is toxic to the brain and unless treated may lead to kernicterus. Exchange transfusion is used both to treat the anaemia and lower the level of bilirubin.

When it is expected that an infant may be severely affected, the paediatricians, haematologist, and the National Blood Service (NBS) should be aware of the likely delivery date so that preparations for an immediate exchange transfusion at birth (if necessary) have been made.

Neonatal alloimmune thrombocytopenia (NAIT)

NAIT is defined as an isolated thrombocytopenia with a count $<150 \times 10^9$/L and caused by maternal IgG alloantibodies against platelet-specific alloantigens. So-called human platelet antigen (HPA) antibodies cause severe thrombocytopenia in approximately 1 per 1200 live births in Caucasians, and this is the most frequent cause of severe thrombocytopenia in the otherwise healthy term infant.

In sharp contrast to HDN, NAIT is *frequently observed in a first pregnancy*. No screening for HPA immunization is in place.

NAIT may present as:
- Venticulomegaly on prenatal USS.
- An infant with thrombocytopenic purpura.
- Petechiae and/or other signs of bleeding.

The main clinical concern is the risk of an intracranial haemorrhage during pregnancy, delivery, or in the neonatal period.

No screening programme is in place. It is important to investigate the HPA antigen status of sisters of childbearing age when the condition has been confirmed in an index case. Families need to be managed in close partnership with a fetal medicine unit and the haematologist and the NBS.

Management
The management of the pregnant woman who is known to be alloimmunized against HPA-1a is complex and must be co-ordinated by the specialist obstetrician.
- The least traumatic route of delivery, generally, a planned Caesarean section, is chosen but there is no good evidence that this reduces the risk of an intracranial bleed in the 'at risk' neonate.
- The paediatrician, haematologist, and transfusion service should be informed prior to delivery so that compatible HPA-matched platelets are available to treat the baby.

Support group
Platelet Disorder Support Association: ♨ www.pdsa.org

Imaging in prenatal diagnosis

Ultrasound scanning (USS)

Detailed fetal anomaly scanning is best interpreted if there is secure dating of the pregnancy. Targeted USS can be very useful in prenatal diagnosis or surveillance of conditions with structural anomalies.

It is important that someone (e.g. PCP, ultrasonographer) discuss with their patient the **limitations of USS**. It can detect many major structural anomalies, but not all (e.g. cleft palate can often be difficult to diagnose), the sonographic signs of some anomalies may present late (hydrocephalus, microcephaly, some renal anomalies), or the condition may have a variable presentation. USS does not give information regarding cognition, vision, or hearing (except when there are obvious gross structural defects present).

Families may treat an ultrasound appointment as a 'fun day out' with older siblings, relatives, and friends; they are often completely unprepared for any abnormal results.

Dating USS

- Is best undertaken at 8–12 weeks' gestation. At this stage in pregnancy there is a tight correlation between crown–rump length (CRL) and gestation.
- It is an important investigation if invasive tests are planned, e.g. chorionic villus sampling (CVS) or amniocentesis, or if scanning will subsequently be used to monitor fetal growth or limb length.

Nuchal scanning

- Is best undertaken at 11–13 weeks' gestation.
- Increased nuchal translucency can be an indication of a chromosomal anomaly or congenital heart disease (CHD), or a wide variety of other syndromes, but many fetuses with a mildly enlarged nuchal translucency measurement are normal at birth (see Fetal anomalies: nuchal translucency, cystic hygroma, and hydrops, p. 351).

Fetal anomaly scanning

- Routine anomaly USS is usually undertaken around 20 weeks.
- High risk for fetal anomalies may be scanned at 16 weeks.
- If there is a past history of specific structural anomalies, or USS is being undertaken for prenatal diagnosis rather than routine obstetric screening, scanning can be arranged in conjunction with a fetal medicine specialist as the appropriate gestational age at which to scan will vary with the particular condition (see Table 9.1).

Three-dimensional USS

New developments in USS technology enable the image to be presented in three dimensions. This may be particularly valuable when assessing facial features and anomalies of the hands and feet, although advances in two-dimensional technology have improved imaging considerably.

Table 9.1 Guidelines for timing of fetal ultrasound scanning (USS) for specific congenital malformations

Feature	Time to start USS (weeks' gestation)
Anencephaly	12
Anterior abdominal wall defects (e.g. gastroschisis/exomphalos)	12
Cleft lip (cleft palate often difficult to visualize)	From 16
Congenital heart disease	11–13 (nuchal scan)
	16 (scan)
	20–22 (review)
Corpus callosum	From 20*
Ear anomalies (only detectable if severe)	20
Eyes and orbital spacing	12–14
Facial profile (e.g. severe micrognathia)	14
Fingers and toes (number of digits)	From 12–14
Gender assignment	From 11+†
Hydrocephalus	20 (serial scanning thereafter)*
Kidneys	From 12–14; readily visualized from 16 weeks
Lissencephaly	From 20+*
Microcephaly	From 20+*
Spina bifida	From 13

*Serial scanning. Fetal MRI may be offered in addition.

†Sometimes gender cannot be assigned with confidence until 20–22 weeks' gestation.

Fetal echocardiography

Routine obstetric anomaly USS includes a minimum of the four-chamber view of the heart but, increasingly, views of the outflow tracts are included. If there is suspicion of a CHD, or scanning is being undertaken because of an increased risk of CHD (e.g. family history or increased nuchal translucency), a more comprehensive study of the fetal heart will be undertaken. Specialist fetal echocardiography includes ventricular outlet views and Doppler assessment of flow.

Fetal sexing

- Up to 11–12 weeks' gestation, the external genitalia appear the same in both sexes (although the orientation of the phallus differs, pointing cranially in males and caudally in females).
- Even up to 20 weeks' gestation it can sometimes be difficult to reliably determine the fetal sex from the appearances of the external genitalia.
- Analysis of maternal blood for free fetal DNA (ffDNA) may enable reliable non-invasive fetal sexing from 8 weeks' gestation in pregnancies at high risk for an X-linked disorder or congenital adrenal hyperplasia (CAH).

Indications for karyotyping

There are a few abnormalities that, when seen in isolation, do not warrant consideration of karyotyping. These include: gastroschisis or unilateral multicystic dysplastic kidney (MCDK). The majority of other anomalies will confer an increased risk for a chromosome anomaly, but the need for karyotyping will be assessed by a geneticist, considering:

- The presence or absence of other USS anomalies.
- The detail of the USS performed.
- Other risk factors (maternal age, nuchal translucency measurement, maternal serum screen result).

Fetal magnetic resonance imaging (MRI)

Fetal MRI requires ultrafast technology to capture images to minimize movement artefact. Currently, fetal MRI is considered for the further delineation of intracranial anomalies, especially neuronal migration defects, and some other complex disorders.

Support group

ARC (Antenatal Results and Choices): ☎ 020 7631 0285; 🖥 www.arc-uk.org

Invasive techniques and genetic tests in prenatal diagnosis

Chorionic villus sampling (CVS) and placental biopsy

CVS was introduced into clinical practice in the UK during the 1980s. The technique enables sampling of the chorion (developing placenta) during the first trimester of pregnancy. In the second and third trimester of pregnancy, the same technique is termed placental biopsy. The trophoblast and embryo are both derived from the fertilized egg, and therefore share the same genetic make-up. This genetic identity is the basis for using CVS as an indirect way of determining the genetic make-up of the fetus. Trophoblast is a highly cellular tissue and ideal for DNA extraction, making this the procedure of choice for many molecular genetic investigations (□ see Fig. 9.3).

- The procedure-associated loss rate is estimated at ~1%.
- In the early 1990s two clusters of babies with limb defects following CVS were reported, raising the possibility of a causal association between early CVS and transverse limb deficiency. The risk of limb deficiency extends through the period of limb morphogenesis and slightly beyond, falling from levels ten- to twentyfold above background at ≤9 weeks, to levels approaching (or only a few-fold above) background at 11 weeks and beyond. Hence CVS is not usually offered before 11 weeks.
- The frequency of vascular disruption defects, e.g. gastroschisis, intestinal atresias, and club-foot, was significantly increased among infants exposed to early CVS compared with a baseline unexposed population.

Amniocentesis

- Mid-trimester amniocentesis became established during the 1970s as the standard technique for the prenatal diagnosis of chromosome abnormalities
- A 22-gauge spinal needle is directed transabdominally under ultrasound guidance through the wall of the uterus, into a pool of amniotic fluid. Usually ~15mL of amniotic fluid is withdrawn (□ see Fig. 9.2).
- Randomized studies of low-risk women have shown a fairly constant risk of around 0.5–1% (fetal loss rate in women after amniocentesis was 1.7% compared with controls, 0.7%).
- The use of ultrasound continuously throughout the procedure, operator experience, and time after gestation are the most important factors determining the risk of postprocedure loss.
- A retrospective case-control study of 1296 children born following amniocentesis showed no increase in registrable disability (hearing impairment, learning disability, visual problems, and limb anomalies) over a follow-up period of 7–18yrs.

Early amniocentesis

- Early amniocentesis (before 13 weeks' gestation) is associated with an increased risk of fetal loss and talipes equinovarus (1.3% versus 0.1%) compared with mid-trimester amniocentesis and should be abandoned.

Pros and Cons of Amnio v. CVS (see Table 9.2)

- The Cochrane review of CVS versus amniocentesis concluded that the increase in miscarriages after CVS compared to amniocentesis appeared to be procedure-related and that second-trimester amniocentesis appeared to be safer than CVS.
- Uncertain results (e.g. mosaicism) are *more frequent with CVS* than mid-trimester amniocentesis. Amniocentesis gives fewer false-positive and false-negative diagnoses.
- The benefits of earlier diagnosis with CVS must be set against the greater risk of pregnancy loss and uncertain results.
- Mid-trimester amniocentesis remains the safest invasive procedure.

CVS is the preferred investigation for most DNA-based prenatal diagnosis, particularly testing for single gene disorders eg. DMD, CF etc. and for pregnancies at high genetic risk.

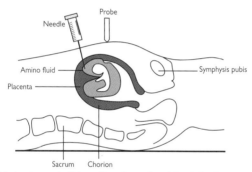

Fig. 9.2 Amniocentesis. (Adapted from Flinter, F. *et al.* (2004) *The Genetics of Renal Disease*, with permission from Oxford University Press.)

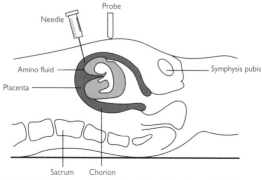

Fig. 9.3 Chorionic villus sampling. (Adapted from Flinter, F. *et al.* (2004) *The Genetics of Renal Disease*, with permission from Oxford University Press.)

Table 9.2 Comparison of chorionic villus sampling (CVS) and amniocentesis

Feature	CVS	Amniocentesis
Gestation	From 11 weeks' gestation; usually 11–13 weeks' gestation	From 15 weeks' gestation; usually 15–17 weeks' gestation
Post-procedural loss rate (miscarriage risk)	1%	0.5–1%
Complications	Vaginal spotting/bleeding (1–4%) especially after transcervical (TC) procedures Intrauterine infection (<0.1%) Amniotic fluid leak after unintentional puncture of amniotic sac (rare)	Amniotic fluid leak causing oligohydramnios Increased risk for respiratory problems, e.g. transient tachypnoea of the newborn Chorioamnionitis (rare)
Culture failure	0.21%*	0.1%*
Maternal contamination	<1% after microscopic selection of the villi	Very low
Mosaicism risk	Confined placental mosaicism in 1.9% and true fetal mosaicism in 0.19%	0.3% (with ~50% of cases representing true fetal mosaicism)
Time scale for results‡	Interphase trisomy FISH or PCR-based common aneuploidy screen, 2–3 days	Interphase trisomy FISH or PCR-based common aneuploidy screen, 2–3 days
	Routine karyotype, around 14 days (cultured cells)	Routine karyotype, around 14 days (cultured cells)
	Molecular genetic analysis. CVS is the procedure of choice as DNA can be extracted directly from the trophoblast sample, e.g. fetal sexing by amelogenin probe§, 2–3 days; routine mutation analysis, 7–14 days; mutation analysis requiring Southern blotting, 10–21 days	Molecular genetic analysis. Amniocentesis is usually substantially slower than CVS since any investigation requiring substantial amounts of DNA requires amniocyte culture (for 10–14 days) prior to DNA extraction. Molecular genetic analysis then takes a further period of time (see CVS column for estimates). It is usually possible to obtain sufficient DNA for a single PCR-based analysis (e.g. cystic fibrosis prenatal diagnosis) from the amniotic liquor

Table 9.2 Comparison of chorionic villus sampling (CVS) and amniocentesis (*continued*)

Feature	CVS	Amniocentesis
	Biochemical diagnosis, e.g. enzyme assay usually within 14–21days	Biochemical diagnosis, e.g. enzyme assay, usually within 14 days
Availability	Specialist centres	Most obstetric units

*Placental biopsy at late gestations, e.g. third trimester, has a higher incidence of culture failure than CVS at 11–13/40. Amniocentesis at late gestations, e.g. third trimester, also has a higher incidence of culture failure than amniocentesis at 15–17/40.

‡ These are intended only as a rough guide. Check with your local laboratory before providing information to patients.

§ Fetal sexing. PCR analysis of the amelogenin locus is sometimes used for fetal sexing in the prenatal diagnosis of X-linked recessive disorders. In the future, a combination of USS of the genital tubercle and analysis of maternal blood for free fetal DNA may enable reliable non-invasive fetal sexing from 8/40.

Consultation plan in primary care

Any woman, or couple, facing amniocentesis will already be concerned about possible problems with the fetus and may need to air those concerns with their PCP in a supportive environment. Although a full clinical assessment of the woman will be done by the person doing the amniocentesis, with full discussion and explanation, the PCP can consider:
- Checking the maternal blood group prior to the procedure.
- Discussing anti-D prophylaxis (offered to all rhesus-negative women).

Multiple pregnancies

- First-trimester ultrasound scan (USS) is necessary to delineate chorionicity, and, hence, zygosity.
- For a monozygotic (MZ) pregnancy, the risk that both twins are affected approximates to the risk for a singleton pregnancy.
- For a dizygotic (DZ) pregnancy, each twin is assessed independently, and the risk that one or both twins might be affected is *twice* that in a singleton pregnancy. Careful consideration needs to be given to the management of the pregnancy if one twin is shown to be affected, whereas the other is normal.
- When an invasive procedure is indicated in twins, CVS has, over amniocentesis, the advantage of allowing selective termination to be performed in the first trimester, when the procedure-related risk of pregnancy loss is less than when performed later in pregnancy. However:
  - CVS has the disadvantage of leading to ambiguous results in up to 2% of cases

- selective termination in mid-trimester carries a 5–10% risk of pregnancy loss or very preterm delivery
- the overall procedure-related risk of miscarriage following sampling of a twin pregnancy is estimated to be ~5% with either CVS or amniocentesis.

Support group

ARC (Antenatal Results and Choices): ☎ 020 7631 0285; 🖰 www.arc-uk.org

Low maternal serum oestriol

Maternal serum unconjugated oestriol (uE_3) is a component of many antenatal maternal serum screening programmes for Down syndrome. Occasionally, serum screening reveals very low levels of uE_3.

In one large study, 0.27% had low uE_3 levels of ≤0.2ng/mL, or 0.15 MoM (multiples of the median). Intrauterine fetal death (IUD) occurred in:
- 57% of women with low uE_3 and positive screening results.
- 6% of women with low uE_3 levels and negative screening results.

In viable pregnancies, the most common cause of a low uE_3 is X-linked ichthyosis.

X-linked ichthyosis (steroid sulphatase (STS) deficiency)

STS-deficiency, or X-linked ichthyosis (XLI), is located at Xp22.3 and affects 1/1300–1/1500 males. Affected males have generalized scaling that usually begins soon after birth. There may be associated corneal opacities that do not affect vision, and there is an increased incidence of cryptorchidism. XLI is often a comparatively mild disorder with the diagnosis in previous generations of the family often only recognized in retrospect.

Perinatal risks in pregnancies affected by XLI include:
- Failure to initiate labour with prolonged gestation (postmaturity).
- A small increased risk of IUD.

Support group

Ichthyosis Support Group: ☎ 020 7461 9034; ✆ www.ichthyosis.co.uk

Male infertility: genetic aspects

World Health Organization (WHO) criteria for 'normal fertility':
- Sperm count of 20×10^6/mL or more.
- Spermatozoa should show 50% progressive motility.
- 30% healthy morphology.

Natural pregnancy is still possible below these cut-off figures, but conception is less likely to occur. A male factor is judged to be the dominant cause of subfertility in 20–26% of couples. Despite advances in the diagnosis of causes of subfertility, inability to conceive remains unexplained in 25–30% of fully investigated couples. Referrals are usually only made to the genetics clinic when a specific diagnosis with genetic implications has been made.

Sperm analysis

The following terminology is used:
- **Azoospermia.** No sperm seen in the ejaculate.
- **Severe oligozoospermia.** Sperm count $<10 \times 10^6$/mL.
- **Oligozoospermia.** Sperm concentration $<20 \times 10^6$/mL.
- **Asthenozoospermia.** <50% of sperm have normal motility or <25% have any motility.
- **Teratozoospermia.** <30% of sperm have a normal morphology.

One or more of abnormalities of sperm count, motility, or morphology is found in almost 90% of infertile males.

- 13.7% of non-obstructive azoospermic and 4.6% of oligozoospermic men have an abnormal karyotype (mainly consist of an XXY constitution or a Robertsonian or reciprocal translocation).

Consultation plan in primary care

History
- If congenital bilateral absence of the vas deferens (CBAVD), detailed enquiry about respiratory symptoms, nasal polyps, chronic sinusitis, pancreatic insufficiency (□ see Chapter 5, Cystic fibrosis, p. 104).
- Mumps as a child, history of chronotherapy.
- Bilateral herniae repair.
- Three-generation family tree.

Examination
- General physical examination.
- Assessment of secondary sex characteristics.
- Testicular size, consistency.
- Presence/absence of vas deferens.

> **Management in primary care**
> Further investigation requires onward referral to a fertility specialist/andrologist.

Investigations in secondary care

- Sperm count (semen analysis).
- Testosterone, follicle-stimulating hormone (FSH), luteinizing hormone (LH), prolactin and thyroid function tests (TFTs).
- Chromosome analysis.
- Possible testing for azoospermia factor (AZF) microdeletions.
- DNA for mutation analysis of the cystic fibrosis (CF) gene (*CFTR*; 70% of males with CBAVD have mutations in both *CFTR* alleles). Consider partner screening if positive (see below).
- If azoospermia with normal karyotype, ultrasound scan (USS) to look for unilateral renal agenesis.

Differential diagnoses

Congenital bilateral absence of the vas deferens (CBAVD)

- Obstructive azoospermia due to absence of the vas deferens can occur as an autosomal recessive (AR) disorder due to mutations in the CF gene, *CFTR*.
- CBAVD is an almost invariable finding in males with CF.
- CBAVD can also occur in association with unilateral (or bilateral) renal agenesis; this condition is not associated with mutations in *CFTR*.
- Advances in reproductive medicine make it possible for some men with CBAVD to father children using percutaneous epididymal sperm aspiration (PESA), intracytoplasmic sperm injection (ICSI), and *in vitro* fertilization (IVF) techniques.

CBAVD due to mutations in CFTR

- There is a risk of classical (or non-classical) CF in offspring.
- Offer CF mutation analysis to partners of CBAVD males.

Chromosome anomalies

Klinefelter syndrome (47,XXY)

This is the most common chromosomal anomaly causing infertility and hypogonadism (📖 see Chapter 8, Klinefelter syndrome (47,XXY), p. 298).

Y chromosome anomalies

- **Microdeletions.** Approximately 10–15% of men with idiopathic azoospermia or severe oligospermia have AZF (azoospermia factor) deletions.
- **Isodicentric Y chromosome—idic(Yp).** Males with an isodicentric Y chromosome have a male phenotype because of the presence of the *SRY* gene, but have azoospermia because they have no copies of the *AZF* genes that are required for spermatogenesis (📖 see Fig. 9.4).

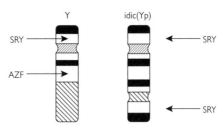

Fig. 9.4 (Left) Normal Y chromosome and (right) isodicentric Y chromosome (idic(Yp)). SRY, Male-determining gene; AZF, azoospermia factor gene. (Reproduced from Firth, Hurst and Hall (2005). *Oxford Desk Reference—Clinical Genetics*, with permission from Oxford University Press.)

- 46,XX males. Prevalence is 1/20 000. This condition is usually due to:
  - cryptic translocations involving *SRY*-bearing Y material and the X chromosomes
  - mosaicism for XX and cell lines involving Y chromosome material
  - true XX hermaphroditism, where both testicular and ovarian tissues persist (findings are variable but may have ovary on one side and testis on the other); may be due to mosaicism or chimerism or to mutations in genes in the pathway downstream of *SRY*.

Hypogonadotrophic hypogonadism
The clinical presentation is often with delayed puberty or lack of masculinisation (voice/sexual hair, etc.) rather than infertility. Adolescent and adult males with hypogonadotrophic hypogonadism require testosterone replacement; infertility may be treatable with gonadotrophins or GnRH.

Kallmann syndrome (KS) is a genetic condition characterized by the association of hypogonadotrophic hypogonadism and anosmia with or without other anomalies. KS affects about 1 in 8000 males and 1 in 40 000 females, with most presentations being of the 'sporadic' type. It can follow autosomal dominant (AD), AR, or X-linked inheritance.

Genetic advice

- The role of the geneticist is to explain the genetic basis of the disorder causing infertility. Depending on the specific diagnosis, if assisted reproductive techniques (ART) could be used to achieve a pregnancy with the patient's own sperm, then advice about reproductive implications is also appropriate.
- Management of the infertility is the remit of a specialist in reproductive medicine.
- The role of the PCP is to explain and co-ordinate and support the couple.

Support group

CHILD: The National Infertility Support Network: ☎ 01424 732361; ✑ www.child.org.uk

Maternal age

Over the past 20yrs very many more women have chosen to delay having children for professional, personal, or financial reasons until their late 30s/ early 40s. Many female PCPs are familiar with the problems of their own biological clocks ticking away.

With advanced maternal age there is an increased risk for the following:

- **Subfertility.** An increasing incidence of chromosomally abnormal conceptuses with advancing age is a major factor in decline in fertility. Chromosomally abnormal embryos have a lower implantation rate than chromosomally normal embryos.
- **Miscarriage.** Increased risk due to increased incidence of chromosomally abnormal conceptuses with advanced maternal age and higher miscarriage rate with advancing age for both chromosomally normal and abnormal conceptions. Risk of early pregnancy loss in a 40-yr-old woman is 30–40%.

Table 9.3 Observed and predicted odds of Down syndrome live birth by maternal age

Maternal age at child's birth (yrs)	Counselling odds*
17	1:1550
20	1:1450
25	1:1350
30	1:950
35	1:350
36	1:260
37	1:200
38	1:150
39	1:110
40	1:85
41	1:70
42	1:55
43	1:45
44	1:40
45	1:35
46	1:30
47	1:30

*Counselling odds are 'rounded' figures for use in the clinic setting.

- **Aneuploidy** (except 45,X; 47,XYY; triploidy; and *de novo* rearrangements). Risks increase exponentially with advancing maternal age for +21, +18, +13, and also for 47,XXX and 47,XXY. In IVF embryos, aneuploidy increased with maternal age, from 3.1% in embryos from 20–34-yr-old patients to 17% in patients 40yrs or older.
- **Dizygotic twinning** (📖 see Twins and twinning, p. 402).

Genetic advice and management

Refer all pregnant women for national antenatal screening (📖 see Antenatal screening for genetic disorders, p. 324).

- The figures in Table 9.3 are for live births. The risk for Down syndrome at CVS or amniocentesis is higher, since a proportion of affected pregnancies result in spontaneous fetal loss (miscarriage or IUD). Approximately 43% of affected pregnancies would be lost spontaneously between the time of CVS and term, and approximately 23% between the time of amniocentesis and term.
- Overall, the risk for *any chromosome aneuploidy* (e.g. +21, +18, +13, 47,XXX, 47,XXY, which are age-dependent, and 45,X, 47,XYY, triploidy and *de novo* arrangements, which are not influenced by maternal age) is *approximately double the risk for Down syndrome.*

Maternal diabetes mellitus and diabetic embryopathy

The key to managing maternal diabetes mellitus is to encourage the woman to gain excellent blood sugar control BEFORE conception, and for her to understand why this is imperative for her future health and for that of the potential fetus.

A pre-conception discussion with her diabetologist or specialist obstetrician will be helpful.

- The incidence of major congenital malformations amongst infants of diabetic mothers (IDMs) is 6–9%, i.e. 2–3 times background rates.
- The risk is limited to patients who are diabetic at the time of conception and is not found amongst gestational diabetics.
- Diabetic women also have an increased risk of first-trimester spontaneous abortion (approximately twofold).
- Risks for both complications can be reduced by improved metabolic control.
- With good to excellent control, risk for malformation remains elevated, whereas risk for miscarriage reduces to background levels.
- The Diabetes in Early Pregnancy study showed that good maternal control is associated with normal neurodevelopmental outcomes.
- Three types of congenital anomaly are all much more common in IDMs:
  - anomalies of the heart and great vessels (transposition of the great arteries (TGA), truncus arteriosus, and tricuspid atresia are overrepresented (×4.5))
  - neural tube defects (NTDs; ×11.5)
  - bilateral renal agenesis (×5).

The mechanism of diabetic embryopathy is not well understood. The diabetic environment appears to simultaneously induce alterations in several interrelated teratological pathways (e.g. disturbances in metabolism of inositol, prostaglandins, and reactive oxygen species). Several clinical studies have not established an association between maternal hypoglycaemia and diabetic embryopathy in humans, but animal studies clearly indicate that hypoglycaemia is potentially teratogenic during embryogenesis.

There is a high incidence of skeletal and vertebral defects in diabetic embryopathy. This group includes a variety of findings, e.g. radial aplasia/hypoplasia, ulnar aplasia/hypoplasia, pre-axial polydactyly. Pre-axial polydactyly of the foot with unusual proximal insertion of the pre-axial digit has been suggested as a marker for diabetic embryopathy.

Caudal regression. Most cases of caudal regression are sporadic or associated with maternal diabetes. The condition is thought to be part of a spectrum including imperforate anus, sacral agenesis, and sirenomelia.

Consultation plan in primary care

History
- Three-generation family tree (to assess whether there is an obvious genetic explanation for any observed malformation).
- Quality of diabetic control periconceptually. What was the glycated haemoglobin (HbA1c) level? Is she experiencing any hypoglycaemic episodes?
- Brief enquiry about other possible teratogenic exposures, e.g. drugs, infection, alcohol.
- If child live born, detailed perinatal history, birth weight, and growth parameters.

Examination
If anomaly identified, examine parents, e.g. if limb defect in fetus/child examine hands/feet of parents; if cardiac defect, likewise.

Investigations in primary care
- Maternal serum screening for NTD (lab must be informed of maternal diabetes because norms for alpha-fetoprotein (AFP) need to be adjusted).
- HbA1c: periconceptual HbA1c > 9% was associated with a high incidence of major anomalies (14.3%).

Management plan in primary care
- Refer any diabetic woman who is contemplating pregnancy to her diabetologist as early as possible.
- Refer a woman to her diabetologist as soon as pregnancy is confirmed.

Investigations in secondary care
- Detailed fetal anomaly ultrasound scan (US should be informed that patient is diabetic). The detection rate for fetal anomalies is lower for diabetic women (30%) than for non-diabetic women (73%), with suboptimal image quality (maternal obesity) a major factor.
- Fetal echocardiography at 20 weeks for patients with insulin-dependent diabetes and those with HbA1c > 6.2 in the first trimester.

Genetic advice and management
Insulin-dependent diabetes mellitus (T1D/IDDM) follows polygenic inheritance with an important role for the immune response genes associated with the HLA complex on chromosome 6.
- 2% offspring risk if mother has T1D.
- 4% offspring risk if father has T1D.

Self-help
Diabetes UK: ☎ 020 7424 1000; 🖥 www.diabetes.org.uk
Also has self-help info. in many other languages: Arabic, Bengali, Chinese, Gujarati, Hindi, Punjabi, Somali, Urdu, and Welsh.

Maternal phenylketonuria (PKU)

PKU is a treatable autosomal recessive (AR) inborn error of metabolism resulting from a deficiency of phenylalanine hydroxylase and characterized by mental retardation when untreated.

In a recent survey, adolescents and young adults generally do not comply with recommendations for the monitoring and control of phenylalanine concentrations.

> Maternal PKU can be teratogenic unless very strict dietary control is resumed prior to conception and maintained during pregnancy: if patient is considering a pregnancy, refer for pre-pregnancy discussion with specialist + expert dietary advice.

Teratogenic effects on the offspring are very similar to those of the fetal alcohol syndrome (FAS):
- Microcephaly from birth.
- Mental retardation. Reduced cognitive function is a virtually constant feature in offspring of untreated maternal PKU. Also striking hyperactivity and emotional problems.
- Congenital heart disease (CHD), especially tetralogy of Fallot, and aortic coarctation.
- Intrauterine growth retardation (IUGR).
- Facial dysmorphism:
  - epicanthic folds
  - maxillary hypoplasia
  - flattened nasal bridge and upturned nose
  - long philtrum and thin upper lip
  - micrognathia.

Consultation plan in primary care

History
- Brief family tree.
- Enquire about pre-pregnancy diet and pre-pregnancy maternal blood phenylalanine levels.

Investigations in primary care

- Maternal phenylalanine levels should be monitored weekly in pregnancy.
- Detailed ultrasound scan (USS) surveillance is usually offered but CHD is the only feature likely to be detectable on mid-trimester scan.

Genetic advice and management

This is an example of a genetic disease (PKU) in the mother that is very harmful (teratogenic) to her unborn infant. The genetic risks are less crucial; the mother is usually a compound heterozygote for mutations in the phenylalanine hydroxylase gene.

- Risk to offspring for PKU if mother's partner is unrelated and has no family history of PKU is 1/100 (1/50 × 1/2).
- Neonatal screening by Guthrie spot on day 5 is a robust and sensitive method of diagnosis of the newborn with PKU. Levels >350μmol/L are diagnostic (levels are usually >1000μmol/L in newborns with PKU). In a high-risk situation, some labs offer a preliminary check on a blood spot and/or serum phenylalanine on day 3 (even if this is normal the routine blood spot on day 5 remains essential). ♒ http://newbornscreening-bloodspot.org.uk
- Close follow-up and counselling for a girl with PKU is essential to make her aware of the risk for fetal damage when pregnant and the methods for prevention.

Presentation in first trimester
In practice many women with PKU present already pregnant. Maternal phenylalanine level at presentation may help to determine the likelihood of problems. Urgent expert advice is required.

Pre-pregnancy counselling
- Women with PKU should receive information about the need for strict dietary control and careful supervision during pregnancy as teenagers.
- Moderate hyperphenylalanaemia (blood level 400–600μM) will need strict dietary control in pregnancy, even though they do not have PKU.

The following information and management programme should be followed.
- Information about teratogenic effects of untreated maternal PKU.
- Stress the need for careful planning of pregnancies with initiation of strict dietary control at least 1 month before conception.
- Stress the need to maintain maternal blood phenylalanine level <360μM (6mg/dL).
- Stress the need for joint supervision by obstetrician/physician with an interest in metabolic disease during pregnancy.
- During pregnancy aim for phenylalanine level of 100–250μM.

Support groups
National Society for PKU (NSKPU): ♒ http://web.ukonline.co.uk/nspku
CLIMB (Children Living with Inherited Metabolic Diseases): ♒ www.climb.org.uk

Miscarriage and recurrent miscarriage

Miscarriage is used to encompass spontaneous early pregnancy loss from a variety of causes, known and unknown:

- **Blighted ovum.** Empty gestational sac seen on ultrasound scan (USS) with no fetal parts.
- **Early pregnancy loss (EPL).** Miscarriage or spontaneous abortion at <12 weeks' gestation (📖 see Tables 9.4 and 9.5).
- **Spontaneous abortion.** Spontaneous pregnancy loss at <24 weeks' gestation.
- **Missed abortion.** Fetal parts identified in gestational sac, but no cardiac activity in pregnancy <24 weeks' gestation.
- **Intrauterine fetal death (IUD).** Fetal death >24 weeks' gestation but before onset of labour.
- **Recurrent abortion.** Three or more consecutive spontaneous abortions.
- 25–30% of all pregnancies end in early pregnancy loss.
- The rate of EPL decreases with gestation.
- Gestation, maternal age, and previous history are the most important determinants of EPL
- Risk of miscarriage increases with maternal age: women aged 40 are twice as likely to miscarry as women aged 20, attributable in part to increased risk of a chromosomally abnormal conceptus with increased maternal age.

At least 50% of miscarriages have a chromosome abnormality.

Table 9.4 Incidence of early pregnancy loss (EPL)

	(%)
Total loss of conceptions (includes biochemical pregnancies)	50–70
Total clinical miscarriages	25–31
Clinical miscarriages <6 weeks' gestation	18
Clinical miscarriages at 6–9 weeks' gestation	4
Clinical miscarriages at >9 weeks' gestation	3
In primigravidas	6–10
Risk after 3 miscarriages	25–30
Risk in a 40-yr-old woman	30–40

Recurrent miscarriage

In a study of products of conception (POCs) from couples with recurrent miscarriage, 46% were cytogenetically abnormal (of which 66.5% were trisomic, 19% were polyploid, 9% were 45,X, 4% were unbalanced translocations, and one was 46,X + 21). The distribution of cytogenetic abnormalities in the recurrent miscarriage group was not significantly different from that in controls when stratified for maternal age, although slightly more unbalanced translocations were identified.

- 5.5% of couples with three or more miscarriages will carry a balanced translocation (~10 × background rate), usually a reciprocal autosomal or a Robertsonian translocation (☐ see Chapter 8, Translocations, p. 306).

Table 9.5 The most common chromosomal abnormalities leading to miscarriage

Chromosome abnormality	Percentage of	
	Chromosome abnormalities	Spontaneous abortions
Autosomal trisomy*	50	25
Triploidy (69,XXX; 69,XXY; 69,XYY)	15	7.5
45,X	10	5
Tetraploidy (92,XXXX or 92,XXYY)	5	2.5
Unbalanced structural chromosome abnormalities†	4	2

*+16 is the most common, accounting for 30% of trisomies.

†50% *de novo*; 50% inherited.

It has been found that the aetiology of trisomy is predominantly a result of meiotic errors related to increased maternal age, regardless of whether the couple has experienced one or multiple aneuploid spontaneous abortions. This is true even when a second spontaneous abortion involves the same abnormality. The overwhelming majority are simply a consequence of the dramatic increase of trisomic conceptions with increased maternal age.

Consultation plan in primary care

History

Three-generation family tree noting history of miscarriage, stillbirth, or neonatal death or unexplained handicap/congenital anomaly.

Examination

Not usually appropriate.

Management in primary care

- Recurrent miscarriage with normal parental chromosomes is not in itself an indication for referral to the genetics clinic.
- ✍ However, if a couple has a significant history of recurrent fetal loss, and especially if cytogenetic abnormalities have been identified in POCs, the couple may be referred to the genetics clinic.

Special investigations in secondary care

- Karyotyping of both partners will be done if they have had three or more miscarriages or if a balanced or unbalanced translocation has been identified in the POC, if the partners wish for this (they may choose not to).
- Other investigations such as antiphospholipid antibodies, lupus anticoagulant and investigations for systemic lupus erythematosus (SLE), protein C, and factor V Leiden are best undertaken in a gynaecological setting.

Genetic advice and management

- If a parental chromosome rearrangement is identified, they will be counselled appropriately (📖 see Chapter 8, Translocations, p. 306).
- If there is no parental chromosome rearrangement, the couple are best managed in a reproductive medicine clinic rather than a genetics clinic.
- If the karyotype of abortus is aneuploid, the chance of a successful next pregnancy is higher (68%) than if the abortus is euploid (41%).
- Recurrent pregnancy loss of affected males can occur in some rare X-linked dominant disorders, such as incontinentia pigmenti, but it is rarely a presenting feature and together they account for only a miniscule fraction of recurrent miscarriages.

Support group

The Miscarriage Association: 🖰 www.miscarriageassociation.org.uk

Neonatal screening

Currently in the UK the neonatal screening programme (🕮 see Fig. 9.1, p. 327) offers:
- Newborn blood spot screening.
- Newborn hearing assessment.
- Newborn physical examination.
- Sickle cell screening (not universal except in England).

Newborn blood spots (formerly known as the Guthrie test)

- The newborn test uses dried blood spots and is taken ideally on postnatal day 5.
- This national newborn screening programme was introduced in 1969 for *phenylketonuria* (PKU) and in 1981 for *congenital hypothyroidism* (CHT). The success of this screening was partly due to the high uptake (99%), but also because these two conditions could be diagnosed and treated before the onset of neurological sequelae.
- All babies in England are now offered screening for a total of five conditions, as screening for *sickle cell disease, cystic fibrosis* and MCADD (*medium-chain acyl-CoA dehydrogenase deficificency*) is now fully implemented.
- Screening in Wales also includes *Duchenne muscular dystrophy*. In Wales, Northern Ireland, and Scotland newborns are not screened for sickle cell disease at present.

Newborn hearing test

The aim of this screen is to detect >40dB hearing loss. A combination of the otoacoustic emission test and automated auditory brainstem response is used. The aim is to offer this within 72h of birth, but in some areas testing is performed in the community where this time frame is not possible.

Newborn physical examination

For babies born in hospital the first examination is at 48–72h by a paediatrician. For those born at home or in midwife-led units, the examination may be by either the PCP or a specially trained midwife. Attention is paid particularly to examination of the hips for dislocation, auscultation of the heart for murmur, eyes for cataract and the testes in males. The examination is repeated by the PCP at 6–8 weeks.

Sickle cell screen

This is performed using the blood spot and complements haemoglobinopathy screening already performed in pregnancy.

Useful resources

℘ www.screening.nhs.uk
℘ www.newbornbloodspot.screening.nhs.uk
℘ www.nsd.scot.nhs.uk

Neural tube defects (NTD)

Includes anencephaly, encephalocele, myelocele or rachischisis, inien-cephaly, meningomyelocele, spina bifida, and spina bifida occulta.

To prevent first occurrence of NTD, women who are planning a preg-nancy should take 400 micrograms daily of folic acid from at least 1 month before conception and continue until the 12th week of pregnancy.

NTDs usually present prenatally after an abnormal triple test and nuchal/anomaly scans.
- Neural tube defects (NTDs) arise from failure of closure of the neural tube, which normally occurs 18–28 days post-fertilization.
- The prevalence of NTDs varies considerably from 1/300 (0.003) in Northern Ireland to <1/1000 (0.001) in parts of the USA.
- Isolated NTDs usually have a multifactorial basis, with contribution from environment (dietary folate) and genetic factors. There is considerable variation in the ethnic prevalence for NTD, with rates generally being high in Celtic populations and Canadian Sikhs.
- Several genes are implicated in the elevation of the neural folds.
- The birth prevalence of NTDs was declining substantially even before the introduction of periconceptual folate supplementation and prenatal screening, perhaps due to improved maternal nutrition.
- Infants of diabetic mothers have an increased risk for NTDs with a relative risk of 11.5.
- Folic acid antagonists, e.g. valproate, are teratogenic early in the first trimester of pregnancy.
- Several studies have shown an increased risk for NTDs associated with pre-pregnancy maternal obesity.
- Of all cases with NTDs, approximately 50% have spina bifida, 40% have anencephaly, 8.5% have encephalocele, and 1.5% have iniencephaly.
- More females are affected than males (1M:1.3F).
- Vertebral anomalies and hydronephrosis are commonly seen in 'isolated' NTDs.

Natural history

In babies with open spina bifida who had their backs surgically closed in the immediate neonatal period, morbidity and mortality were strongly correlated with the level of the sensory deficit; with the best outcome in those with the lowest defects. On review 35yrs later, of the survivors with a sensory level in infancy below L3, 54 were still alive, 71% had a cerebrospinal fluid (CSF) shunt, 88% had an intelligence quotient (IQ) = 80, 67% were able to walk ≥50m with aids if required, 33% were continent, 58% were living independently and able to drive, and 38% were in open employment.

Definitions (🔲 see Fig. 9.5)

- *Anencephaly:* failure of fusion of the caudal folds of the neural tube 18–28 days after ovulation (4.5–6 gestational weeks). The forebrain fails to develop and the defect is lethal.

- ***Chiari II malformation.*** Downward protrusion of the medulla below the foramen magnum to overlap the spinal cord (can cause lower cranial nerve palsies and central apnoea). It is present in >70% of cases with meningomyelocele. Increasing symptoms with age.
- ***Diastematomyelia.*** The presence of a sagittal cleft that divides the spinal cord into two halves, each surrounded by its own pia mater. Plain radiographs show abnormalities in most cases. These include abnormal vertebral segmentation, spina bifida, and scoliosis.
- ***Dysraphism.*** Continuity between posterior neuroectoderm and skin.
- ***Encephalocele.*** Outpouching of the brain through a bony defect. Sometimes anterior or lateral, but most are occipital. Occipital defects usually project through an apical defect of the occipital bone or enlarged posterior fontanelle.
- ***Iniencephaly/craniorachischisis.*** Developmental abnormality of the skull and upper spine.

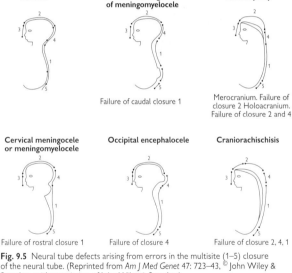

Fig. 9.5 Neural tube defects arising from errors in the multisite (1–5) closure of the neural tube. (Reprinted from *Am J Med Genet* 47: 723–43, © John Wiley & Sons Inc., with permission of John Wiley & Sons Inc.)

Spina bifida

Spina bifida cystica

Failure of fusion of the rostral folds of the neural tube between days 18 and 28 of embryonic development (4.5–6 gestational weeks). Lesions may occur anywhere along the length of the spine, but most commonly in the lumbosacral region. In a **meningocele** there is no neural tissue present in the cystic lesion; in a **myelomeningocele** the spinal cord is a component of the cyst wall. Hydrocephalus complicates 90% of cases with lumbosacral meningomyelocele.

Spina bifida occulta

A hairy patch of pigmented or abnormal skin, subcutaneous mass, dimple, or sinus over the lumbosacral spine associated with failure of fusion of the dorsal vertebral arches (usually at L5/S1). As a radiological finding only, in the absence of cutaneous or neurological findings, it is fairly common (5% of the population) and not thought to confer an increased risk of NTD to offspring.

Differential diagnoses/conditions to consider

- **Folic acid antagonists.** Maternal exposure to folic acid antagonists early in the first trimester, e.g. anticonvulsants (📖 see Fetal anticonvulsant syndrome, p. 360) (sodium valproate, carbamazepine, phenytoin, phenobarbitone, or primidone) or sulfasalazine, triamterene, or trimethoprim. Valproate-induced NTDs affect predominantly the lower lumbar and sacral region.
- **Meckel syndrome.** Lethal autosomal recessive (AR) syndrome with occipital encephalocele, bilaterally large kidneys with multicystic dysplasia and fibrotic changes of the liver, and postaxial polydactyly.

Genetics

Inheritance and recurrence risk (📖 see Table 9.6)

Table 9.6 Anencephaly and spina bifida: approximate recurrence risks (%) without folate supplementation in relation to population incidence

Relationship of affected individual to 'at risk' pregnancy	Population incidence of NTD		
	0.005	0.002	0.001
One sibling	5%	3%	2%
Two siblings	12%	10%	10%
One 2nd degree relative	2%	1%	1%
One 3rd degree relative	1%	0.75%	0.5%
One parent	4%	4%	4%

- In non-syndromal NTD a recurrence may be of a different type.

To prevent recurrence of NTD, women who are planning a pregnancy should take 5mg daily of folic acid from at least 1 month before conception and continue until the 12th week of pregnancy.

- High-dose folate prevents approximately 70% of recurrences.
- No known or suspected adverse effects of folic acid at the proposed 5mg daily dose have been recorded, and it has no contraindications, although women with epilepsy should have their anticonvulsant treatment reviewed.
- Where a recurrence occurs on high-dose folate, the clinical geneticist will reconsider whether there is a syndromal association. High-dose folate supplementation is continued in a subsequent pregnancy, but with little expectation of benefit and, therefore, a 10% recurrence risk is appropriate.

Other situations where high-dose folate (5 mg per day) may be appropriate:

- One or other parent has spina bifida occulta with a hairy patch or abnormal skin over the lumbosacral spine.
- The mother needs to continue with anticonvulsant therapy during pregnancy.
- One or other parent has a neural tube defect.

Consultation plan in primary care

History

- Three-generation family tree with enquiry about stillbirths and neonatal deaths.
- Enquiry about pre-conceptual folic acid.
- Detailed pregnancy history including enquiry about drug exposure, e.g. folic acid antagonists, and maternal diabetes.

Management in primary care

Ensure high-dose folic acid, 5mg/day, for women at increased risk of NTD.

Examination in secondary care

Affected individual

The affected individual with be referred to the paediatric team. Additional anomalies are present in 20% but, if additional anomalies are found, the possibility of a syndrome or chromosomal anomaly will be re-examined.

Parents or intervening relative

Will be examined for signs of spina bifida occulta.

Prenatal diagnosis

- **Ultrasound scanning (USS).** Anencephaly is detectable on USS from 11–12 weeks' gestation; spina bifida is detectable with fetal anomaly scanning from 16 weeks' gestation; large defects may be visible earlier, e.g. from 13 weeks' gestation. The sensitivity of prenatal diagnosis by USS in an unselected population is 98% for anencephaly and 75% for spina bifida. Sensitivity higher than this may be possible when USS is specifically targeted because of an increased risk.
- **Maternal serum screening for alpha-fetoprotein (AFP).** Serum screening using a cut-off of 2.5 MoM (multiple of the median) at

16 weeks' gestation is a reliable method of screening, with a detection rate for spina bifida of 82% for a false-positive rate of 1.9%. It does not detect closed defects (i.e. those covered by intact skin); hence it is wise to use it in conjunction with detailed anomaly USS if monitoring a subsequent pregnancy.

AFP screening is less sensitive in women taking valproate, which is unfortunate since the risk of NTDs is increased in valproate-exposed pregnancies.

- *Amniocentesis.* Due to the efficacy of detailed USS in combination with maternal serum screening, amniocentesis is nowadays rarely used for the sole indication of prenatal diagnosis of NTD.

Support group

Association for spina bifida and hydrocephalus: ♒ www.asbeh.org

Radiation exposure, chemotherapy, and landfill sites

Radiation-induced heritable diseases have not been demonstrated in humans, and estimates of genetic risks for protection purposes are based on mouse experiments. The most comprehensive epidemiological study is of the Japanese atomic bomb survivors and their children, which found little evidence for inherited defects attributable to parental radiation. Studies of workers exposed to occupational radiation or of populations exposed to environmental radiation appear too small and exposures too low to convincingly detect inherited genetic damage.

Diagnostic radiation

Radiation exposure after diagnostic imaging in pregnancy is too small to cause developmental problems. The main risk is an incremental added risk for childhood cancer.

- The background risk for childhood cancer is 1/650 (all (fatal and non-fatal) cancers in the first 15yrs of life).
- Added risk of childhood cancer per millisievert (mSv) exposure is 1/17 000.
- Fetal exposure from a chest X-ray or mammogram is <0.01mSv.
- Background radiation in Cambridge, UK is about 2.5mSv per annum.

Therapeutic radiation

A study of over 25 000 survivors of childhood cancer who gave birth to or fathered over 6000 children (doses to gonads are being reconstructed from radiotherapy records with 46% over 100mSv and 16% over 1000mSv) reassures that cancer treatments, including radiotherapy, do not carry much, if any, risk for inherited genetic disease in offspring conceived after exposure.

Offspring risks to survivors of childhood cancer

Female survivors

- Pregnancy outcomes among surviving female participants in the Childhood Cancer Survivor Study showed 63% live births, 1% stillbirths, 15% miscarriages, 17% abortions, 3% unknown or in gestation.
- There were no significant differences in pregnancy outcome by treatment.
- A higher, but not statistically significant, risk of miscarriage was present among women whose ovaries were in the radiation therapy field.
- The rate of live births was not lower for the patients treated with any particular chemotherapeutic agent, and the study did not identify adverse pregnancy outcomes for female survivors treated with most chemotherapeutic agents.
- The offspring of the patients who received pelvic irradiation were more likely to weigh <2500g at birth (RR, 1.84; $P = 0.03$).

Male survivors
- For surviving male participants in the Childhood Cancer Survivor Study who sired pregnancies, pregnancy outcomes of their partners were: 69% live births, 1% stillbirths, 13% miscarriages, 13% abortions, 5% unknown or in gestation.
- This large study did not identify adverse pregnancy outcomes for the partners of male survivors treated with most chemotherapeutic agents. (The male:female ratio was slightly altered compared with offspring of siblings of survivors and concerns about procarbazine warrant further investigation.)

Landfill sites
- In a survey of >1 million live births in the UK, the relative risk for a woman resident within <2km of a landfill site for all congenital anomalies was 1.01 (adjusted for confounders), i.e. there is a very small excess risk of congenital anomalies.
- Adjusted risks were 1.05 for neural tube defects (NTDs), 1.07 for hypospadias and epispadias, 1.19 for gastroschisis and exomphalos, 1.05 for low birth weight (<2.5kg), and 1.04 for very low birth weight (<1.5kg).
- There was no excess risk for stillbirth.
- In reality what this means is: 'this 1% higher rate of birth defects would represent about 100 cases of birth defects each year across England and Wales. This is out of a total of ~12 000 cases of birth defects expected each year in England and Wales.'

Hazardous waste
- There is a 33% increase in the risk of non-chromosomal congenital anomalies for residents living within 3km of a *hazardous waste* landfill site.
- A similar effect was found for chromosomal anomalies, with an odds ratio of 1.41 for chromosomal anomalies in people who lived close to the sites (0–3km) compared with those who lived further away (3–7km) after adjustment for confounding by maternal age and socio-economic status.

Reproductive options

After the diagnosis of a genetic disorder that confers a significant risk of recurrence to a sibling or offspring, many families are faced with a difficult choice about future pregnancies. It may be helpful for them to be introduced to the range of reproductive options available to them for future pregnancies. This is not always easy as such decisions are very personal. It may help to introduce the topic by explaining that some of the choices available may include options that they would *not* consider choosing.

Accepting the risk of another affected child

Once they are fully informed, after seeing a consultant geneticist, for some families this will be the option of choice. For others it is an option they cannot bear to contemplate.

Electing against further pregnancies

The burden of caring for a child with a severe genetic disorder may be such that the family feel that they do not wish to extend their family because all of their energy is channelled into caring for their existing child(ren).

Adoption

Although this process can be frustrating and lengthy, some couples are successful in locating a baby or child to join their family. (Some couples may choose to adopt another affected child as in achondroplasia and Down syndrome—📖 see Chapter 1, Adoption, p. 4.)

Donor gamete

- **AID** (artificial insemination by donor) is an option that can be used to minimize the risk of recurrence of an autosomal recessive (AR) disorder for which both parents are carriers, or to evade the risk of a dominant disorder present in the father, or the risk of unbalanced products of a balanced translocation present in the father.
- **A donor ovum** can also be used to minimize the risk of recurrence of an AR disorder, and has the advantage that both parents play a biological role in bringing the baby into the world—technically this is much more demanding and the shortage of donor eggs means that, in practice, AID is usually the more pragmatic option. A donor ovum is also an option to avoid the risk of a dominant disorder present in the mother, or a mitochondrial encoded disorder carried by the mother, or the risk of unbalanced products of a balanced translocation present in the mother.

Prenatal diagnosis

For many couples facing a high risk of recurrence for a serious disorder this is the option of choice, but for others (particularly those with religious or moral objections to termination of pregnancy) it is ethically unacceptable. Prenatal diagnosis by chorionic villus sampling (CVS) or amniocentesis is possible for cytogenetic disorders, monogenic disorders in which the pathogenic mutation is known, and the great majority of biochemical disorders. Prenatal diagnosis by ultrasound can be used to exclude many conditions that may cause major structural malformations.

Pre-implantation genetic diagnosis (PGD)

At first sight this seems the most attractive option to many couples. In reality, PGD is only available in a very few specialist centres and for a few severe genetic diseases (predominantly those in which single-cell diagnosis is technically feasible, e.g. fluorescent *in situ* hybridization (FISH), for diagnosable conditions such as chromosome translocations or trisomies, or where there is a commonly occurring mutation such as the exon 7, 8 deletion in spinal muscular atrophy (SMA)).

PGD entails ovarian hyperstimulation (and its attendant risks), egg retrieval, *in vitro* fertilization, embryo biopsy, and implantation of screened embryos. For single-gene disorders, a pregnancy rate of 21% per egg retrieval and 25% per embryo transfer procedure has been reported. The costs are often prohibitive. (See Assisted reproductive technology, p. 328.)

The recent application of SNP genotyping to PGD (known as pre-implantation genetic haplotyping (PGH)) may facilitate diagnosis of rare monogenic conditions.

Adopt-out or foster-out an affected child

If the family does not feel they can care for another affected child, but also have religious or other objections to contraception and prenatal diagnosis, this option may need to be considered.

Further information

British Association for Adoption and Fostering: ꝏ www.baaf.org.uk

Support group

Adoption UK: ꝏ www.adoption.org.uk

Twins and twinning

Twins occur in 1 in 80 live births. They have a special place in Greek mythology, ancient legends and Shakespeare's plays (he was father of boy/girl twins). Classical twin studies have played a key role in defining the 'heritability' of a trait by studying the concordance in monozygotic (MZ) versus dizygotic (DZ) twins. Many aspects of twin pregnancies, including prematurity and maternal physiology, make them different from singleton pregnancies.

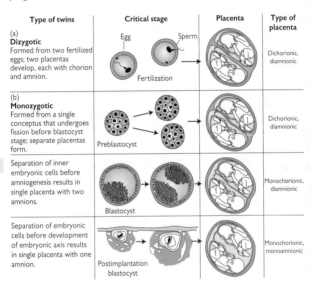

Type of twins	Critical stage	Placenta	Type of placenta
(a) **Dizygotic** Formed from two fertilized eggs; two placentas develop, each with chorion and amnion.	Egg · Sperm · Fertilization		Dichorionic, diamnionic
(b) **Monozygotic** Formed from a single conceptus that undergoes fission before blastocyst stage; separate placentas form.	Preblastocyst		Dichorionic, diamnionic
Separation of inner embryonic cells before amniogenesis results in single placenta with two amnions.	Blastocyst		Monochorionic, diamnionic
Separation of embryonic cells before development of embryonic axis results in single placenta with one amnion.	Postimplantation blastocyst		Monochorionic, monoamnionic

Fig. 9.6 Development of (a) dizygotic and (b) monozygotic twins. (Reproduced from Firth, Hurst and Hall (2005), *Oxford Desk Reference—Clinical Genetics*, with permission from Oxford University Press.)

'Vanishing' twin

Only 29% of women with a twin pregnancy on ultrasound scan (USS) at <10 weeks' gestation will give birth to twins. Hence there is an ~70% loss rate in twin pregnancies.

Congenital anomalies

- Congenital anomalies occur in at least 10% of all twin pregnancies.
- The congenital anomaly rate is higher in MZ than in DZ twins, partly due to the increased burden of anomalies arising from vascular disruption and possibly because, in the earliest phase of embryonic development, the cytoplasm of a single egg cell supports the nutritional requirements of two embryos prior to implantation.
- Both MZ and DZ twins have an increased risk for deformational congenital anomalies, associated with constraint and intrauterine crowding, such as greater moulding of the head, craniosynostosis, dislocated hips, bowing of legs, and club-feet.
- Disruptions in MZ twins, including hemifacial microsomia, limb reduction defects, and amyoplasia and bowel atresia, are probably related to the shared placental circulation unique to MZ twins with differences in vascular flow leading to vascular compromise.

Dizygotic (DZ) twins ('non-identical twins')

- DZ twins share the same genetic similarity as siblings, i.e. they have 50% of their nuclear DNA in common.
- They have a 25% risk to be concordant for autosomal recessive (AR) disorders.
- DZ twins have separate placentas and membranes (dichorionic diamniotic (🕮 see Fig. 9.6a), although they might be fused and even have vascular connections.
- The introduction of artificial reproductive technologies (ART) has led to an 'epidemic' of DZ twins.
- Factors increasing DZ twinning rate:
  - **Raised gonadotrophin levels.** Older, taller, heavier mothers and nulliparas. The peak incidence is at 37yrs.
  - **Fertility drugs,** e.g. clomifene. These promote superovulation with a markedly increased risk for DZ twinning.
  - **Familial factors.** Women with a family history of DZ twinning are more likely to have DZ twins.
  - **Ethnicity.** The rate of DZ twinning varies widely between different populations. It is low in Asian populations with an incidence of 4/1000, intermediate in Europeans and North Americans at 10–14/1000, and high in Africans at 26–40/1000.

Table 9.7 Placentation of MZ twins in relationship to timing of twinning after fertilization

Placentation of MZ twins	Time of twinning after fertilization	% of all MZ pregnancies surviving to term	Comment
Dichorionic diamniotic	Separation by day 3	25	Early separation leads to completely separate placentation
Monochorionic diamniotic	4–8 days	70–75	Single placenta with separate amniotic sacs
Monochorionic monoamniotic	9–12 days	1–2	Risk of tangled cords
Conjoined twins	13–14 days	Rare	75% are female

Monozygotic (MZ) twins ('identical twins') (📖 see Table 9.7)
- MZ twins are genetically identical.
- MZ twinning occurs at the same rate worldwide.
- In MZ twinning a single egg is fertilized by a single sperm.
- MZ twins account for 3–4/1000 births in the UK.
- Manipulation of the environment around the time of conception can induce MZ twinning in animals; the MZ twinning rate is increased threefold in *in vitro* fertilization (IVF) pregnancies.
- The placentation of MZ twinning is thought to be determined by the time at which twinning occurs following fertilization.
- 25–30% of MZ twins have completely separate placentas and membranes.
- 70–75% share one placenta with monochorionic diamniotic membranes.
- 1–2% have one set of membranes and one placenta (monochorionic, monoamniotic).
- Monochorionic placentas of all types are prone to have vascular connections that can lead to twin–twin transfusion syndrome, twin reverse arterial perfusion sequence (TRAP), and to disruptive congenital anomalies.

Discordance
Discordance between MZ twins has been noted for chromosomal anomalies, single-gene disorders, skewed X inactivation, genomic imprinting defects, mitochondrial disturbances, and minisatellites. These factors need to be borne in mind during prenatal diagnosis, since MZ twins could be discordant for chromosomal anomalies and chromosomal mosaicism.

Vascular shunts
MZ twins are at risk of placental vascular anastomoses that may be arterioarterial, venovenous, or arteriovenous. They predispose to a variety

of congenital anomalies due to vascular disruption: microcephaly; poren-cephaly; hydranencephaly; gastroschisis; intestinal atresia; and transverse limb reduction defects. If the co-twin dies in the second or third trimester, the surviving MZ twin is at greatly increased risk of cerebral palsy (perhaps due to embolization or disturbance of the coagulation balance arising from the dying/dead twin).

Consultation plan in primary care

History
- Family tree with history of twinning and determine ethnicity.
- Pregnancy and delivery. Were there separate placentas? Were there separate amniotic sacs?
- Subsequent growth and development. How similar are the twins? Can strangers tell them apart?

Management in primary care
- Health visitors have a major role in supporting exhausted parents with newborn twins, as does the wider community. Mutual support from parents of other 'twins' can be very beneficial.
- Parents of a recently confirmed pregnancy may benefit from advice that effecting 'twins insurance' must be done before any initial USS takes place.
- Code the twin patients' notes.
- Code the parents' notes and suggest their siblings ask for their notes to be coded too.

Management in secondary care

Examination
- Careful examination of MZ (monochorionic) twins for congenital anomalies.
- Growth parameters.
- Examine as for the issue in question. Are the twins concordant or discordant for the problem?

Genetics
Zygosity testing sufficient for clinical practice can usually be accomplished using a relatively small number (e.g. 7 or more) of highly polymorphic microsatellite markers. Microsatellite polymorphisms are based on short tandem repeats usually di-, tri-, or tetranucleotides that can be typed by polymerase chain reaction (PCR) and give a discrete allele with a precise repeat number.

DNA for such testing may need to come from a buccal swab or skin fibroblasts if single placenta.

Support groups
Multiple Births Foundation: ☎ 020 8383 3519; 🖰 www.multiplebirths.org.uk
TAMBA (Twins and Multiple Births Association): ☎ 0870 770 3305; 🖰 www.tamba.org.uk

The future

Education for primary care

The knowledge and skills in genetics acquired as a medical student are now to be reinforced by the embedding of the Royal College of General Practitioners (RCGP) Genetics Curriculum:

ॐ www.rcgp-curriculum.org.uk/PDF/curr_6_Genetics_in_Primary_Care.pdf into general practice training in the UK. The content is easily transferable to similar training in the USA, Canada, Australia, etc.

Beyond the training years, ongoing training of general practitioners is left to individuals to identify their own learning needs in a personal learning plan. However, genetics is not high on many PCP learning agendas for some of the following reasons:

• Not yet seen as relevant to day-to-day practice.
• There are competing learning needs.
• Perceived as 'difficult'.
• Too much science and not enough practical application.

An individual PCP who does identify genetics as a learning need will easily identify the fact that they need:

• Genetic knowledge, e.g. patterns of inheritance, vocabulary, significance of specific symptoms and signs.
• Genetic skills, e.g. taking and recording a family tree.
• Genetic resources.

Two excellent resources are:

• National Genetics Education and Development Centre (NGEDC):
ॐ www.geneticseducation.nhs.uk
• Genetic Tools—Genetics through a primary care lens:
ॐ www.genetests.org—click on 'Educational materials' and select 'Genetic Tools'.

More excellent resources are listed in 📖 Chapter 11, Primary Care Education, p. 428.

Future developments

Genetics in primary care is here to stay, maintained and built on by:
- The sequencing of the human genome.
- Continuing research to define structural variation in the human genome.
- Rapidly increasing knowledge of the genetic basis of disease.
- Greater use of genetic testing in diagnosis and management of disease.
- Media-fuelled patient interest.
- Increased connectivity between primary care and genetic services (see Fig. 10.1).

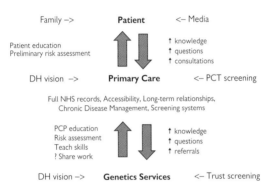

Fig. 10.1 Modelling the future.

Here we briefly examine the help that is available to PCPs in terms of:
- Developing the knowledge and skills required to care for patients with genetic disorders.
- Looking over the horizon to personalized medicine.

Personalized medicine

The ultimate goal of personalized medicine is to comprehensively identify genetic differences among persons and to correlate specific genetic features (or combinations of genetic features) with the differential risk of human diseases or the efficacy of certain therapeutic interventions.[1]

As we near the end of the first decade of the new millenium, we are only at the very start of this process. In order to achieve this goal it will be necessary to identify all relevant forms of human genetic variation and be able to interpret this information in a clinically meaningful manner.

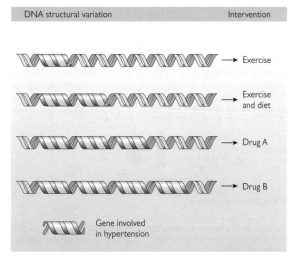

DNA structural variation   Intervention

→ Exercise

→ Exercise and diet

→ Drug A

→ Drug B

Gene involved in hypertension

Fig. 10.2 A model of copy-number variation and treatment of hypertension. A hypothetical scenario is shown. In this model, four approaches to treating hypertension depend on the number of copies of a gene conferring a risk of hypertension that are carried by the affected person. The optimal clinical intervention for a person with one, two, three or four copies of this gene is exercise, exercise and diet, administration of drug A, or administration of drug B, respectively. Reproduced from Lee C, Morton CC (2008). Structural Genomic variation and personalized Medicine. *NEJM* **358**: 740–41. Copyright © 2008 Massachussets Medical Society. All rights reserved.

Fig. 10.2 shows how treatment modalities could potentially be personalized based on knowledge of an individual's genetic results. Although testing for inherited susceptibility on the basis of common risk alleles is premature for most diseases the situation may well change over the next few years.

1 Lee, C. and Morton, C.C. (2008). Personalised medicine. Clinical implications of basic research. *New England Journal of Medicine*, **357**: 740–1.

Resources

Antenatal and neonatal screening timeline

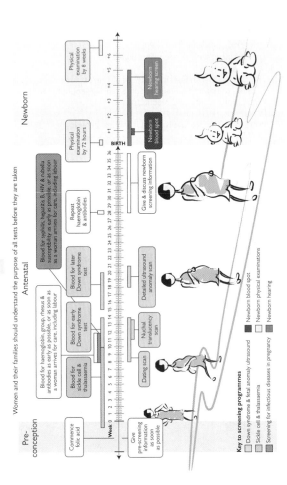

Fig. 11.1 Screening timeline—optimum times for testing. Screening timeline version 2, March 2008. (Reproduced with permission of the UK National Screening Committee ℘ www.screening.nhs.uk/an Copyright 2008) (🔲 Also see Fig. 9.1, p. 327)

Breast cancer family history primary care management algorithm (NICE)

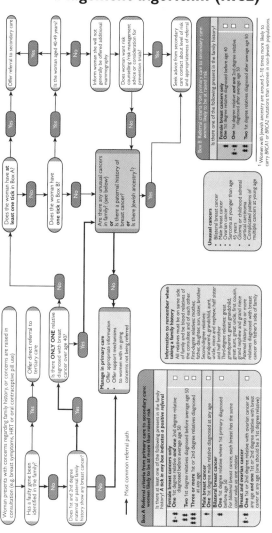

Fig. 11.2 Primary care management algorithm. (From National Institute for Health and Clinical Excellence (2006). *CG 41 Familial breast cancer: the classification and care of women at risk of familial breast cancer in primary, secondary and tertiary care*. NICE, London. Available from ⊘ www.nice.org.uk/GG41. Reproduced with permission.)

Breast cancer surveillance

	Mammography	MRI
20–29 years	Should not be available for women younger than age 30.	Should be available only for those at exceptionally high risk (that is, annual risk greater or equal to 1%), for example TP53 carriers.

30–39 years	Should be available to women satisfying referral criteria for secondary or specialist care:
	• only as part of a research study (ethically approved) or nationally approved and audited service.
	Individualized strategies should be developed for exceptional cases, such as:
	• women from families with BRCA1, BRCA2 or TP53 mutations (or women with equivalent high risk).
		+/− Should be available annually to:
		• women with a 10-year risk of greater than 8%
		• TP53, BRCA1 and BRCA2 mutation carriers
		• women who have not been tested but have a high chance of carrying a BRCA1 or TP53 mutation, specifically:
		  – those at a 50% risk of carrying a BRCA1 or TP53 mutation in a tested family
		  those at 50% risk of carrying a BRCA1 or TP53 mutation from untested or inconclusively tested families with at least a 60% risk of a BRCA1 or TP53 mutation (that is, a 30% chance of carrying a mutation themselves).

40–49 years	Should be available annually to:
	• women at raised and high risk satisfying referral criteria for secondary or specialist care.
		+/− Should be available annually to:
		• women with a 10-year risk of greater than 20%
		• women with a 10-year risk of greater than 12% whose mammography has shown a dense breast pattern†
		• TP53, BRCA1 and BRCA2 mutation carriers
		• women who have not been tested but have a high chance of carrying a BRCA1 or TP53 mutation, specifically:
		  – those at 50% risk of carrying a BRCA1 or TP53 mutation in a tested family
		  – those at 50% risk of carrying a BRCA1 or TP53 mutation from untested or inconclusively tested families with at least a 60% risk of a BRCA1 or TP53 mutation (that is, a 30% chance of carrying a mutation themselves).

Aged 50 and over	Should be available every 3 years as part of the NHS Breast Screening Programme. • more frequent mammographic surveillance should take place only as part of a research study (ethically approved) or nationally approved and audited service. Individualized strategies should be developed for exceptional cases, such as: • women from families with BRCA1, BRCA2 or TP53 mutations (or women with equivalent high risk).	Should not be available for women older than age 50.

†As defined by the 3-point mammographic classification used by UK breast radiologists (Breast Group of the Royal College of Radiologists 1989)

Supporting information

An 8% risk aged 30–39 and a 12% risk aged 40–49 years would be fulfilled by women with the following family histories:
• 2 close relatives diagnosed with average age < 30 years*
• 3 close relatives diagnosed with average age < 40 years*
• 4 close relatives diagnosed with average age < 50 years*.
*All relatives must be on the same side of the family and one must be a mother or sister of the consultee.
A genetic test would usually be required to determine a 10-year risk of 20% or greater in women aged 40–49 years.

For the purposes of these calculations, a women's age should be assumed to be 30 years of age for a women in her thirties and 40 years of age for a women in her forties. A 10-year risk should then be calculated for the period 30–39 and 40–49 years, respectively.

Fig. 11.3 NICE professional guidelines. From National Institute for Health and Clinical Excellence (2006). *CG 41 Familial breast cancer: the classification and care of women at risk of familial breast cancer in primary, secondary and tertiary care.* NICE, London. Available from 🔗 www.nice.org.uk/GG41. (Reproduced from NICE guidelines with permission.) (📖 See also Fig. 7.2, p. 237.)

Directory of UK and Ireland Genetics Centres

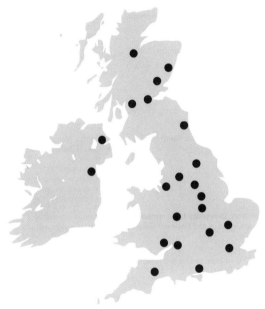

Fig. 11.4 Map showing location of regional genetics services in the UK.
(Reproduced with permission from the British Society for Human Genetics.)

Directory of UK and Ireland Genetics Centres

Name and address	Services offered

East Anglian Medical Genetics Service
 	
East Anglian Medical Genetics Service
Box 134
Level 6, Addenbrooke's Treatment Centre
Addenbrooke's Hospital
Cambridge
CB2 0QQ
☎ 01223 216446
Fax: 01223 217054
⌨ http://www.addenbrookes.org.uk/serv/clin/genetics/genetics_index.html
	• Genetic counselling
	• Clinical and genetic laboratory services
	  • cytogenetics
	  • molecular genetics
	  • molecular cytogenetics

Leicestershire Genetics Centre
 	
Leicester Royal Infirmary
(NHS Trust)
Leicester
LE1 5WW
	• Genetic counselling
	• Clinical and genetic laboratory services
	  • cytogenetics
	  • cancer cytogenetics
	  • molecular genetics
	  • molecular cytogenetics

Manchester University Department of Medical Genetics and Regional Genetic Service
 	
St Mary's Hospital
Central Manchester Healthcare Trust
Hathersage Road
Manchester
M13 0JH
⌨ http://www.mangen.co.uk/
	• Genetic counselling
	• Clinical and genetic laboratory services
	  • cytogenetics
	  • molecular genetics
	  • molecular cytogenetics

Medical Genetics Services for Wales
 	
Institute of Medical Genetics
University Hospital of Wales
Heath Park
Cardiff
CF14 4XW
☎ 02920 744028/744036
Fax: 02920 747603
⌨ http://www.wales.nhs.uk/awmgs
	• Genetic counselling
	• Clinical and genetics laboratory services
	  • cytogenetics
	  • cancer cytogenetics (primarily haematological)
	  • molecular genetics (UKGTN network laboratory, and member of the SCOBEC consortium)
	  • molecular cytogenetics

Merseyside Regional Clinical Genetics Service
 	
Royal Liverpool Children's Hospital
Alder Hey
Eaton Road
Liverpool
L12 2AP
⌨ http://www.lwh.me.uk/html/genetics.php
	• Genetic counselling/clinical and genetic laboratory services
	  • cytogenetics
	  • cancer cytogenetics
	  • molecular genetics
	  • molecular cytogenetics

Name and address	Services offered

North Thames (East) Regional Genetics Service
 	
Institute of Child Health
30 Guilford Street
London
WC1N 1EH
☎ 0207 242 2608
Fax: 0207 813 8141
🖰 http://www.ich.ucl.ac.uk/gosh/
clinicalservices/Clinical_genetics/Homepage
	• Genetic counselling
	• Clinical
	  • cytogenetics
	  • cancer cytogenetics
	  • molecular genetics
	  • molecular cytogenetics

North Thames (West) Regional Genetics Service
 	
The Kennedy Galton Centre
Northwick Park and St Mark's NHS Trust
Watford Road
Harrow
HA1 3UJ
🖰 http://www.nwlh.nhs.uk/nwthamesgenetics/
	• Genetic counselling
	• Clinical
	  • cytogenetics
	  • cancer cytogenetics
	  • molecular genetics
	  • molecular cytogenetics

Northern Genetics Service
 	
Institute of Human Genetics International
Centre for Life
Central Parkway
Newcastle upon Tyne
NE1 3BZ
☎ 0191 2418600
Fax No: 0191 2418799
🖰 http://www.newcastle-hospitals.org.uk/
directorates/northern-genetics-service
	• Genetic counselling
	• Clinical and genetic laboratory service
	  • cytogenetics
	  • molecular genetics

Nottingham Centre for Medical Genetics
 	
H-Block
City Hospital NHS Trust
Hucknall Road
Nottingham
NG5 1PB
☎ 0115 962 7728
Fax: 0115 962 8042
	• Genetic counselling
	• Genetic laboratory services
	  • cytogenetics
	  • cancer cytogenetics
	  • molecular genetics
	  • molecular cytogenetics

Oxford Regional Genetics Service
 	
The Churchill
Old Road
Oxford
OX3 7LJ
☎ 01865 226066
Fax: 01865 226011
🖰 http://www.oxfordradcliffe.nhs.uk/
forpatients/departments/genetics/home.aspx
	• Genetic counselling
	• Clinical and genetic laboratory services
	  • cytogenetics
	  • cancer cytogenetics
	  • molecular genetics
	  • molecular cytogenetics

Name and address	Services offered
Sheffield Regional Genetics Services Sheffield Children's NHS Trust Western Bank Sheffield S10 2TH	• Genetic counselling • Cytogenetics • Molecular genetics

South Thames (East) Regional Genetics Service
 	
Clinic:
7th Floor
New Guy's House
Guy's Hospital
St Thomas's Street
London
SE1 9RT
Laboratories:
5th Floor Guy's Tower
Guy's Hospital
St Thomas's Street
London
SE1 9RT
	• Genetic counselling
	• Clinical
	  • cytogenetics
	  • biochemical genetics
	  • molecular genetics

South Thames (West) Regional Genetics Service
 	
Medical Genetics Unit
St George's Hospital Medical School
Cranmer Terrace
London
SW17 0RE
☎ 020 8725 0574
Fax: 0208 725 3444
🖰 http://www.southwestthamesgenetics.nhs.uk/
	• Genetic counselling
	• Clinical
	  • cytogenetics
	  • cancer cytogenetics
	  • molecular genetics
	  • molecular cytogenetics

South Western Regional Genetics Service—Bristol, Bath, Somerset, and Gloucestershire
 	
St Michael's Hospital
St Michael's Hill
Bristol
BS2 8DT
☎ 0117 9285652
	• Genetic counselling
	• Clinical and genetic laboratory services
	  • cytogenetics
	  • cancer cytogenetics
	  • molecular genetics
	  • molecular cytogenetics
	  • clinical services

South Western Regional Genetics Service—Devon and Cornwall
 	
Clinical Genetics Department
Royal Devon & Exeter Hospital (Heavitree)
Gladstone Road
Exeter
EX1 2ED
☎ 01392 405726
Fax: 01392 405739
🖰 http://www.peninsulaclinicalgeneticsservice.co.uk/
	• Genetic counselling
	• Clinical and genetic laboratory services
	  • cytogenetics
	  • cancer cytogenetics
	  • molecular genetics
	  • molecular cytogenetics
	  • clinical services

Name and address	Services offered

Wessex Clinical Genetics Service
 	
Clinic:
Princess Anne Hospital
Southampton
SO16 5YA
⌂ http://www.wcgs.nhs.uk/
Laboratories:
Salisbury District Hospital
Salisbury
Wiltshire
SP2 8BJ
	• Genetic counselling
	• Clinical and genetic laboratory services
	  • cytogenetics
	  • cancer cytogenetics
	  • molecular genetics
	  • molecular cytogenetics

West Midlands Regional Genetics Services
 	
Birmingham Women's Hospital
Edgbaston
Birmingham
B15 2TG
⌂ http://www.bwhct.nhs.uk/genetics-index.htm
	• Genetic counselling/clinical and genetic laboratory services
	  • cytogenetics
	  • cancer cytogenetics
	  • molecular genetics
	  • molecular cytogenetics

Yorkshire Regional Genetics Service
 	
Department Of Clinical Genetics
Ashley Wing
St James's University Hospital
Leeds
LS9 7TF
☎ 0113 206 5143
Fax: 0113 246 7090
⌂ http://www.leedsteachinghospitals.com/patients/service_directory/index.php
	• Genetic counselling
	• Clinical and genetic laboratory services
	  • cytogenetics
	  • molecular genetics

Dundee—Human Genetics
 	
Pathology Department
Ninewells Hospital
Dundee
DD1 9SY
	• Genetic counselling
	• Clinical and genetic laboratory services
	  • cytogenetics
	  • cancer cytogenetics
	  • molecular genetics
	  • molecular cytogenetics

North of Scotland Regional Genetics Service
 	
Department of Medical Genetics
Medical School
Foresterhill
Aberdeen
AB25 2ZD
☎ 01224 552120
Fax: 01224 559390
	• Genetic counselling/clinical and genetic laboratory services
	  • cytogenetics
	  • cancer cytogenetics
	  • molecular genetics
	  • molecular cytogenetics

Name and address	Services offered
South East Scotland Clinical Genetics Service Western General Hospital Crewe Road Edinburgh EH14 1JF 🖰 http://www.mmc.med.ed.ac.uk/research/clingen/	• Genetic counselling • Clinical and genetic laboratory services • molecular genetics

West of Scotland Regional Genetics Service
 	
Institute of Medical Genetics
Yorkhill Hospital
Glasgow
G3 8SJ
☎ 0141 201 0365 (Reception)
Fax: 0141 357 4277
	• Genetic counselling
	• Clinical and genetic laboratory services
	  • cytogenetics,
	  • cancer cytogenetics,
	  • molecular genetics,
	  • molecular cytogenetics,
	  • biochemical genetics (enzymes)
	  • antenatal biochemical screening

Northern Ireland Regional Genetics Centre
 	
A Floor
Belfast City Hospital
Lisburn Road
Belfast
BT9 7AB
☎ 028 9026 3874
Fax: 028 9023 6911
🖰 http://www.belfasttrust.hscni.net/
	• Genetic counselling/clinical and genetic laboratory services
	  • cytogenetics
	  • cancer cytogenetics
	  • molecular genetics
	  • molecular cytogenetics

Republic of Ireland Genetics Service
 	
National Centre for Medical Genetics (NCMG)
Our Lady's Hospital for Sick Children
Crumlin
Dublin 12
Republic of Ireland
☎ 01409 6737 (General information)
Fax: 01456 0953
🖰 http://www.genetics.ie
	• Clinical genetics
	  • cytogenetics
	  • molecular genetics

Further reading and on-line resources about genetics

Books

Medical Genetics
Ian D. Young (2005)
ISBN 0-19-856494-5
Oxford University Press   ℘ http://www.oup.com

Oxford Desk Reference—Clinical Genetics
H.V. Firth, J.A. Hurst, with advisory editor J.G. Hall (2005)
ISBN 0-19-262896-8
Oxford University Press   ℘ http://www.oup.com

On-line resources

GeneClinics and GeneReviews
℘ http://www.geneclinics.org
Primarily designed for physicians in the USA to find appropriate genetics specialists and testing facilities, this site contains helpful teaching tools for primary care, including such subjects as:
- Taking a family history (with downloadable pdfs).
- Genetic diagnosis red flags (using a mnemonic).
- Understanding genetic tests.

It is also an excellent resource for information about rare disorders (📖 see GeneReviews ℘ www.genereviews.org).

OMIM—Online Mendelian Inheritance in Man
℘ http://www.ncbi.nlm.nih.gov/omim/
Edited at Johns Hopkins University School of Medicine, this database was initiated in the early 1960s and, with daily updating, is a catalogue of all known Mendelian traits and disorders and over 12 000 genes. An extensive chapter on each gene gives:
- Disease description.
- Gene locus.
- Clinical and biochemical features.
- Mode of inheritance.
- Molecular genetics.

Orphanet
℘ http://www.orpha.net
Orphanet aims to provide rare disease information to healthcare professionals, patients, and their relatives, in order to contribute to improving the diagnosis, care, and treatment of these diseases.

Further information and resources

Adoption

Adoption UK	✍ www.adoption.org.uk
British Association for Adoption and Fostering	✍ www.baaf.org

Alpha1-antitrypsin deficiency

Alpha1 (UK)	✍ www.alpha1.org.uk
Alpha1 (USA)	✍ www. alpha1.org

Alzheimer disease

Alzheimer's Society	✍ www.alzheimers.org.uk

Antenatal results and choices

ARC (Antenatal Results and Choices) ☎ 020 7631 0285	✍ www.arc-uk.org

Autism

The National Autistic Society	✍ www.nas.org.uk

Breast cancer

Breakthrough Breast Cancer	✍ www.breastcancergenetics. org.uk

NICE

Breast cancer genetic algorithm	✍ www.nice.org.uk
Useful resource for families and primary care workers: Familial breast cancer CG 41 2006	✍ www.nice.org.uk

Cancer

Cancerline UK	✍ www.cancerlineuk.net/index.asp

Cardiac anomalies

Little Hearts Matter	✍ www.lhm.org.uk

Cardiomyopathy

Cardiomyopathy Association	✍ www.cardiomyopathy.org

Club foot (talipes)

STEPS ☎ 0871 717 0044	✍ www.steps-charity.org.uk

Colon cancer

Hereditary Colon Cancer	✍ www.mtsinai.on.ca/familialgi cancer/Diseases/HNPCC/ default.htm

Cystic fibrosis

Cystic Fibrosis Trust	✍ www.cftrust.org.uk

Deafness

National Deaf Children's Society (NDCS)	www.ndcs.org.ukw
Royal National Institute for the Deaf	www.rnid.org.uk
	www.deafplus.org
National Newborn Hearing Screening Programme (NHSP)	http://hearing.screening.nhs.uk/surveillance

Diabetes

Diabetes UK	www.diabetes.org.uk

Down syndrome

Down Syndrome Association	www.downs-syndrome.org.uk
MDS UK—Mosaic Down Syndrome Support Group	www.mosaicdownsyndrome.org
US National Down Syndrome Society	www.ndss.org
Down syndrome growth charts	www.growthcharts.com

Ehlers–Danlos syndrome

The Ehlers–Danlos National Foundation	www.ednf.org
The EDS support group (UK)	www.ehlers-danlos.org

Epilepsy

Epilepsy Action	www.epilepsy.org.uk
The National Society for Epilepsy	www.epilepsynse.org.uk
Epilepsy Foundation of America	www.efa.org

Familial adenomatous polyposis (FAP)

FAP support group	www. fapsupportgroup.org

Fetal alcohol syndrome

Fetal Alcohol Syndrome Trust	www.medicouncilalcol.demon.co.uk/FAST/fast. htm

Fetal anticonvulsant syndrome

National Fetal Anti-convulsant Syndrome Association	www.facsline.org

Fragile X syndrome

Fragile X Society
☎ 01424 813147	www.fragilex.org.uk
National Fragile X Foundation (US)	www.fragileX.org

Glaucoma

International Glaucoma Association
☎ 020 7737 3265	www.iga.org.uk

Haemochromatosis

The Haemochromatosis Society	www.ghsoc.org
Hemochromatosis Foundation	www.hemochromatosis.org

Haemoglobinopathies

UK Thalassaemia Society   ✍ www.ukts.org

The Sickle Cell Society   ✍ www.sicklecellsociety.org

Advice for carriers   ✍ www.chime.ucl.ac.uk/APoGI/menu.htm

Haemophilia

Haemophilia Society (UK)   ✍ www.haemophilia.org.uk

National Hemophilia Foundation (USA)   ✍ www.infonhf.org

The Haemophilia Alliance is a national partnership whose aim is to advance and promote high levels of care for people with haemophilia and related disorders   ✍ www.haemophiliaalliance.org.uk

Hereditary motor sensory neuropathy (HMSN/CMT) / Charcot–Marie–Tooth disease (CMT)

CMT UK   ✍ www.cmt.org.uk

Huntington disease

Huntington Disease Association (UK)   ✍ www.hda.org.uk

Huntington's Disease Society of America   ✍ hdsa.mgh.harvard.edu

Hypercholesterolaemia

Heart UK   ✍ www.heartuk.org.uk
☎ 01628 628638

Ichthyosis

Ichthyosis Support Group   ✍ www.ichthyosis.co.uk
☎ 020 7461 9034

Infertility

Müllerian aplasia   rosagroup@yahoo.co.uk

CHILD: The National Infertility Support Network   ✍ www.child.org.uk
☎ 01424 732361

Klinefelter's syndrome

Klinefelter's Syndrome Association UK   ✍ www.ksa-uk.co.uk

Klinefelter's Syndrome and Associates   ✍ www.genet.org/ks

Long QT/Brugada

SADS UK (The Sudden Arrhythmic Death Syndrome Foundation UK)   ✍ www.sadsuk.org

The Cardiac Arrhythmia Research and Education Foundation   ✍ www.longqt.org

Marfan syndrome

Marfan Association UK   ✍ www.marfan.org.uk

National Marfan Foundation (US)   ✍ www.marfan.org

MedicAlert Foundation
Bridge Wharf
156 Caledonian Road
London
N1 9UU
Freephone: 0800 581420
☎ 020 7833 3034
Fax: 020 7278 0647
Email: info@medicalert.org.uk

🖱 www.medicalert.org.uk

Metabolic diseases
CLIMB (Children Living with
  Inherited Metabolic Diseases)

🖱 www.climb.org.uk

Miscarriage
The Miscarriage Association

🖱 www.miscarriageassociation.
  org.uk

Multiple Endocrine Neoplasia
Association for Multiple Endocrine
Neoplasia Disorders (AMEND)

🖱 www.amend.org.uk

Muscular dystrophies
Muscular Dystrophy Campaign

🖱 www.muscular-dystrophy.
  org

Duchenne Family Support Group
Parent Project UK—Muscular
  dystrophy

🖱 www.dfsg.org.uk
🖱 www.ppuk.org

Myotonic dystrophy
Myotonic Dystrophy Support Group

🖱 www.mdsuk.org

Neurofibromatosis
The Neurofibromatosis Association
National Neurofibromatosis
  Foundation (US)

🖱 www.nfa.zetnet.co.uk
🖱 www.nf.org

Osteoporosis
National Osteoporosis Society
WHO Fracture risk assessment
  (FRAX) calculator

🖱 www.nos.org.uk
🖱 www.shef.ac.uk/FRAX

Parkinson disease
Parkinson's Disease Society
☎ 0808 800 0303

🖱 www.parkinsons.org.uk

Phenylketonuria
National Society for PKU (NSKPU)

🖱 www.web.ukonline.co.uk/
  nspku

Platelet disorders

Platelet Disorder Support Association   ♫ www.pdsa.org

Polycystic disease

Polycystic Disease Charity   ♫ www.pkdcharity.co.uk
☎ 01388 665004

Premature ovarian failure

Premature Ovarian Failure   ♫ www.pofsupport.org
Support Group

Retinitis pigmentosa

British Retinitis Pigmentosa Society   ♫ www.brps.org.uk
☎ 01280 860363

Foundation Fighting Blindness (US)   ♫ www.blindness.org

Retinoblastoma

Retinoblastoma Society   ♫ www.rbsociety.org.uk
☎ 020 7600 3309

Syndromes—general

Contact a family   ♫ www.cafamily.org.uk

Teratology

UK: National Teratology   ♫ www.ncl.ac.uk/pharmsc/
Information Service (NTIS)   entis.htm
☎ 0191 232 1525

Europe: European Teratology   ♫ www.entisorg.com
Information Services (ENTIS)

Canada: Motherisk Program   ♫ www.motherisk.org
☎ (416) 813 6780

USA: OTIS Organisation of Teratology   ♫ www.otispregnancy.org
Information Services
☎ (866) 626 6847

Thrombophilia

Thrombophilia: information for   ♫ www.bcshguidelines.com
patients and their relatives·

Thrombophilia support   ♫ www.fvleiden.org

Tuberous sclerosis

UK Tuberous Sclerosis Association   ♫ www.tuberous-sclerosis.org
☎ 01527 871898

Tuberous Sclerosis Alliance (US)   ♫ www.tsalliance.org

Turner syndrome

Turner Syndrome Support Society   ♫ www.tss.org.uk

Unique
Unique—The Rare Chromosome
 Disorder Support Group
☎ 01883 330766

🖱 www.rarechromo.org

von Hippel–Lindau
VHL Family Alliance

🖱 www.vhl.org

Primary care education

National Genetics Education and Development Centre (NGEDC)

🖰 www.geneticseducation.nhs.uk

Funded by the Department of Health as one of the major initiatives of the 2003 Genetics White Paper, *Our Inheritance, Our Future*, the centre is committed to improving the understanding of genetics throughout the NHS. The web pages in the 'Learning Genetics' are subdivided according to profession, i.e. medical or nursing, and contain articles on:
- Understanding genetics
- Patterns of inheritance
- Family history
- Genetic testing and screening
- Ethical, legal, and social implications of genetics
- Communicating genetic information.

They can also provide a plastic template for drawing family history charts, with a printed reminder of how to format the chart.

PEGASUS (Professional Education for Genetic Assessment and Screening)

🖰 www.pegasus.nhs.uk

Here, although the main focus is on screening for haemoglobinopathies, they are used as a springboard for basic genetic learning. With subsections on:
- A medical or nursing practitioner's role in screening for genetics disorders.
- Key clinical information.
- Genetics.
- Responding to diversity.
- Newborn bloodspot screening for sickle cell disorders and cystic fibrosis.

A further aim of the organization is to train up a workforce of genetic trainers

Primary Care Genetics Society (PCGS)

🖰 www.pcgs.org.uk

Founded in 2007, the Primary Care Genetics Society (PCGS) was to support primary care professionals (PCPs) in dealing with the increasing demand from their patients who are becoming more aware of the potential impact of genetics on their lives. Its primary aim is to support and facilitate the educational needs of PCPs. This is achieved through its regional conferences and an increasing list of resources accessible through its website, covering:
- The genetic basis of diseases such as cancer, reproductive medicine, diabetes, and heart disease.
- The management of patients with genetic disorders.
- Advice on screening.
- Genetic testing.
- Ethical dilemmas in primary care.

Public Health Genetics Foundation
🕮 www.phgfoundation.org

An international, independent charity whose aims include:
- The identification of biomedical science that may benefit health and disseminate that knowledge for the public's benefit.
- Contributing to the integration of biomedical science into mainstream medicine and health services.
- The promotion and provision of education and training to support the responsible and effective application of biomedical science for health.

As well as a helpful resource for standard genetics, including:
- Basic genetics
- Genetic technology
- Genetics and disease
- Basic epidemiology.

The site also contains an excellent series of web-based interactive tutorials, including:
- Moral theories
- Pharmacogenomics
- DNA test methods
- Disease susceptibility
- Informed consent.

Other e-Learning
UK PCPs already use a variety of accredited educational e-resources, and modules on genetics in primary care can be found on:
- 🕮 www.learning.bmj.com/learning/main.html
- 🕮 www.doctors.net.uk/

The US site 'GeneTests' 🕮 www.genetests.org includes a tab entitled 'Educational Materials' that enables you to access the web-site **Genetic Tools: Genetics Through a Primary Care Lens**. This site provides resources for primary care teaching, presenting genetics information and concepts in the context of primary care. It includes four main sections:
- Genetic Concepts and Skills (inheritance, genetic testing, family history, and public health implications).
- Teaching cases (41 primary care presentations of genetic conditions).
- Ethical, legal, social, and cultural issues.
- Other resources (including references and web resources for patients).

Professional bodies involved in UK clinical genetics

British Society for Human Genetics (BSHG)
℘ www.bshg.org.uk

BSHG is largely a forum for clinical and research professionals in genetics, but has accessible policy statements that are relevant to primary care. For an example 📖 see Chapter 1, Confidentiality and consent, p. 8.

Ethox
℘ www.ethox.org.uk

Ethox is dedicated to enhancing patient care by improving ethical understanding and ethical standards. Approaching the study of ethics across many subject areas, there is a separate section focusing on ethical dilemmas in genetics.

Genetic Interest Group (GIG)
℘ www.gig.org.uk

The Genetic Interest Group (GIG) is a UK alliance of patient organizations, including more than 130 charities supporting children, families, and individuals affected by genetic disorders. Largely devoted to effective and practical dissemination of genetic knowledge from scientists, through policy setters down to practitioners and, through them, their patients, GIG provides a series of informative resources, including videos, showing how people live and cope with genetic disease within their family.

Human Genetics Commission
℘ www.hgc.gov.uk

The HGC is the UK Government's advisory body on new developments in human genetics and their impact on individual lives, with a particular focus on the social, ethical, and legal issues, rather than the specifics of genetics as a science. It monitors such areas as:
- Identity testing
- Genetic discrimination
- Intellectual property and genetics
- Databases
- Genetic services.
Recent working groups have been looking at:
- Genetics and reproductive decision making.
- Genetically profiling babies at birth.

Rare Disease UK
℘ www.raredisease.org.uk

The national alliance for people with rare diseases and all who support them. Rare Disease UK is an alliance of key stakeholders brought together to develop a national plan for rare diseases in the UK.

Regional Genetics Services (UK)
📖 See Directory of UK and Ireland Genetics Centres, p. 415 for a map and contact details of genetic centres in the UK and Ireland.

Samples for genetic tests

Occasionally, PCPs may be asked to obtain samples from patients for genetic testing.

Before samples are obtained, practitioners must:
- Check that the appropriate consents are in place.
- Be clear that their patient is aware of the possible implications of the test.
- Label sample tubes clearly using three-point patient references, preferably including their name, DoB, and NHS number on both request form and sample bottles.

Samples of venous blood should be taken as follows:
- **DNA** analysis into an EDTA tube (5mL)—this is usually the same type of tube as that used for a Full Blood Count (FBC).
- **Chromosome analysis** into a lithium heparin tube (2–5mL) (this may change to an EDTA sample in the near future as the approach to chromosome analysis changes from light microscopy to genomic array). Occasionally tests may be possible on buccal swabs or mouthwashes. In these cases the equipment will be supplied. Most PCPs will be familiar with the types of kits supplied by private firms who offer paternity testing.

Read the request form carefully and if in doubt phone the laboratory.

Glossary of terms

Acrocentric A chromosome where the centromere is near one end. The gene coding material is usually located only on the long arm. The human acrocentric chromosomes are 13, 14, 15, 21, and 22.

Allele One of several alternative forms of a gene occupying a given locus on a chromosome.

Allele drop-out (ADO) The failure, for technical reasons, to detect an allele that is present in a sample; the failure to amplify an allele during a polymerase chain reaction.

Allele frequency The frequency in a population of each allele at a polymorphic locus.

Aneuploidy In *full aneuploidy* there is an abnormal chromosome number differing from the usual diploid or haploid set by loss or addition of one or a small number of chromosomes, e.g. 45,X or 47,XY + 21. It can be the result of non-disjunction in (i) a premeiotic mitotic division in the germline of either parent, (ii) a first or second meiotic division in either parent, or (iii) an early embryonic mitotic (postzygotic) division in an affected individual. In *partial aneuploidy*, the imbalance involves the gain or loss of part of a chromosome.

Anticipation Worsening of disease severity in successive generations. Characteristically occurs in triplet repeat disorders where there is expansion of the triplet repeat in the maternal or paternal line, e.g. myotonic dystrophy.

Apoptosis Programmed cell death.

Array-CGH Microarray-based comparative genomic hybridization (*see* Microarray and Comparative genomic hybridization).

ART (assisted reproductive technologies) Assisted reproductive technology, e.g. *in vitro* fertilization (IVF) and intracytoplasmic sperm injection (ICSI), has revolutionized the treatment of infertility. In conjunction with single-cell genetic analysis based on polymerase chain reaction (PCR) or fluorescent *in situ* hybridization (FISH) it has also made pre-implantation genetic diagnosis (PGD) possible for some genetic disorders. 📖 See Chapter 9, Assisted reproductive technology.

Autosome A chromosome that is not an X or Y chromosome. There are 22 pairs of autosomes in the human chromosome complement.

Band/banding Differential staining of a chromosome leading to distinction of chromosomal segments. A Giemsa-stained (G-banded) karyotype has 850 bands visible at prometaphase.

Birth prevalence The number of cases of disorder/condition per number of live births (usually per 1000).

bp (base pair) In DNA a purine and pyrimidine base on each strand that interact with each other through hydrogen bonding.

cDNA DNA complementary to, and copied from, an RNA molecule. cDNA libraries of living cells therefore represent the RNA content of those cells, and thereby represent expressed gene sequences.

Centimorgan (cM) Unit of genetic map distance corresponding to a recombination fraction of 0.01.

Centromere The constricted region of a chromosome that includes the site of attachment to the mitotic or meiotic spindle.

Chimerism The presence in an organism of two or more cell lines that are derived from different zygotes. Such an organism is termed a chimera. Chimerism is extremely rare in humans.

Chip (📖 see Microarray).

Chromatid A chromosome that has undergone replication has two identical sister chromatids that are joined at the centromere before they separate into two distinct chromosomes during cell division.

Chromatin The DNA helix is wrapped around core histones to form a simple 'beads on a string' configuration, where the beads represent nucleosomes. This is then folded into higher-order chromatin. Chromatin can be modified by processes such as DNA methylation and histone modification (acetylation, phosphorylation, methylation, and ubiquitylation). The regulation of higher-order chromatin structures is crucial for genome reprogramming during early embryogenesis and gametogenesis, and for tissue-specific gene expression and global gene silencing.

Chromosome A thread-like structure composed mainly of chromatin that carries a highly ordered sequence of linked genes and resides in the nucleus of eukaryotic cells.

Cloning Production of genetically identical cells (or organisms from a single ancestral cell (or nucleus)). Also a technique used in molecular biology to propagate single or discrete DNA fragments of interest.

Coding strand The coding strand of DNA has a complementary sequence to mRNA since it serves as the template for mRNA synthesis.

Comparative genomic hybridization (CGH) Reference and test DNA samples are fluorescently labelled, e.g. one with green probes, the other with red probes. After hybridization of labelled probe mixes to metaphase chromosome spreads, the ratio of green to red fluorescence along each chromosome is compared in an attempt to identify genomic imbalance in the test DNA.

Compound heterozygote An individual that has altered gene function because each copy of the gene is altered by different mutations, e.g. an individual with cystic fibrosis may have the *CFTR* genotype deltaF508/G542X, i.e. there are two mutations in both alleles at the *same* locus. (NB A double heterozygote is an individual who is heterozygous at two different loci).

Concordance Presence of the same trait in both members of a pair (as in twins) or in all members of a set of similar individuals.

Consanguinity Parents are related (i.e. have a recent common ancestor) and share a proportion of their genetic material. In practice, a consanguineous relationship is often considered as one between individuals who are second cousins or closer.

Consultand An individual seeking advice about a genetic disorder.

Copy number The number of copies present of a given chromosomal locus.

Cumulative risk Cumulative risk of a disease by age n is the probability of an individual being diagnosed with that disease by their nth birthday

Deletion Loss of part of a chromosome, or part or all of a gene or DNA sequence.

Digenic inheritance Two genes are involved, with at least one mutation at both loci needed, in order to produce the phenotype, e.g. connexin 26 and 30 in sensorineural deafness.

Diploid (2n) A paired set of chromosomes comprising two of each autosome and two sex chromosomes. Diploid chromosome sets occur in somatic cells, e.g. 46,XX and 46,XY. Often used as diploid cell or diploid organism.

Discordance A twin pair or set of individuals in which the members differ in whether they exhibit a certain trait.

Dizygotic twins (DZ) Two individuals born together derived from two separate eggs fertilized by two separate sperm.

Domain A discrete portion of a gene or protein with its own function.

Dominant A trait in which the mutant allele is dominant to the wild-type allele, i.e. the disease or disorder is manifest when one copy of the mutant allele is inherited, e.g. achondroplasia.

Dominant negative mutation A mutation in one copy of a gene resulting in a mutant protein that has not only lost its own function, but also prevents the wild-type protein of the same gene from functioning normally. Commonly acts by producing an altered polypeptide (subunit) that prevents the assembly of a multimeric protein.

Double heterozygote An individual who is heterozygous at two *different* loci. (NB An individual who is a compound heterozygote has two different mutations at the same locus.)

Downstream A region of DNA that lies 3′ to the point of reference.

Embryonic stem cell Cell derived from the inner cell mass of an early embryo that can replicate indefinitely and differentiate into many cell types.

Empiric risk Risk of recurrence that has been observed based on family studies—often used for complex multifactorial disorders.

Epigenetic Any heritable influence (in the progeny of cells or of individuals) on chromosome or gene function that is not accompanied by a change in DNA sequence, e.g. X-chromosome inactivation, imprinting, centromere inactivation, and position-effect variegation.

Exon A segment of an interrupted gene that is represented in the mature RNA product.

Expressivity Variation in the severity of a disorder in individuals who have inherited the same disease alleles. Note the difference from *penetrance*, which is the percentage of individuals expressing the disorder to any degree, from the most trivial to the most severe.

FISH (fluorescence *in situ* hybridization) *In situ* hybridization in which the DNA-probe is labelled with a fluorophore. Using fluorescence microscopy, the probe can be visualized binding to a specific chromosomal region. The efficacy of FISH is limited in some applications by low-resolution sensitivity.

Founder effect A high prevalence of a genetic disorder in an isolated or inbred population due to the fact that many members of the population are derived from a common ancestor who harboured a disease-causing mutation. Founder effects are seen both for dominant and recessive disorders and, if the disorder is due to a founder effect, the affected individuals in a given population carry the same mutation (founder mutation). Examples include the recessive disorders Meckel syndrome, hydrolethalus syndrome, Cohen syndrome, and congenital Finnish nephropathy, which all occur with disproportionately high incidence in Finland compared with other European populations.

Founder mutation A disease-causing mutation that is found repeatedly in a given population and is derived from a common ancestor who harboured that mutation.

Frameshift mutation Deletion or insertion of a number of bases, that is not a multiple of three, leading to alteration of the reading frame.

Gamete An egg or sperm cell.

Gene The fundamental unit of heredity. A sequence of DNA involved in producing a polypeptide chain—it includes coding segments (exons) and intervening sequences (introns) together with regulatory elements, e.g. promoter. A gene is functionally defined by its product.

Genetic counselling The process by which individuals or relatives at risk of a disorder that may be hereditary are advised of the consequences of the disorder, the probability of developing or transmitting it, and the ways in which this may be prevented, avoided, or ameliorated.

Genome The entire genetic complement of a prokaryote, virus, mitochondria or chloroplast, or the haploid nuclear genetic complement of a eukaryotic species. The human genome contains about 32 000 genes.

Genome-wide scan A systematic survey to discover if a phenotypic trait or genetic disease is linked to a genetic mapping marker(s) used to try and identify the gene(s) responsible for a given disease.

Genotype The genetic constitution of an individual, at one or more gene loci.

Germline mosaicism The presence in a gonad of genetically distinct populations of cells, usually implying that the mosaicism is confined to the ovary/testis. If both parents appear unaffected, but one parent is a germline mosaic, this can result in recurrence of affected children, e.g. tuberous sclerosis.

Haploid (n) A set of chromosomes comprising one of each autosome and one sex chromosome. Haploid chromosome sets (n) occur in the gametes, e.g. 23,X and 23,Y.

Haploinsufficiency Situation in which the product of only one allele is produced and is insufficient for normal function. It arises when the normal phenotype requires the protein product of two alleles, and reduction of 50% of the gene product results in an abnormal phenotype.

Haplotype A set of closely linked alleles on a single chromosome that tend to be inherited *en bloc*, i.e. not separated by recombination at meiosis.

Hedgehog genes A highly conserved family of genes that encode signalling molecules.

Hemizygote The usual situation in males, with one copy of genes on the X chromosome (see below).

Hemizygous The presence of only one copy of a gene. Males are hemizygous for most genes on the X chromosome (with the exception of the pseudoautosomal regions, which are also represented on Y).

Heritability The proportion of the variation in a given characteristic or state within a particular population that can be attributed to genetic factors.

Heteroplasmy The existence of more than one mitochondrial DNA (mtDNA) type in the same cell, tissue, or individual, e.g. mitochondria containing a mixture of mtDNA carrying the MELAS 3243 point mutation and mtDNA with the wild-type sequence. In mitochondrial disorders, because of the thousands of mitochondria in each cell, there are often variable percentages of mutant and wild-type mtDNAs between different cells and especially between different tissues (⌨ see Homoplasmy).

Heterozygote An individual who has two different alleles at one specified locus. Heterozyotes may also be described as carriers.

Heterozygote advantage The increase in reproductive fitness observed in unaffected heterozygotes (carriers) compared to affected homozygotes.

Heterozygous The presence of two different alleles at a specified locus.

Histones Small, highly conserved basic proteins that associate with DNA to form a nucleosome (the basic structural subunit of chromatin).

Homoplasmy The existence of only one mitochondrial DNA (mtDNA) type in the same cell, tissue, or individual, e.g. mitochondria containing only mtDNA carrying the A1555G sensorineural deafness sequence (see Heteroplasmy).

Homozygote An individual with two identical alleles at a specified locus on homologous chromosomes.

Homozygous The presence of two identical alleles at a specified locus.

Hybridization The artificial pairing of two complementary strands of DNA (or one strand of DNA and one of RNA) to form a double-stranded molecule. One strand is often labelled and used as a probe to detect the presence of the other.

ICSI (intracytoplasmic sperm injection) Used as an adjunct to IVF to overcome infertility due to oligospermia and/or immotile sperm and for polymerase chain reaction (PCR)-based pre-implantation genetic diagnosis (PGD) techniques, to avoid the risk of extra sperm buried in the zona pellucida contaminating the assay.

Incidence The number of new cases arising in a specified population over a given period of time.

Imprinting A genetic mechanism by which genes are selectively expressed from the maternal or paternal homologue of a chromosome. This expression may be time specific and even tissue specific. For a small number of genes, epigenetic mechanisms can determine expression from one generation of the organism to the next. Imprinting invokes a variety of mechanisms that distinguish the maternal and paternal homologues and affect the chromatin structures that determine transcriptionally silent and active states. The inactive allele is epigenetically marked by histone modification, cytosine methylation, or both. Imprints, once established, are erased during the early development of the male and female germ cells and then reset prior to germ cell maturation. In humans about 50 genes are imprinted, i.e. differentially expressed according to their origin in either the oocyte or spermatozoa. These imprinted genes have roles in growth and development as well as in tumour suppression.

Incest Incest is defined as sexual intercourse between close relatives. In English law it is the crime of sexual intercourse between parent and child or grandchild, or between siblings or half-siblings (*Shorter Oxford English Dictionary*).

Informed choice 'An informed choice is one that is based on relevant knowledge consistent with the decision maker's values and behaviourally implemented' (Marteau 2001).

In-frame mutation Deletion or insertion of multiples of three bases that lead to a deletion or insertion to the encoded protein, but not to early termination.

Intron A segment of DNA that is transcribed, but removed from within the transcript by splicing together the coding sequences (exons) on either side of it.

IVF (*in vitro* fertilization) An assisted reproductive technology (ART) procedure that involves collecting eggs from a woman's ovaries (egg retrieval) and fertilizing them in the laboratory. The resulting embryos are then transferred back into the uterus through the cervix. Hormone therapy is administered to stimulate ovulation prior to egg collection, and to prepare the endometrium to facilitate implantation of the embryo(s). Usually a maximum of two embryos are implanted to minimize the risk of triplets and higher-order multiple births.

Karyotype The chromosome complement of a cell or species. In humans, the karyotype of a normal male is 46,XY and that of a normal female is 46,XX.

kb (kilobase) 10^3 base pairs of DNA.

Lambda (λ) The ratio of the frequency of a multifactorial disease in the relative of an affected person compared with its rate in the general population; e.g. in sib-pair studies, $lambda_s$ is the ratio of the frequency of the disease in siblings compared with the general population. $Lambda_s$ is a measure of relative risk and hence disease heritability.

Linkage disequilibrium Linkage disequilibrium occurs when the probability of the occurrence of particular DNA variants at two sites physically close to one another on the chromosome is significantly greater than that expected from the product of the observed allelic frequencies at each site independently, i.e. the DNA variants occur together more frequently on individual chromosomes in the population than expected by chance.

Locus A unique chromosomal region that corresponds to a gene or some other DNA sequence.

Locus heterogeneity The disease phenotype caused by mutation in one gene can also be caused by mutations in another gene at a different location in the genome, e.g. tuberous sclerosis can be caused by a mutation in *TSC1* on 9q or by a mutation in *TSC2* on 16p.

LOD (logarithm of the odds ratio) score A measure of genetic linkage, defined as the log_{10} ratio of the probability that the data would have arisen if the loci are linked, to the probability that the data could have arisen from unlinked loci. The conventional threshold for declaring linkage is a LOD score of 3.0, i.e. a 1000:1 ratio (which must be compared with the 50:1 probability that any random pair of loci will be linked).

LOF (loss of function) Referring to a type of mutation resulting in inactivation of the gene product.

Mb (megabase) 10^6 base pairs of DNA.

Meiosis The process by which haploid (n) germ cells are produced by two successive cell divisions without an intervening round of DNA replication. The first meiotic division (MI) is called the reduction division because it reduces the chromosome number from $2n$ to n. Sister chromatids separate from each other only at the second meiotic division (MII). This yields haploid cells that differentiate into ova or sperm. Recombination occurs in the prophase of MI.

Microarray (chip) A high-density miniaturized array of oligonucleotides spotted on to a glass slide. Expression arrays hybridize mRNA to quantify gene expression Genomic arrays hybridize DNA to identify cryptic deletions and duplications.

Microsatellite A stretch of DNA in which a short motif (usually 1–5 nucleotides long) is repeated several times, e.g. a polyA tract $(A)_{13}$. The most common microsatellite in humans is a $(CA)_n$ repeat which occurs in tens of thousands of places in the genome.

Microsatellite instability (MSI) The situation in which germline microsatellite alleles (see above) gain or lose repeat units during mitosis. This generates a variety of repeat lengths for specific microsatellites in different somatic cells of the same individual. Microsatellite instability is a feature of hereditary non-polyposis colorectal cancer (HNPCC).

Mismatch repair Nucleotide mismatches occur normally when two strands of DNA replicate, but almost all such errors are quickly corrected by a molecular proofreading mechanism (encoded by the mismatch repair genes, e.g. *MSH2* and *MLH1*). Defective mismatch repair facilitates malignant transformation by allowing the rapid accumulation of mutations that inactivate genes that ordinarily have key functions in the cell.

Missense mutation Nucleotide substitution that results in an altered amino acid residue in the encoded protein.

Mitosis The process by which the genetic material in a cell is duplicated and divided equally between two daughter cells. Each chromosome undergoes duplication to produce two closely adjacent sister chromatids that separate from each other to become two daughter chromosomes.

Modifier gene A gene whose expression can influence a phenotype resulting from mutation at another locus.

Monogenic A trait or disease governed by the individual action of a single gene (as in classical Mendelian disorders).

Monosomy One copy of a chromosome. Usually two copies are present in a somatic cell ($2n$). Autosomal monosomy is invariably lethal in early pregnancy. Females with Turner syndrome are typically monosomic for X, i.e. 45,X.

Monozygotic twins (MZ) Two individuals born together derived from one sperm and one egg.

Mosaicism The presence of two or more cell populations derived from the same conceptus, but in which has subsequently acquired a genetic difference, either by mitotic non-disjunction, trisomy rescue, or occurrence of a somatic new mutation. Examples include trisomy 21 mosaicism arising either from a normal conceptus with mitotic non-disjunction in the early zygote or from a trisomy 21 conceptus with subsequent trisomy rescue establishing a euploid cell line 47,XY + 21/46,XY, or segmental neurofibromatosis type 1 (NF1) in which cells in just a few dermatomes have acquired a neurofibromin mutation.

Multifactorial disease A disease caused by the interaction of several genes and the environment.

Multiplex ligation-dependent probe amplification (MLPA) A new method for the relative quantification of up to 40 different DNA sequences. Each MLPA probe consists of two oligonucleotides that are ligated by a thermostable ligase if they bind to the target sequence. Target sequences are small (50–70 nucleotides). The ligated probe is then amplified by polymerase chain reaction (PCR) (rather than the target sequence as in conventional assays). Each MLPA probe is designed to have a specific size so that, when the amplification products of the PCR are run on a gel, the product of each probe can be identified by its size. This technique can be used to identify exon deletions and duplications, and, potentially, the copy number of any unique sequence.

Multiplex polymerase chain reaction (PCR) In this test PCR is used with a mixture of different primer pairs. Each primer pair is designed to amplify a single region of interest (e.g. an exon of dystrophin) using genomic DNA as a template.

Mutation A permanent change in the genetic material that can be transmitted to offspring. A pathogenic mutation results in an alteration in the function of the gene product.

Non-disjunction The failure of homologous chromosomes to segregate at meiosis, resulting in one daughter cell with two copies, and one daughter cell with no copies of the chromosome in question. Trisomy 21 usually arises by non-disjunction in maternal meiosis.

Nonsense mutation A mutation resulting in the introduction of a stop codon that causes the premature truncation of a protein.

Nucleosome The basic structural subunit of chromatin, consisting of 200bp of double-helical DNA and an octamer of histone proteins, comprising two of each core histone (H2A, H2B, H3, and H4).

Nucleotide A purine or pyrimidine base to which a sugar and phosphate groups are attached.

Null mutation/allele A mutation which leads to absence or complete loss of function of the gene product, in contrast to a hypomorphic mutation which leads to impaired function of the gene product.

Offspring risk The risk that an affected parent will have an offspring with the same genetic condition. For a fully penetrant autosomal dominant condition, this risk will be 50%.

Oligogenic A trait or disease governed by the simultaneous action of a few (23) gene loci.

Oligonucleotide (oligo) A short fragment of single-stranded DNA that is typically 550 nucleotides long.

Oncogene A gene normally involved in promoting cell proliferation or differentiation, whose overactivity contributes to carcinogenesis. Oncogenes usually act dominantly at the cellular level, i.e. an activating mutation in just one copy of the gene is sufficient to drive carcinogenesis.

PCR (polymerase chain reaction) A technique in which cycles of denaturation, annealing with primer, and extension with DNA polymerase are used to amplify the number of copies of a target DNA sequence by $>10^6$ times.

Penetrance The probability of the carrier of a germline mutation showing signs of the disease, from the most trivial to the most severe. If all individuals who have a disease genotype show the disease phenotype, then the disease is said to be 'fully penetrant' or to have a penetrance of 100%.

PGD (pre-implantation genetic diagnosis) IVF (*in vitro* fertilization) techniques are used (ovarian hyperstimulation, oocyte retrieval, and *in vitro* fertilization) to obtain fertilized embryos. Twelve cells are removed for genetic analysis from several cleavage stage embryos at the 816-cell stage (day 3). Only embryos in which genetic testing predicts that the developing embryo will not develop the genetic disorder under test are then implanted in the mother.

Phenotype The appearance or other characteristics of the organism, resulting from the interaction of its genetic constitution with the environment.

Polygenic A trait or disease governed by the simultaneous action of many (>3) gene loci.

Polyploid (3n or 4n) Multiple sets of chromosomes, e.g. triploid (69,XXX or 69,XXY, or 69,XYY) or tetraploid (92,XXXX or 92,XXYY) sometimes found in spontaneous abortions.

Polymorphism The existence of two or more variants (alleles, sequence variants, chromosomal variants) that are non-pathogenic, the less common variant occurring at a frequency of >1% in a normal population.

Predictive testing Determining the genotype of an individual at risk for an inherited disorder who, at the time of testing, has no symptoms or features of the disorder. Usually contemplated in the context of adult-onset degenerative disorders, e.g. Huntington disease, or disorders for which burdensome screening will be undertaken in at-risk individuals, e.g. familial amyloid polyneuropathy, retinoblastoma.

Premutation A mutation that has no phenotypic effect, but that pre-disposes to a pathogenic mutation in subsequent generations, e.g. triplet repeat expansions in fragile X syndrome.

Primers Oligonucleotides that anneal to template DNA to prime synthesis mediated by DNA polymerase.

Private mutation A mutation unique to a given individual or family.

Proband The first person in a pedigree to be identified clinically as being affected by a genetic disorder.

Promotor A region of DNA involved in the binding of RNA polymerase to initiate transcription of a gene.

Proteome The set of all expressed proteins for a given organism.

Pseudoautosomal region (PAR) The homologous section of the X and Y chromosomes that pair and recombine during male meiosis. The genes in this part of the X chromosome escape X inactivation. Conditions caused by mutation in genes within the pseudoautosomal region appear to be dominantly inherited.

Recessive A trait in which the mutant allele is recessive to the wild-type allele, i.e. the disease is manifest only when two mutant alleles are inherited, e.g. cystic fibrosis.

Recurrence risk The chance of an event happening again. In genetic counselling this term is usually used when advising parents who have experienced the birth of a child with a specific problem about the chance of that problem occurring again in a subsequent pregnancy. For a Mendelian condition following autosomal recessive inheritance, the recurrence risk will be 25% for each pregnancy.

Relative risk (RR; or risk ratio) The ratio of the risk of developing a disease in individuals who have been exposed to (or inherited) a risk factor to that in individuals who have not been exposed (or not inherited) the risk factor. An RR > 1 means a person is estimated to be at an increased risk, while an RR < 1 represents a decrease in risk. An RR of 1.0 means there is no apparent effect on risk.

Repeat sequences Roughly half of the human genome is composed of repeat sequences. The majority of repeated sequences are transposable 'parasitic' elements such as long interspersed elements (LINEs) and short interspersed elements (SINEs) (e.g. Alu elements). Together LINE1 and Alu account for >60% of all repeated sequences in our genome. About 5% of the genome is made up of large duplicated regions, e.g. chromosome-specific low-copy repeats (LCRs).

Reproductive cloning The use of cloning technology to create a new organism. A reproductive clone is an organism that develops from the genetic information contained in one somatic cell of its parent and is genetically identical to that parent.

Satellite DNA Consists of many tandem repeats (identical or related) of a short basic repeating unit.

Screening 'The systematic application of a test or enquiry in order to identify individuals at sufficient risk of a specific disorder to warrant further investigation or to direct preventive action among persons who have not sought medical attention on account of symptoms of that disorder' (UK National Screening Committee).

Sensitivity The frequency with which a test result is positive when the disorder/disease is present.

Silent substitution (synonymous change) A nucleotide substitution that does not result in an amino acid substitution in the encoded protein because of the redundancy of the genetic code.

SNP (single nucleotide polymorphism, pronounced 'snip') The occurrence in a population of different nucleotides at particular sites in the genome. SNPs are not disease causing and are present at an appreciable frequency. They can be used in association studies, and several adjacent SNPs can be combined into a haplotype.

Somatic mosaicism The presence in a given individual of genetically distinct populations of somatic cells that have derived from one zygote, usually implying that the germline is not affected by the genetic change.

Southern blotting Procedure for transferring denatured DNA that has been cut with restriction enzymes from an agarose gel to a nitrocellulose filter where it can be hybridized with a radioactively labelled probe (complementary nucleic acid sequence). Used to size high-copy repeats, e.g. in Huntington disease, myotonic dystrophy, fragile X.

Specificity The frequency with which a test result is negative when the disorder/disease is absent.

Splice acceptor site Junction between the dinucleotide AG at the end of an intron and the start of the next exon.

Splice donor site Junction between the end of an exon and the dinucleotide GT at the start of the next intron.

Splicing The process by which introns are removed from the primary transcript, and the exons are joined together. Some genes have alternative splice variants, where a single gene gives rise to more than one mRNA sequence which may have different tissue distributions.

Stem cell A cell of a multicellular organism that is pluripotent and capable of giving rise to indefinitely more cells of the same type, and that retains the potential to undergo terminal differentiation, e.g. into a neuron or an oligodendrocyte, or into a red blood cell or a white blood cell.

Telomere The tip of a chromosome.

Trisomy Three copies of a chromosome. Usually two copies are present in a somatic cell ($2n$). The most common human trisomy surviving to live birth is Down syndrome, e.g. 47,XY + 21.

Truncating mutation A deletion or insertion of one or more bases (but not multiples of three) that disrupt the open reading frame, or a substitution leading to the creation of a stop codon. All result in premature termination of translation.

Tumour suppressor gene A gene normally involved in inhibition of cell proliferation or differentiation, whose inactivation contributes to carcinogenesis. Tumour suppressor genes usually act recessively at the cellular level, i.e. inactivating mutations in both copies of the gene are necessary to drive carcinogenesis.

Upstream A region of DNA that lies 5' to the point of reference.

Wild type The term used to indicate the normal allele (often symbolized as +) or the normal phenotype.

X-inactivation The process by which most of the genes on one of the X chromosomes in female somatic cells are inactivated or turned off during embryonic development. Also termed Lyonization.

Zygote A diploid cell resulting from the fusion of two haploid gametes; a fertilized ovum.

Index